Reconstructive Oral and Maxillofacial Surgery

Carlos Navarro Vila
Editor

Reconstructive Oral and Maxillofacial Surgery

Springer

Editor
Carlos Navarro Vila
Hospital General Universitario Gregorio Marañón
Madrid
Spain

ISBN 978-3-319-35968-7 ISBN 978-3-319-20487-1 (eBook)
DOI 10.1007/978-3-319-20487-1

Springer Cham Heidelberg New York Dordrecht London

Softcover reprint of the hardcover 1st edition 2015

Printed on acid-free paper

Springer International Publishing AG Switzerland is part of Springer Science+Business Media
(www.springer.com)

Preface

Reconstruction of head and neck defects after tumor resection is one of the main challenges facing the maxillofacial surgeon.

Such complex defects require not only cosmetic reconstruction but also functional reconstruction that enables patients to return to their family, social, and professional life under optimal conditions and as quickly as possible.

While resection surgery has developed little in recent years—with the exception of new techniques, such as navigation, that enable safer and more adapted procedures—reconstruction has advanced considerably, with the incorporation of free flaps and virtual planning, which makes it possible to model flaps and customize prostheses to the defect.

These advances are evident in reconstruction of the mandible.

Various pedicle flaps have been used to provide bone. The outcome has generally been unsatisfactory, except for Demergasso's trapezius osteomyocutaneous flap, which proved to be a very acceptable option for cosmetic and functional reconstruction.

The advent of free fibula flaps and scapula flaps revolutionized reconstruction and enabled defects to be repaired with high-quality bone and abundant soft tissue.

The placement of dental implants in transferred bone makes it possible to insert prostheses that restore chewing and phonation and considerably improve labial competence.

Software-based virtual surgery enables more accurate anatomical reconstruction using customized plates and cutting guides for the flap bone, which can be adapted exactly to the defect left by resection and to the patient's original facial structure.

Similarly, pedicle flaps and microsurgical flaps have transformed the reconstruction of defects of the maxilla and the middle third.

Each chapter of this book covers a specific area on the spectrum of head and neck reconstruction: mandibular reconstruction, reconstruction of the middle third, reconstruction of the cranio-orbital region, reconstruction of soft tissue defects, treatment of facial paralysis, dental implants, and regional flaps, which continue to be extremely useful.

We present our experience in the Maxillofacial Surgery Department of Hospital General Universitario Gregorio Marañón, Madrid, Spain, where these techniques have been taught to numerous specialists from Spain, Europe, and South America.

Madrid, Spain Carlos Navarro Vila

Contents

Contributors

Julio Acero Sanz, MD, DDS, PhD, FEBOMS Head of Oral and Maxillofacial Surgery Department, Ramón y Cajal University Hospital, Madrid, Spain

Associate Professor of Alcalá University, Madrid, Spain

Teresa González Otero, MD, PhD, FEBOMS Consultant at Oral and Maxillofacial Surgery Department, La Paz University Hospital, Madrid, Spain

Ana María López López, MD, DDS, FEBOMS Consultant at Oral and Maxillofacial Surgery Department, Miguel Servet University Hospital, Zaragoza, Spain

Cristina Maza Muela, MD, DDS, FEBOMS Consultant at Oral and Maxillofacial Surgery Department, Gregorio Marañón General University Hospital, Madrid, Spain

Carlos Navarro Cuellar, MD, DDS, PhD, FEBOMS Associate Professor Medical Faculty, Complutense University of Madrid, Madrid, Spain

Consultant at Oral and Maxillofacial Surgery Department, Gregorio Marañón General University Hospital, Madrid, Spain

Ignacio Navarro Cuellar, MD, DDS, FEBOMS Consultant at Oral and Maxillofacial Surgery Department, Virgen de la Salud Hospital, Toledo, Spain

Carlos Navarro Vila, MD, DMD, PhD, FEBOMS Full Professor Medical Faculty, Complutense University of Madrid, Madrid, Spain

Head of Oral and Maxillofacial Department Surgery, Gregorio Marañón General University Hospital, Madrid, Spain

Académico Correspondiente of the Royal National Academy of Medicine of Spain, Madrid, Spain

Santiago José Ochandiano Caicoya, MD, DDS, FEBOMS Consultant at Oral and Maxillofacial Surgery Department, Gregorio Marañón General University Hospital, Madrid, Spain

José Alfonso Ruiz Cruz, MD, DDS, FEBOMS Consultant at Oral and Maxillofacial Surgery Department, University Hospital del Sur, Madrid, Spain

José Ignacio Salmerón Escobar, MD, PhD, FEBOMS Associate Professor Medical Faculty, Complutense University, Madrid, Spain

Consultant at Oral and Maxillofacial Surgery Department, Gregorio Marañón General University Hospital, Madrid, Spain

Mandibular Reconstruction

1

Carlos Navarro Cuellar, Cristina Maza Muela, Santiago José Ochandiano Caicoya, and Carlos Navarro Vila

Abstract

Mandibular reconstruction involves restoration of the functions of chewing, swallowing, phonation, and facial expression. Until relatively recently, the only reconstruction options available were pedicle flaps, bone grafts, and reconstruction plates. Microsurgery has provided us with better options for reconstruction. Pedicle flaps and microsurgical flaps can provide sufficient bone and soft tissue to resolve these problems.

Reconstruction of the mandible and associated soft tissue can be performed during the ablation procedure (primary reconstruction) or during a subsequent procedure (secondary reconstruction).

The optimal approach is one that attempts to reconstruct the original contour as much as possible using bone and soft tissue for extraoral and intraoral tissue defects where applicable.

C. Navarro Cuellar, MD, DDS, PhD, FEBOMS (✉)
Associate Professor Medical Faculty, Complutense University of Madrid, Madrid, Spain

Consultant at Oral and Maxillofacial Surgery Department, Gregorio Marañón General University Hospital, Madrid, Spain
e-mail: cnavarrocuellar@gmail.com

C. Maza Muela, MD, DDS, FEBOMS • S.J. Ochandiano Caicoya, MD, DDS, FEBOMS
Consultant at Oral and Maxillofacial Surgery Department, Gregorio Marañón General University Hospital, Madrid, Spain
e-mail: crismazamuela@gmail.com; sochandiano@hotmail.com

C. Navarro Vila, MD, DMD, PhD, FEBOMS
Full Professor Medical Faculty, Complutense University of Madrid, Madrid, Spain

Head of Oral and Maxillofacial Department Surgery, Gregorio Marañón General University Hospital, Madrid, Spain

Académico Correspondiente of the Royal National Academy of Medicine of Spain, Madrid, Spain
e-mail: cnavarro.vila@clinicanavarrovila.com

C. Navarro Vila (ed.), *Reconstructive Oral and Maxillofacial Surgery*,
DOI 10.1007/978-3-319-20487-1_1

1.1 Introduction

Reconstructive surgery dates back to the sixth century, when Sushruta Samhita [1, 2] performed the first reconstructions of the nose and ears in India. However, it was not until the time of the Romans that Celsus recorded the use of advancement flaps for the reconstruction of the head and neck. Mandibular reconstruction has a shorter history, since most clinical experience and research dates from the treatment of injuries from the First and Second World Wars. In the United States, two hospitals were built to care for patients with these injuries, and emphasis was placed on the development of head and neck units, where specialists in maxillofacial surgery were trained. Laboratories were also established for the manufacture of devices such as arch bars, ferrules, and wires, all of which are necessary for the treatment of traumatic and oncologic lesions of the face.

The angiosome is a key concept in mandibular reconstruction that was introduced in 1987 by the plastic surgeons Taylor and Palmer [3, 4]. An angiosome is a three-dimensional block of tissue that involves the muscular, cutaneous, and subcutaneous territories that are supplied by an artery and a vein. This discovery made it possible to apply both free and pedicle osteomyocutaneous flaps for mandibular reconstruction.

Mandibular reconstruction involves not only restoration of continuity with cosmetic objectives in mind but also restoration of the functions of chewing, swallowing, phonation, and facial expression. Thus, maxillofacial surgery has evolved over time with the introduction of muscle transfer techniques, nerve anastomosis, and osseointegrated implants, all of which help to restore mandibular function.

When part of the mandible is missing, generally as a result of ablative surgery for the treatment of tumors, the major sequelae in bone and soft tissue have both a cosmetic and a functional effect. In cosmetic terms, we can observe retrusion of the lower third, which is more remarkable when the part of the mandible affected is the parasymphysis or symphysis, and eversion of the lower lip. When resection affects the body of the mandible, we observe asymmetry with sinking of the affected side and retraction of the soft tissue that leads to deviation of the remnant mandible to the missing area. In functional terms, missing structure in the anterior area leads to labial and salivary incontinence and phonation disorders. When the body of the mandible is affected toward the condyle, we observe the occlusal plane canted with crossbite, which hinders mouth opening, chewing, and swallowing. The absence of some areas of the mandible generates overload on the remnant mandible and other structures of the oral cavity with altered proprioception leading to incoordination of mandibular movement.

Analysis of the possible sequelae arising from partial or total mandibular bone loss clearly illustrates the serious difficulties faced by patients in leading a normal social and working life.

As Wong et al. [5] reported, there is no ideal biomechanical solution for mandibular reconstruction. The mechanical resistance and forces acting on the reconstructed mandible are complex and not fully understood. Excessive pressure on traditional bone grafts and metal plates can lead to fracture of the plate, loosening of the screws, and bone resorption, which could in turn lead to potential fracture of the mandible. New approaches in mandibular reconstruction attempt to distribute forces evenly in the remnant mandible.

The aim of mandibular reconstruction is to return cosmetic and functional integrity and thus ensure quality of life. Until relatively recently, the only reconstruction options available were pedicle flaps, bone grafts, and reconstruction plates. Microsurgery has provided us with better options for reconstruction.

1.2 Bone Grafts

Publications on mandibular reconstruction with free bone grafts date from as early as the end of the eighteenth century and beginning of the nineteenth century. Bardenheuer [6] and Skyoff [7] reported the first cases of mandibular reconstruction with autologous bone grafts harvested from the iliac crest, tibia, and rib.

Considerable experience treating traumatic mandibular defects was gained during the First World War. Ivy and Epes [8] followed a delayed approach to reconstruction of the mandible using solid blocks of tibial bone or mandibular bone pedicle grafts. The authors reported mandibular continuity in 76 % of cases and a long period of intermaxillary fixation.

The Second World War saw the advent of new approaches in this type of reconstructive surgery. These included internal blocks for stabilizing the graft, use of the iliac crest as the donor site, and administration of antibiotics. Studies from this period by Blocker and Stout [9] reported the use of bone grafts for mandibular reconstruction harvested from the tibia, ribs, and iliac crest. Graft survival was 90 % in approximately 1000 grafts. These successes made autologous bone grafts the main option for reconstruction of both traumatic and oncologic defects during the 1950s and 1960s.

Despite these promising beginnings, problems with bone grafts began to appear, mainly when contouring the symphysis. Brown et al. [10] and Millard et al. [11] reported difficulties shaping the symphysis with iliac crest grafts.

In other series, the rate of complications and graft loss was greater. Wersal et al. [12] performed 23 mandibular reconstructions with rib grafts, and although the author indicated that the grafts were for lateral and anterior defects, 22 % of the grafts failed. Hamaker [13, 14] used delayed reconstruction with bone grafts in 15 patients who had undergone mandibulectomy and radiation therapy. The graft failed in 33 % of cases because of radionecrosis and superinfection.

Cummings and Leipzig [15] reported the use of a cryogenically devitalized autograft for mandibular reconstruction. DeFries et al. [16] used cadaver mandible grafts with autologous bone from the iliac crest and reported 10 failures in 14 patients who had undergone radiation therapy. The main problem of bone grafts is their low tolerance of infection, particularly in cancer patients. This problem did not affect traumatic defects, since surgery was delayed and based on an extraoral approach, thus preventing contamination of the oral cavity. Therefore, most surgeons recommended delaying reconstructive surgery and, if the graft survived locoregional recurrence, using an extraoral approach.

Bone grafts continue to be the subject of debate. Although the maximum length indicated to ensure viability is 3 cm, recent publications [17] report the vascularization of free bone grafts in 11 patients measuring up to 7 cm in length in a single block and 14 cm when blocks are combined.

1.3 Alloplastic Materials

Alloplastic materials are inert (nonorganic) materials normally implanted inside the body to remodel and create volume or replace a given anatomic area. They have the advantage that no donor site is necessary and no antigen response to foreign proteins occurs. The main alloplastic materials used are iron, titanium, hydroxyapatite, chrome-cobalt, methyl methacrylate, and other polymers.

Titanium was first used in 1983 by Luckey and Kubli [18] for implants and prostheses. It is the material of choice for medical devices because it is light in weight, resistant, and biocompatible. In addition, it does not interfere with diagnostic techniques such as nuclear magnetic resonance or computed tomography.

Several materials have been described in the literature. Castermans et al. [19] reported a failure rate of 70 % in a series of patients undergoing mandibular reconstruction with Kirschner wires. Joyce and McQuarrie [20] reported a 25 % failure rate in their series of patients undergoing reconstruction with a silicone and metal prosthesis. Bowerman [21] used titanium plates in patients who had not undergone radiation therapy to reconstruct the symphysis, with losses of 35 %, and Conley [22] and Cook [23] used vitallium plates, with losses of 33 % at 5 years. A-O plates have also been used to reconstruct the mandible [24], with failure rates of 4 % in the first year, increasing exponentially with time and radiation therapy.

As these authors show, alloplastic materials have high rates of exposure and superinfection, especially in patients undergoing radiation therapy.

Prostheses are currently being made from polyether ether ketone, hydroxyapatite, and polyethylene, which can be prepared using computer-assisted design (CAD)/computer-assisted manufacture (CAM) systems [25] before surgery to provide a more adapted approach to defects. However, the number of patients necessary to perform feasibility studies is insufficient, and not enough time has passed to determine long-term survival and resistance to radiation.

1.4 Combination of Bone Grafts and Alloplastic Material

During the 1960s, surgeons began to think that the reasons for graft failure were incorrect fixation and poor vascularization. Supporting trays made of metal or Dacron were used to improve fixation by filling them with cancellous bone, thus enhancing neovascularization. In 1944, Moulem [26] first demonstrated the osteogenic capacity of cancellous bone chip grafts. Boyne and Zarem [27] were the first to use a wire mesh tray with cancellous bone chips for mandibular reconstruction. The mesh had to be removed in 11 % of 53 cases.

Lawson et al. [28] reported a series of 54 cases of mandibular reconstruction performed using metal trays and cancellous bone in which the failure rate was 54 % for immediate reconstructions compared with 19 % in delayed procedures. Infection of the intraoral wound was the factor that most contributed to the failure of the reconstruction. Albert et al. [29] used Dacron trays with cancellous bone and reported a 24 % failure rate.

Branemark et al. [30] used titanium mesh with and without cancellous bone in mandibular reconstruction procedures. In patients whose graft was with mesh only, the failure rate was 40 %, and the graft was reabsorbed in 60 %.

In 1987, Klotch and Prein [31] performed reconstruction in 60 patients with A-O reconstruction plates. Regional pedicle grafts were used to cover the plates and thus fully seal the soft tissue. The authors reported a success rate of 86 % with exposure of the plate in 25 % of patients who received radiation therapy, multiple salivary fistulas, and late fractures in 8 %.

In 1990, Komisar [32] studied series with plates used for primary and deferred reconstruction, whether combined or not with bone, and found that 82 % of primary reconstructions were complicated by infection and that, when a bone graft was used, the reabsorption rate was more than 50 %.

In 1990, Saunders et al. [33] presented a series of 27 patients who underwent primary reconstruction with titanium plates not combined with bone graft. The success rate was 78 %, although none of the patients who underwent reconstruction of the symphysis could wear dentures after surgery. The results reported by Gullane [34] were similar, with a 78 % success rate during the first year.

Almost 40 years later, the combination of bone grafts with alloplastic material remains controversial. Studies continue to show integration and corticalization of iliac crest grafts packed in titanium mesh [35].

No multicenter studies have analyzed reconstruction of mandibular defects in cancer patients who undergo radiation therapy. Yagihara et al. [36] recently published the results of a study in which they combined poly-L-lactide mesh with cancellous bone grafts. As this material descomposes after 6 months to 2 years in the body, the authors reported a success rate of 84 % and concluded that the frequency of excellent or good regeneration tended to be better in primary reconstruction, benign lesions, and marginal resections, in patients not undergoing radiation therapy, and in procedures that do not involve reconstruction of associated soft tissue. A separate analysis of patients receiving radiation therapy showed that classic concepts remained unchanged, with poor bone regeneration in 27.4 % of cases compared with 13.3 % in those who did not receive radiation therapy.

Therefore, mandibular reconstruction would not be the technique of choice for defects resulting from cancer, although such techniques are associated with low morbidity and could be considered in patients who cannot undergo other procedures.

1.5 Distraction Osteogenesis

Techniques for the reconstruction of the lower third (both soft tissue and bone) are very varied. Each has its indications and risks.

Distraction osteogenesis was first described in 1957 by Ilizarov and involves a process in which bone is formed between two segments that are gradually separated by progressive traction using a device known as a distractor. This separation generates both bone and the surrounding tissue. The technique has been used by orthopedic surgeons for more than 40 years. Distraction osteogenesis of the mandible was first described in 1998 by McCarthy et al. [37].

We can distinguish between two types of distraction osteogenesis. The first is performed without bone transport and is used to treat bone malformations in maxillofacial and orthopedic surgery. This technique makes it possible to lengthen the bone and adjacent soft tissue. The second type involves bone transfer and is used to treat bone defects by filling the defect without altering the original length of the bone.

Mandibular bone is distracted by means of bone resection and placement of the distractor. This is followed by the latency period, which is the time necessary for the bone to lengthen, generally between 5 and 7 days. The distraction period then begins, with growth of 0.8–1 cm per day. When the planned length is reached, the distractor must be kept in place for the so-called consolidation period, which usually lasts about 3 months.

The associated mortality of this technique is low and results are good. However, it is not the technique of choice in mandibular reconstruction after tumor resection, because the application time is too long, thus preventing coadjuvant radiation therapy from being administered within the effective window period (4–6 weeks). In addition, the likelihood of osteoradionecrosis is increased. If possible, the technique should be applied after other bone reconstructions, for example, using microsurgical fibular flaps, for vertical lengthening in order to gain sufficient height and fit implants.

1.6 Primary Reconstruction vs Secondary Reconstruction

Reconstruction of the mandible and associated soft tissue can be performed during the ablation procedure (primary reconstruction) or during a subsequent procedure (secondary reconstruction).

We favor primary reconstruction for several reasons. It is technically easier than secondary reconstruction, there is no fibrosis or retraction, and anatomic relationships can be maintained (e.g., with intermaxillary fixation or by molding and fixing before resection of mandibular reconstruction plates to maintain the mandibular arch). Furthermore, a second procedure is obviated, the cost is lower, and the patient can return more quickly to his/her social and working life. Since the patient does not have to face the functional and cosmetic sequelae of ablative surgery, psychological recovery is much quicker and complete after oncologic surgery.

We do not agree with the reasons against primary reconstruction, mainly poor control of subsequent relapses. Today, imaging techniques such as computed tomography or magnetic resonance enable relapses—even those involving only a few millimeters—to be detected very quickly.

Similarly, we do not agree with the other reason against primary reconstruction, namely, the recommendation to avoid exertion, because 50 % of patients were lost to follow-up during the first year. We believe that the quality of life patients gain during the remainder of their lives is more than sufficient reason to perform immediate reconstruction.

In our department, we limit secondary reconstruction to those cases where primary reconstruction was not successful and for patients who underwent procedures at other centers, where, for whatever reason, no reconstruction was performed during the first intervention.

1.7 Type of Reconstruction: Pedicle Flaps and Microvascular Flaps

The optimal approach is one that attempts to reconstruct the original contour as much as possible using bone and soft tissue for extraoral and intraoral tissue defects where applicable. Pedicle flaps and microsurgical flaps can provide sufficient bone and soft tissue to resolve these problems. Several factors must be taken into consideration when deciding which technique to choose.

Many factors come into play when deciding on reconstruction and selecting a specific flap. The most important are the following:

1. Type, size, and position of the defect
2. Quantity and quality of the remnant bone
3. Size and defect of the soft tissue
4. Intraoral and extraoral defects
5. Quality of local vascularization (compromised by previous radiotherapy, diabetes mellitus, arteriosclerosis)
6. State of the maxilla, tongue, and floor of the mouth, as well as lip competence
7. Previous surgery: functional or radical neck dissection, failed reconstructions
8. Previous local surgery: functional or radical neck dissection
9. General status of the patient

1.7.1 Pedicle Flaps

In the 1980s, myocutaneous flaps began to be used for soft tissue defects. Bone was later included in these flaps for mandibular reconstruction. The flaps were taken from the pectoralis major with the fifth or sixth rib, as described by Cuono and Ariyan [38] in 1980, the trapezius muscle with the spine of the scapula, the sternocleidomastoid muscle with the clavicle, and the latissimus dorsi with the iliac crest.

In 1979, Demergasso and Piazza [39] reported for the first time the use of the trapezius osteomyocutaneous flap for mandibular reconstruction. Panje and Cutting [40, 41] used this flap in 24 patients, and the flap failed in 13 %. Little et al. [42]

used a pectoralis major flap with the fifth rib for mandibular reconstruction and reported complications in two cases, although the rib was viable in a further three patients.

Kudo et al. [43] reconstructed the mandible of five patients using a pectoralis major flap with rib and sternum. Two patients experienced pneumothorax, and the rib had to be withdrawn in a further two cases.

The results of our experience with this reconstruction have not been good, since the rib is largely reabsorbed after radiation therapy.

1.7.2 Microvascular Flaps

The first microsurgery-based mandibular reconstruction was reported in 1971 by Strauch et al. [44]. The subsequent studies by Ostrup and Fredrickson [45], Daniel [46], and Taylor [47] show that both the rib and the iliac crest can be transferred to the mandible using microsurgery. Thanks to these techniques, flap failure is much reduced, although surgical time and morbidity increase.

Franklin et al. [48] performed six mandibular reconstructions with the iliac crest flap of which one failed (16 %). The author reported problems such as the large size of the flap, the lack of sensitivity of the skin paddle, and surgical time.

MacLeod and Robinson [49] published a series of 12 reconstructions of the anterior mandible. The flap used was the second metatarsal based on the dorsalis pedis vein and artery. They reported only one case of flap loss.

In 1986, Soutar and Widdowson [50] reported on the use of the radius as a radial osteofasciocutaneous flap for mandibular defects associated with a soft tissue defect. The flap failed in only 1 of the 14 patients who underwent surgery.

Cordeiro and Hidalgo [51] compared mandibular reconstructions performed with free flaps and those performed with reconstruction plates combined with pedicle flaps to seal soft tissue. The authors reported a greater number of complications, longer hospital stay, and greater number of reoperations in the series that underwent reconstruction with plates and pedicle flaps.

Schusterman et al. [52] also compared reconstruction with plates and free flaps. The free flaps survived in most cases and could be used to reconstruct any segment, whereas plates were exposed and superinfected in the symphysis in 66 % of cases.

Hoffmeister et al. [53] combined an iliac crest free flap and a jejunal free flap to reconstruct the mandible and mucosa in a series of 22 patients.

1.8 Microvascular Flaps

1.8.1 Fibula Flap

The microsurgical fibula flap was first described by Taylor et al. [47] in 1975. Hidalgo [54] was the first to use this flap for mandibular reconstruction in 1988. The fibula is a long thin non-weight-bearing bone. It has a constant tubular cross section along its length, with a thick cortex (66 % of the section [55]), thus making it one of the strongest bones for transfer. The fibula provides approximately 25 cm of bone, which is sufficient to reconstruct any mandibular defect [56]. Both a bone flap and an osteocutaneous flap can be obtained.

The main advantages of this flap are that it is very long and enables two teams to work simultaneously. Furthermore, its rich periosteal vascularization makes it possible to perform several osteotomies for remodeling. The skin paddle can be reinnervated to provide sensation, and morbidity in the donor area is minimal. We prefer the fibula flap to the iliac crest flap in obese patients, because the bone is easy to harvest. According to Moscoso et al. [55], the main disadvantage of this flap is that 15 % of men and a somewhat higher percentage of women cannot receive implants owing to the size of the bone. In addition, multiple osteotomies are necessary for remodeling, thus necessitating a large quantity of osteosynthesis material and preventing immediate fitting of implants. The fibula lacks sufficient height in segmental defects in dentulous patients; therefore, there is some discrepancy between the height of the flap and the remnant mandible, which leads to a poor crown-implant ratio. Horiuchi et al. [57] and Siciliano et al. [58] resolved this issue with a double-strut fibula or secondary vertical distraction of the fibula. The main disadvantage of this flap is the very variable number of septocutaneous perforators that irrigate the skin paddle. Wei et al. [59] provided the clearest explanations of the vascularization of the skin paddle, which is supplied by 4–7 branches, of which between 1 and 4 are septocutaneous (inconstant, may be missing) and the remainder musculocutaneous. Two septocutaneous branches feed an area of skin measuring 20 × 25 cm. Futran et al. [60, 61] proposed Doppler imaging to locate the perforators and prepare the preoperative sketch of the skin paddle based on these perforators and achieved excellent results; in our opinion, this technique is the approach of choice when attempting to ensure maximum viability of the skin paddle. In 1994, Hidalgo [62] proposed obtaining a very broad skin paddle by de-epithelializing any surplus skin. Thus, we can ensure vascularization of the skin paddle, whose viability ranges between 95.5 % and 100 %. In order to ensure this viability, it is a good idea to design a skin paddle based on the intermuscular septum and the distal third of the bone and to include a wedge of muscle (soleus and flexor hallucis longus) to ensure that the musculocutaneous perforators are included. The last main disadvantage of the fibula flap is that it requires preoperative confirmation by arteriography or Doppler imaging that there is sufficient circulation to supply the skin once the fibular artery has been resected, because some arterial disorders can lead to ischemic necrosis.

The main characteristics of the fibula flap are its maximum length (25 cm, mean length of 17–18 cm), pedicle length (2–3 cm at the origin, increasing via subperiosteal dissection to 12 cm), artery caliber (1.8–3 mm), and vein caliber (2–4 mm).

The fibula flap is indicated in the following situations:

- Reconstruction of total or subtotal mandibular defects: when the defect is greater than 14 cm, only the fibula provides sufficient bone.
- The main application of the fibula is reconstruction of mandibular segment defects: the strength of the bone can resist the forces of mastication, and implants can be placed. In defects measuring less than 14 cm, the iliac crest has lost ground in favor of the fibula, which is today the main flap in mandibular reconstruction.

- Secondary reconstructions that affect the ramus and condyle. The thin bone of the fibula flap is easy to insert in the tunnel created by the fibrous soft tissue without damaging the facial nerve.
- Reconstruction of mandibular defects accompanied by major defects of intra-oral soft tissue, which advise against using the iliac crest and in which we cannot use the trapezius osteomyocutaneous flap for the reasons specified above.
- Microsurgical reconstruction of the mandible in children [63].

As for functional recovery of the teeth, the fibula accepts small-to-medium implants. Given the number of miniplates and screws necessary to fix osteotomies and ensure a good cosmetic outcome, we place implants in this flap during a secondary procedure.

If the patient undergoes radiation therapy after surgery, we wait until 9–12 months have passed. The screws and miniplates are removed and the implants inserted. The percentage of osteointegration of the implants in the patients we treat was 96.6 %, which decreases to 92 % in the long term (more than 3 years) [64] (Figs. 1.1, 1.2, 1.3, 1.4, 1.5, 1.6, 1.7, 1.8, 1.9, 1.10, 1.11, and 1.12).

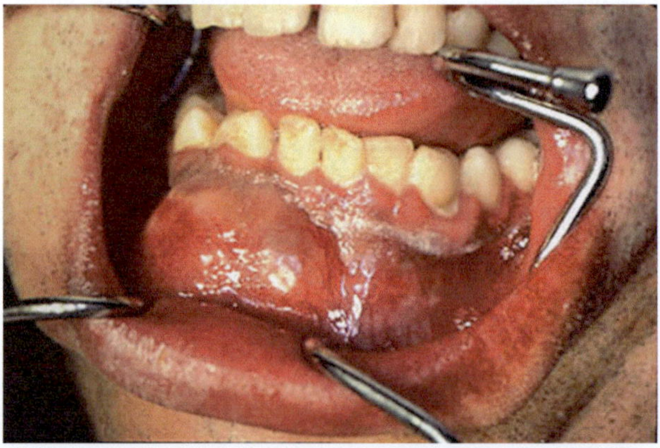

Fig. 1.1 Mandibular tumor (ameloblastoma)

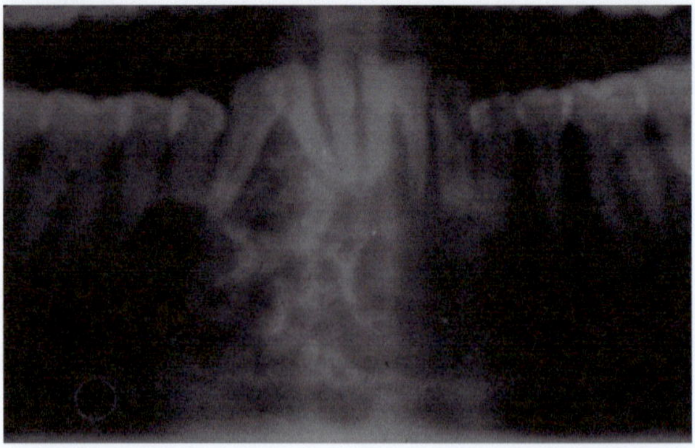

Fig. 1.2 Preoperative OPT

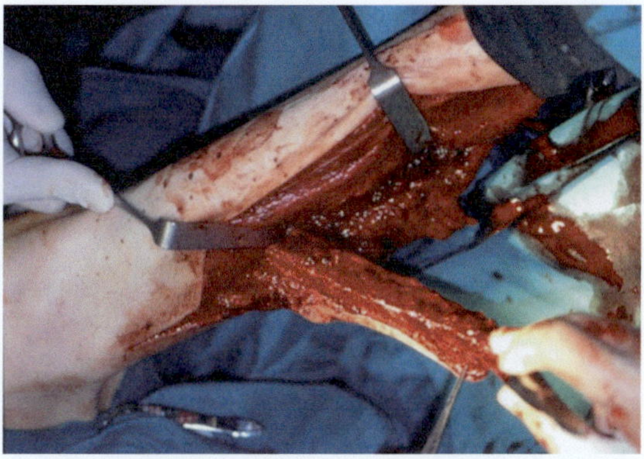

Fig. 1.3 Fibula flap dissection

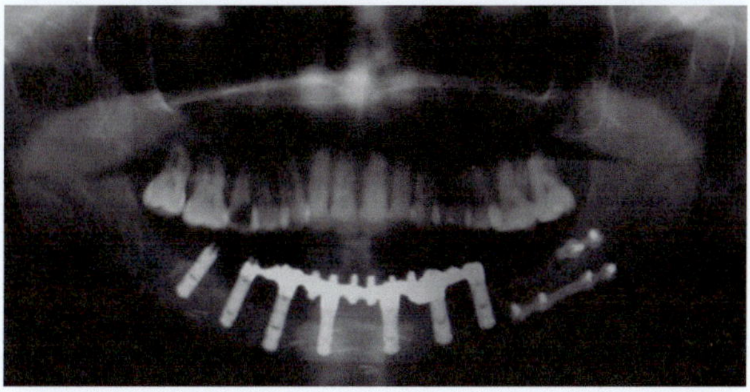

Fig. 1.4 Postoperative OPT with dental implants

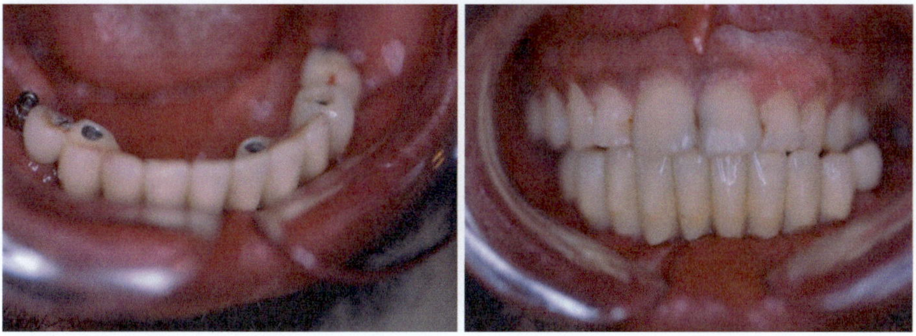

Fig. 1.5 Dental prosthesis and occlusion

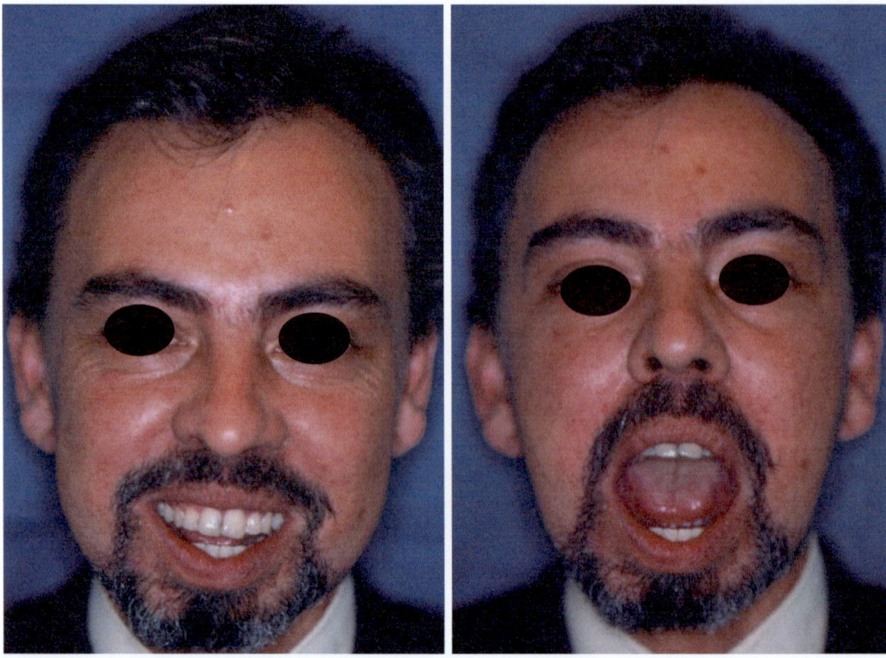

Fig. 1.6 Postoperative view

Fig. 1.7 Ablative resection

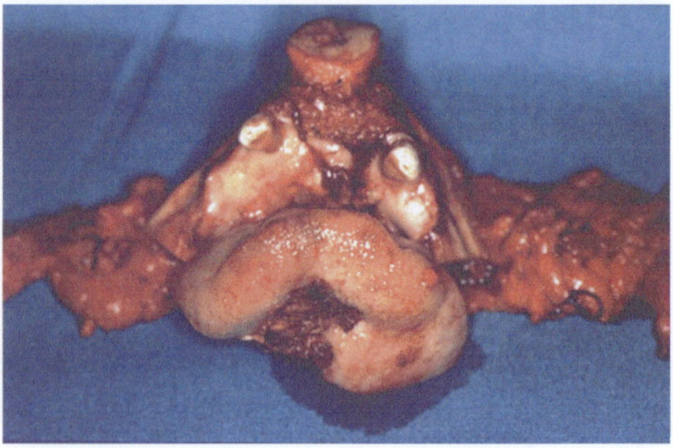

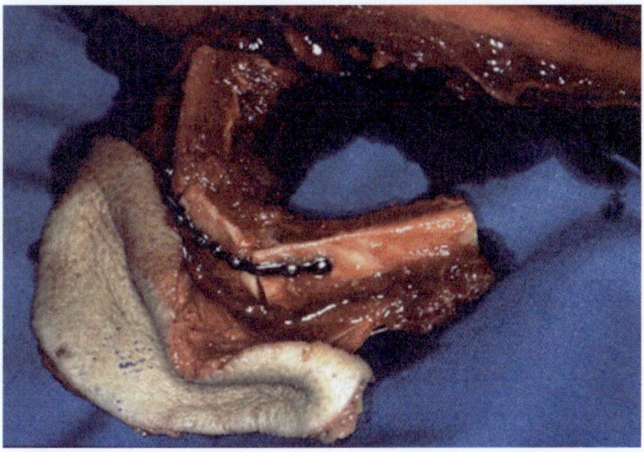

Fig. 1.8 Fibula flap intraoperative design

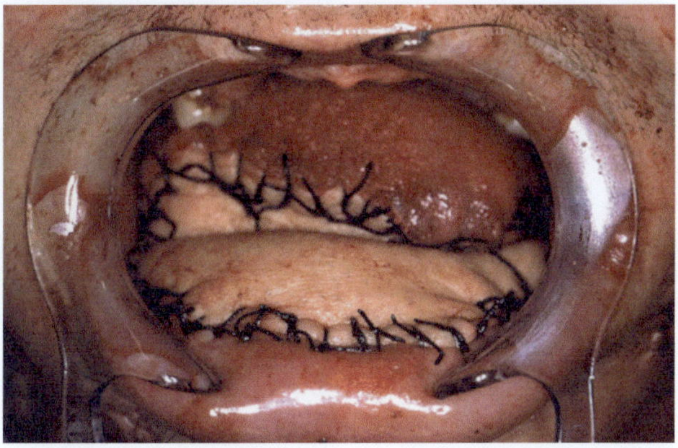

Fig. 1.9 Immediate postoperative reconstruction

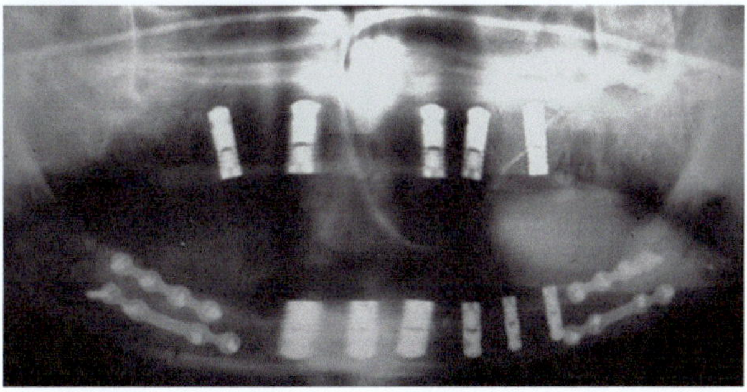

Fig. 1.10 Postoperative OPT

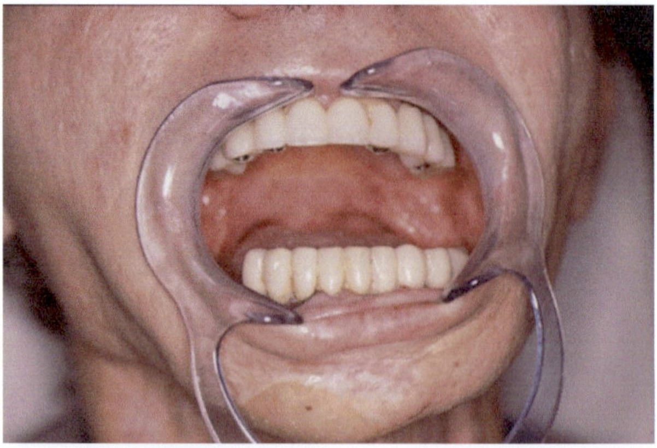

Fig. 1.11 Definitive occlusion

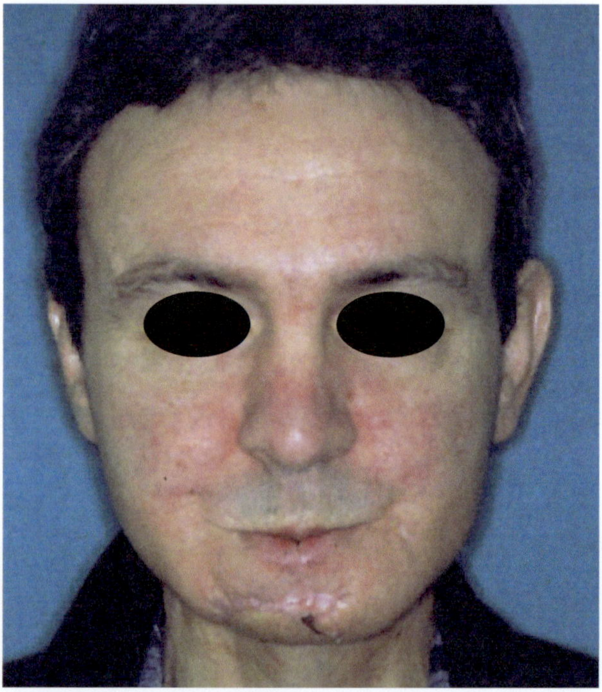

Fig. 1.12 Postoperative view

1.8.2 Iliac Crest Flap

The iliac crest flap is based on the deep circumflex iliac artery, which arises from the external iliac artery 1–2 cm cranially to the inguinal ligament. It runs toward the anterosuperior iliac spine, internal face of the iliac bone, and between the iliacus and transversus abdominis muscles. It gives off an ascending branch, which supplies the lesser oblique muscle, periosteal and endosteal branches that supply the bone, and musculocutaneous perforating branches toward the skin.

Venous drainage is from the deep circumflex iliac vein, which is usually a double vein, into the external iliac vein.

Skin is obtained via the perforators along the internal part of the crest that cross the three muscles of the abdominal wall. Therefore, a considerable part of the major and minor oblique muscles and the transversus abdominis must remain attached to the internal portion to carry the perforators. It is also necessary to design a wide skin flap to incorporate as large a number as possible of perforators (between three and nine in a field that extends longitudinally 9 cm posterior to the anterosuperior iliac spine and 2.5 cm medial to the crest). The wide mesentery of the skin flap limits the relative mobility of the skin.

The anatomical characteristics of this flap are as follows: short vascular pedicle (5–7 cm); 1.5–3 mm diameter at its origin; bone length, 14–16 cm; lesser oblique muscle of 10 × 15 cm; and skin surface of 15 × 25 cm.

Its main indications are as follows:

- Mandibular bone defects. We think that the iliac crest has the best quality, height, and thickness for mandibular reconstruction of all the bone flaps; however, as it is only 10–12 cm long, larger defects require a fibular flap. It takes the thickest and longest osseointegrated implants, which can be inserted during the same procedure.
- In defects of the symphysis, the flap can be molded to the form of the defect using osteotomies and preserving the periosteum of the internal surface to maintain the supply to the bone. When the defect includes the body and ascending ramus of the mandible, the ramus can be contoured by designing an "L"-shaped flap.
- Bone defects associated with extraoral soft tissue defects. In this case, the cutaneous part of the flap is used to reconstruct the defect, although inguinal skin is considerably paler in color. The cutaneous part can also be used to monitor the flap
- Bone defects associated with intraoral soft tissue defects. In these cases, the flap is only feasible if it contains internal oblique muscle. The large volume of soft tissue renders it inadequate for this type of reconstruction. We prefer other types of osteocutaneous flap, such as the fibula, scapula, and trapezius osteocutaneous flaps.

The excellent quality of the bone in an iliac crest flap makes it possible to fit a sufficient number of implants for the rehabilitation of most patients with an implant-supported prosthesis. Since the height of the flap is similar to that of the remnant mandible, for dentulous patients the crown-implant ratio obtained is optimal (1:3; the crown accounts for 33 % of the total length of the crown-pillar-implant complex). Implants can be fitted during mandibular reconstruction with a balanced occlusal relationship. We obtained a 94 % osseointegration success rate with Mozo Grau implants (MG osseous) and, in the long term, a 12 % failure rate [64].

In our opinion, the iliac crest flap is the best flap for mandibular bone reconstruction when we do not need to reconstruct soft tissue and for the reconstruction of the symphysis and mandibular body up to 10 cm (Figs. 1.13, 1.14, 1.15, 1.16, 1.17, 1.18, and 1.19).

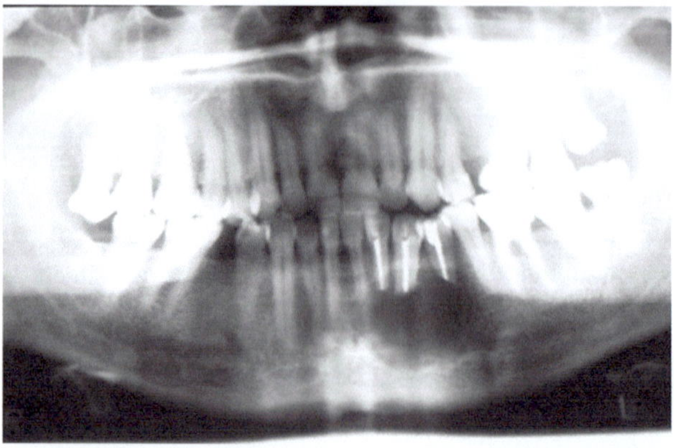

Fig. 1.13 Preoperative

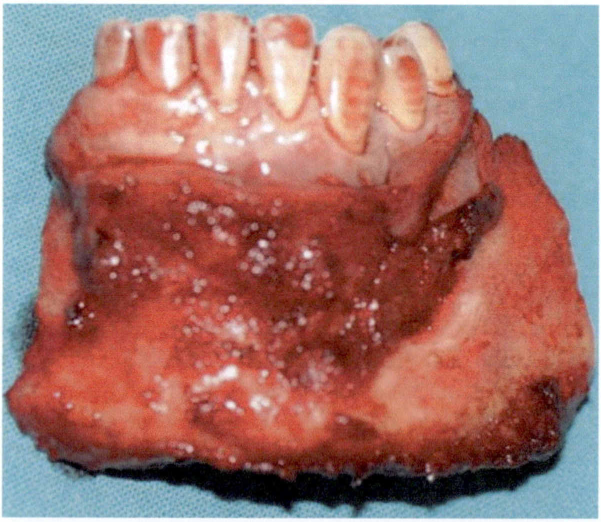

Fig. 1.14 Tumor resection

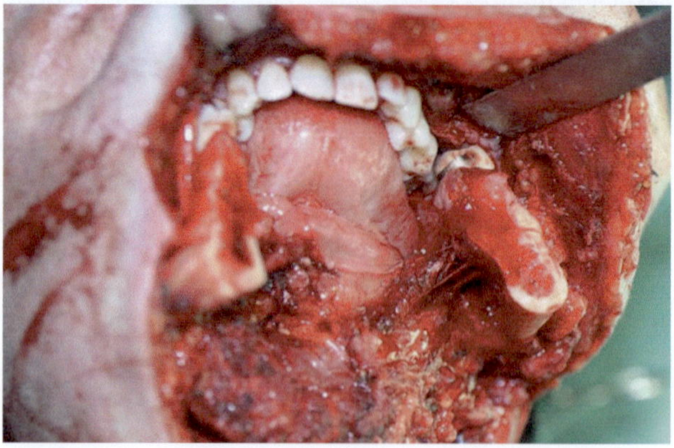

Fig. 1.15 Defect after ablative surgery

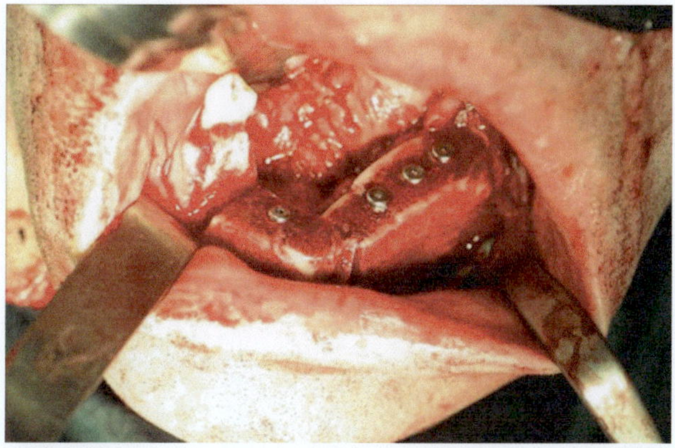

Fig. 1.16 Intraoperative reconstruction with iliac crest free flap and MG osseous implants

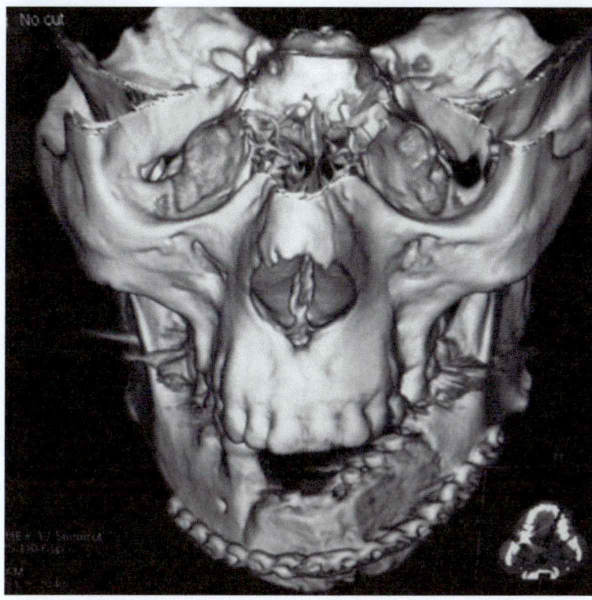

Fig. 1.17 Postoperative CT

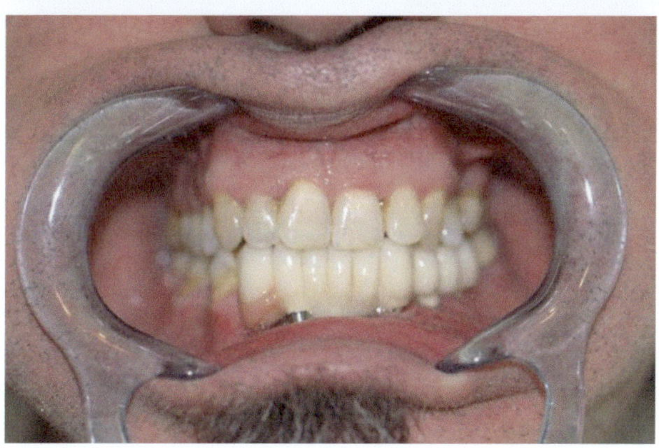

Fig. 1.18 Final occlusion

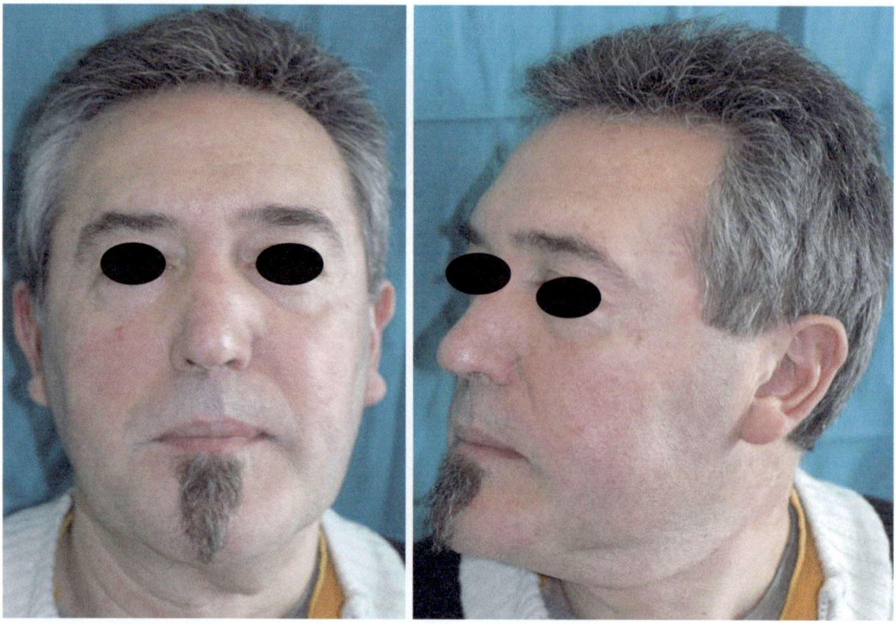

Fig. 1.19 One year postoperative views

As shown in the indications (see above), reconstruction of soft tissue requires the use of the internal oblique muscle, which is excessively bulky. Navarro Cuellar et al. [65] present an alternative technique that enables mandibular reconstruction using an iliac crest flap combined with one or two nasolabial flaps to reconstruct intraoral soft tissues. This technique combines the advantages of mandibular reconstruction and insertion of osseointegrated implants (MG osseous) using an iliac crest flap in combination with reconstruction of anatomically adapted intraoral soft tissue defects, avoiding the dissection of internal oblique muscle (Figs. 1.20, 1.21, 1.22, 1.23, 1.24, and 1.25).

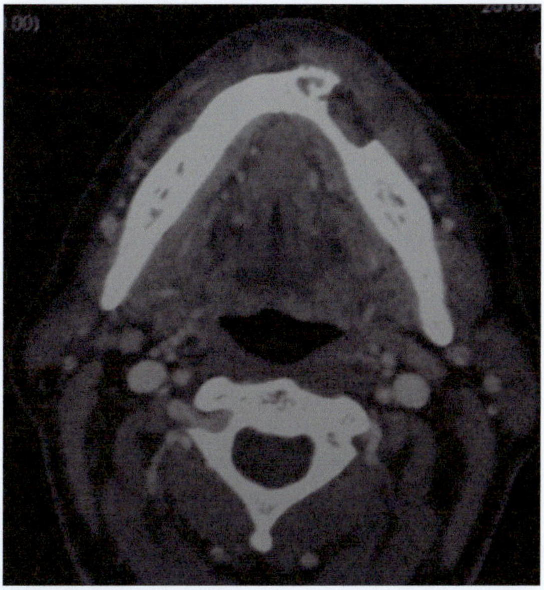

Fig. 1.20 Preoperative CT

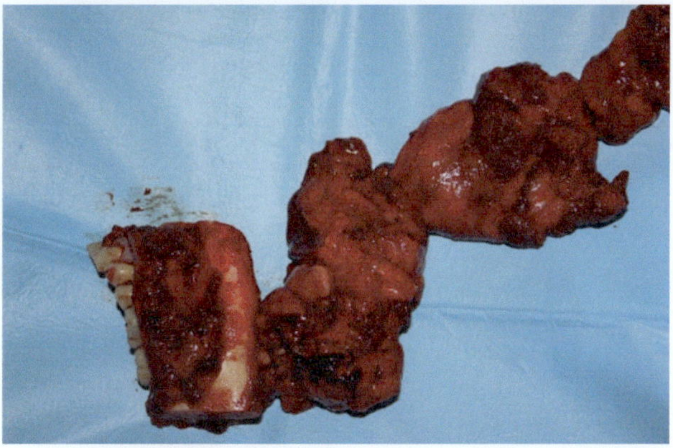

Fig 1.21 Squamous cell carcinoma resection with cervical dissection

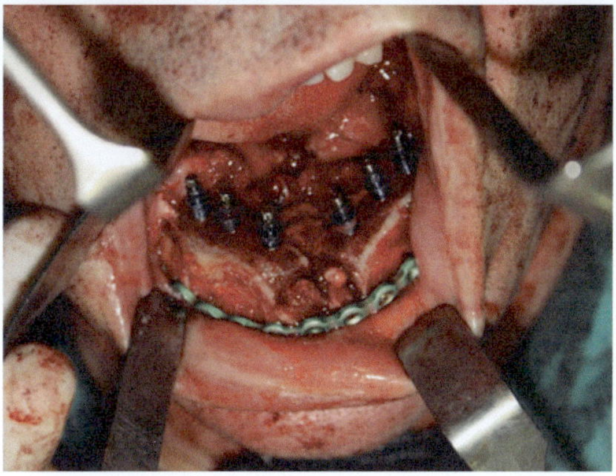

Fig. 1.22 Iliac crest free flap reconstruction with MG osseous implants

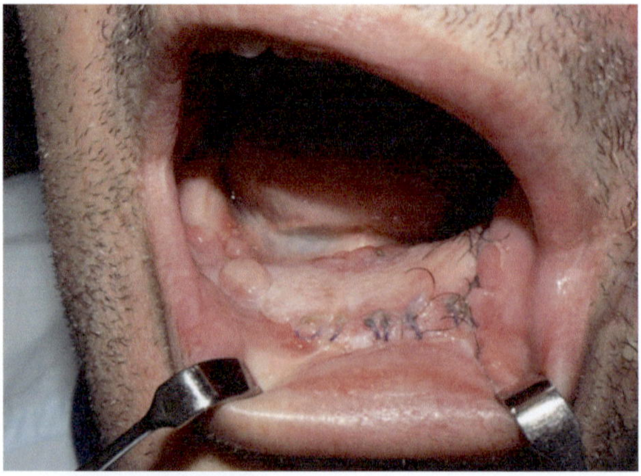

Fig. 1.23 Nasolabial flap covering iliac crest flap

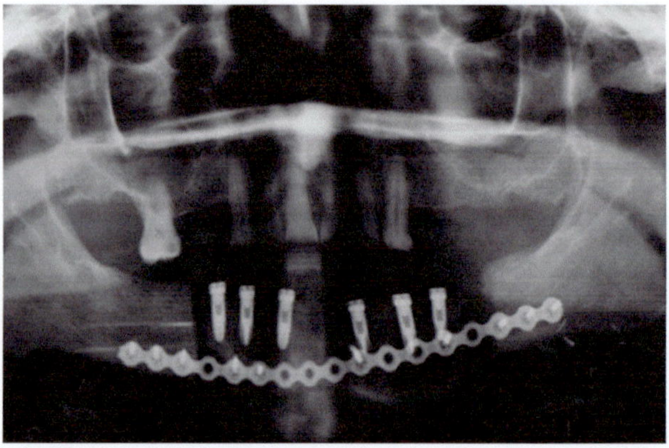

Fig. 1.24 Postoperative OPT

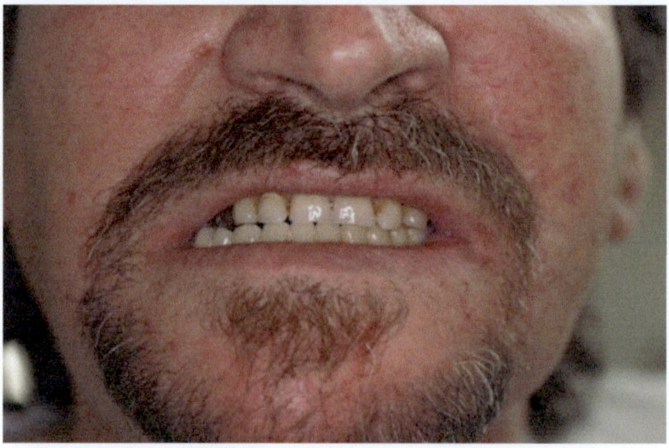

Fig. 1.25 Final occlusion

1.8.3 Scapular Flap

In 1981, Teot et al. [66] described the scapular and parascapular osteomyocutaneous flap. Swartz et al. [67], Baker and Sullivan [68], and Sullivan et al. [69] subsequently reported the use of the scapular osteocutaneous free flap for immediate mandibular reconstruction.

The skin covering the posterior surface of the scapula and the periosteum of the lateral border of the scapula are vascularized by the scapular circumflex artery, a branch of the subscapular artery.

The circumflex artery exits the triangular space and divides into a horizontal branch (scapular flap) and a vertical branch (parascapular flap), which supply the skin field (14 × 21 cm) covering the scapula.

The specific anatomical distribution of the vessels means that the bony part of the flap can be placed independently in three dimensions with respect to the skin flap. The mobility of the soft tissue with respect to the bone makes it possible to reconstruct complex orofacial defects in which soft tissue requirements are as important as the bone defect itself.

Many options are available for reconstruction using this flap, since it can be exclusively muscular, musculocutaneous, osteomyocutaneous, or combined with the latissimus dorsi and serratus anterior (megaflap).

In addition, the skin covering the scapula is thin, hairless, pliable, and similar in color to facial skin [70].

The flap provides well-vascularized corticocancellous bone (1.5–3 cm wide and 10–14 cm long). We can also obtain a further 3–4 cm from the angle of the scapula if we include the angular branch of the thoracodorsal artery.

The disadvantages of this flap are the need to rotate the patient, thus preventing two surgical teams from working simultaneously. It has been suggested that this disadvantage could be avoided by placing the patient on his/her side, although it is still difficult for two teams to work simultaneously. Furthermore, the amount of bone is limited, thus hindering reconstruction of large defects and placement of implants. The resulting scar is usually unsightly, and sensory reinnervation of the flap is not possible.

The characteristics of the scapular flap are as follows: pedicle diameter, 3–4 mm; length, according to Swartz et al. [67] and Neukam et al. [71], is 4–6 cm from the scapular border to the axillary artery (6–9 cm if bone is not taken; if bone is included, the pedicle is shortened); bone length, 14 cm in men and 10 cm in women (if we include the tip, we gain a further 3–4 cm); bone thickness, 1.5 × 3 cm; and skin surface, 14 × 21 cm (sizes greater than 12 cm hinder direct closing).

The scapular flap is our last option for mandibular reconstruction. We think it has very specific indications, as follows:

- Three-dimensional orofacial defects with large defects of bone and soft tissue (intraoral and extraoral), since the mobility between these parts is considerable
- If the patient has peripheral vascular disease involving the iliofemoral and tibiofibular system and the defect cannot be reconstructed using a trapezius osteomyocutaneous flap

As reported by Deschler and Hayden [72], the contralateral scapula is usually shaped to the defect for two reasons. First, removal of the scapular flap requires disinsertion of several muscles from the upper edge (long part of the triceps, teres major and minor, and subscapular muscle), thus weakening the arm. If we proceed to radical dissection, the shoulder will be even more limited. Therefore, in order to prevent weakening of the arm and of the shoulder, the contralateral scapula is shaped to the defect and radical dissection performed. Second, by using the contralateral scapula and moving the lateral border of the scapula downward in the neomandible, we ensure that the pedicle emerges distally, in the area of the angle. Thus, the orientation of the pedicle in the neck is optimal.

Weakness of the upper arm is minimized by immobilization for a few days after surgery and rigorous physiotherapy [70] (Figs. 1.26, 1.27, 1.28, 1.29, and 1.30).

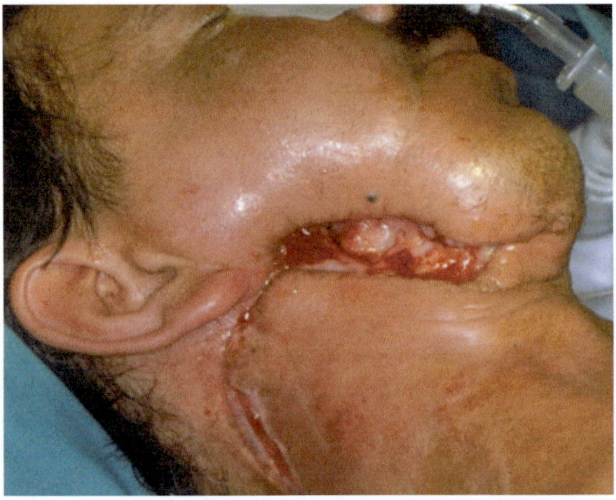

Fig. 1.26 Mandible tumor [87]

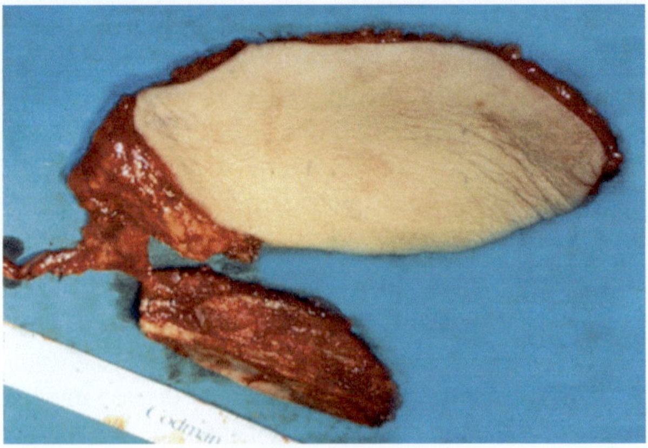

Fig. 1.27 Scapular free flap dissection

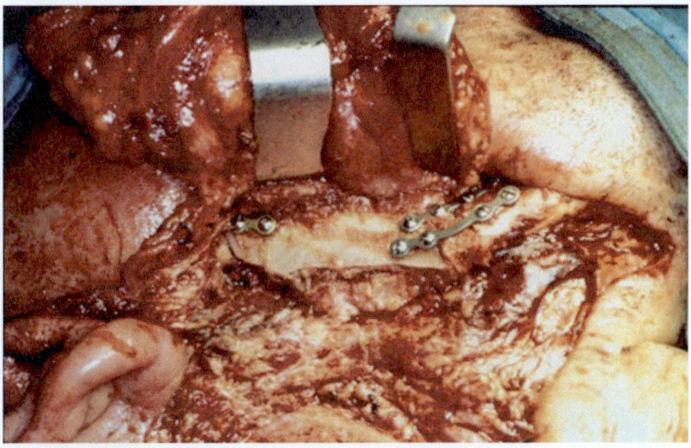

Fig. 1.28 Scapular free flap adapted at the defect

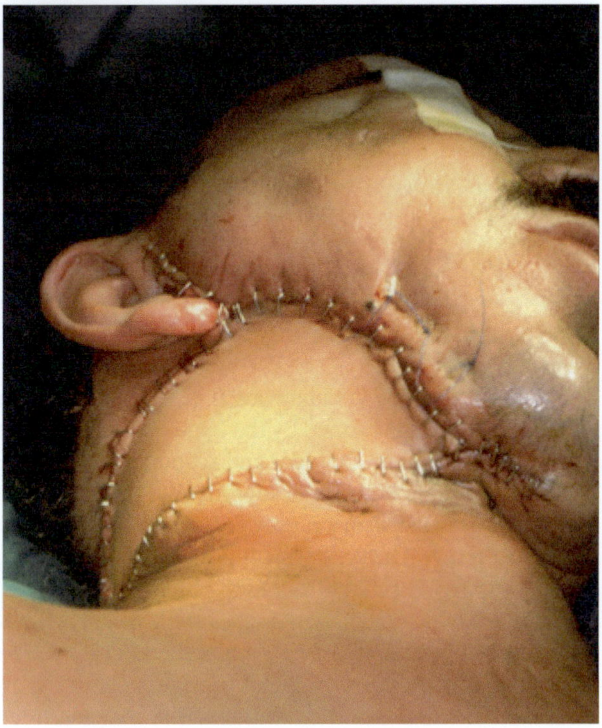

Fig. 1.29 Immediately postoperative view

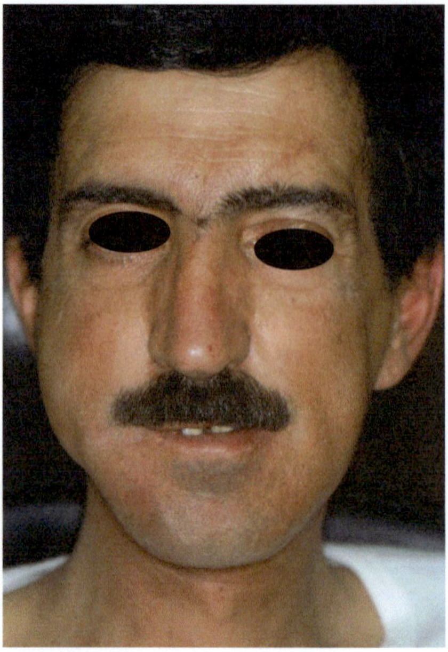

Fig. 1.30 Final appearance

1.9 Pedicle Flaps

1.9.1 Trapezius Osteomyocutaneous Flap

The trapezius osteomyocutaneous flap was first described in 1977 by Demergasso and Piazza [73]. It is formed by the upper and middle portion of the trapezius muscle, a skin island from the shoulder and scapular spine, and the acromion of the scapula.

The flap is supplied by the superficial transverse cervical artery, its main pedicle, and receives an accessory supply from the dorsal scapular artery, the occipital artery, and the intercostal arteries.

This supply makes it possible to obtain three different myocutaneous flaps [74]: the superior trapezius myocutaneous flap, which is based on the occipital artery and the intercostal paraspinal perforators; the lateral trapezius osteomyocutaneous flap, which is based on the superficial transverse cervical artery; and the inferior trapezius flap, which is based on the dorsal scapular artery and the deep branch of the transverse cervical artery.

We only discuss the lateral trapezius osteomyocutaneous flap (trapezius island flap), since it is the only one of the three that includes richly vascularized scapular bone [75].

It is based on the superficial transverse cervical artery and vein. In 80 % of cases, the superficial transverse cervical artery arises in the thyrocervical trunk; in the remaining 20 %, it arises in the subclavian artery [76]. When the artery arises directly from the subclavian artery, it can course deeply or via the brachial plexus, thus seriously limiting the arc of rotation of the pedicle and necessitating the use of another flap (10 % of cases) [74].

Venous anatomy is much more variable than arterial anatomy. The transverse cervical vein drains into the medial subclavian system in two-thirds of cases and into the external jugular vein (close to its union with the subclavian vein) in the remaining third [77] (Fig. 1.31).

In our experience, the skin paddle and anatomical references must be drawn with the patient seated and arms tight to the trunk. We center the paddle on the acromio-clavicular joint. The paddle can be as long as 12–20 cm from the back and up to 10 cm from the shoulder [78].

Including the acromion, the scapular spine measures about 13.5 cm in length and 0.7 cm in height at its medial border and up to 4 cm at its lateral border. Its width ranges between 1 and 2.4 cm.

Depending on the location of the mandibular defect, we use the acromion, spine, or both, as follows:

1. Symphyseal defect: can be reconstructed exclusively with the acromion and respecting the scapular spine
2. Lateral defect: can be reconstructed with the scapular spine respecting the acromion at its anatomical site
3. Mixed anterior and lateral defect: requires both the acromion and the scapular spine

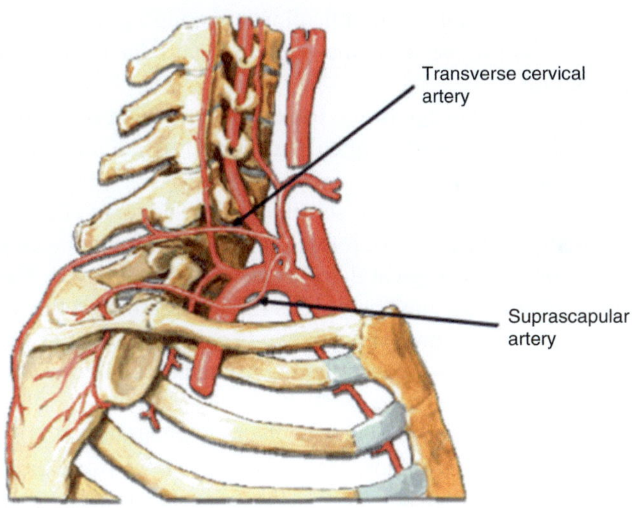

Fig. 1.31 Vascular pedicle [88]

In order to prevent functional sequelae, the muscle at the donor site must be reconstructed at closure: the supraspinatus muscle is sutured to the infraspinatus muscle. Once joined, both muscles are sutured to the deltoid, and the anterior group is anchored to the clavicle by nonabsorbable suture through purpose-made openings. The skin island is closed with a posterior rotation flap.

One of the reasons this flap has fallen into disuse was the fact that it was impossible to insert dental implants, without which only 10 % of patients could wear stable prostheses. In their study of cadaver scapulas, Navarro Vila et al. [74] showed that the acromion can take 13-mm implants in 100 % of cases, whereas the lateral border of the spine can do so in 80 % and the medial border in 20 %.

The trapezius island flap is indicated for mandibular reconstruction in patients with intraoral bone and soft tissue defects who simultaneously undergo radical ipsilateral dissection. The acromion and the scapular spine can be used to reconstruct the mandibular bone defect, while the skin island is used to repair the intraoral soft tissue defect. This flap makes it possible to repair bone defects of up to 10–12 cm. In some cases, the skin paddle has been unfolded to repair intraoral and extraoral tissue. The main contraindications are exclusively bone defects (iliac crest or fibula free flaps are preferred) and situations where cervical dissection is functional rather than radical. Using the trapezius muscle for the flap limits external rotation of the scapula, which is necessary for raising the shoulder and elevation and separation of the arm by 180°. It is also necessary to resect the sternocleidomastoid muscle to leave space in the neck so that the flap can be passed through to the mouth. If the dissection is radical, the nerves of the trapezius are always cut (XI pair) and the sternocleidomastoid is resected; therefore, the trapezius flap does not involve added morbidity. A final contraindication is secondary reconstruction after previous cervical dissection, because the pedicle could have been damaged during the first procedure.

A clear advantage of the trapezius flap is that it is a regional flap; consequently, morbidity is reduced, surgical time is shortened, and there is no need for two surgical teams.

Since this flap is more sensitive to the adverse effects of radiation therapy than microsurgical flaps [79], implants must always be placed immediately.

Before microsurgical flaps began to be widely used, Navarro Vila et al. [74] used the trapezius osteomyocutaneous flap to reconstruct the mandible in 78 cases, most of which (52 %) involved squamous cell carcinoma of the floor of the mouth. The cosmetic results were excellent, and the percentage of total/partial failures for this flap at all sites was only 14 %.

Today, this flap is only used when severe arteriosclerosis prevents reconstruction with microsurgical flaps, since the superficial transverse cervical vessels are not usually involved. In addition, as the reconstruction is with a pedicle, there is no need for anastomosis (Figs. 1.32, 1.33, 1.34, 1.35, and 1.36).

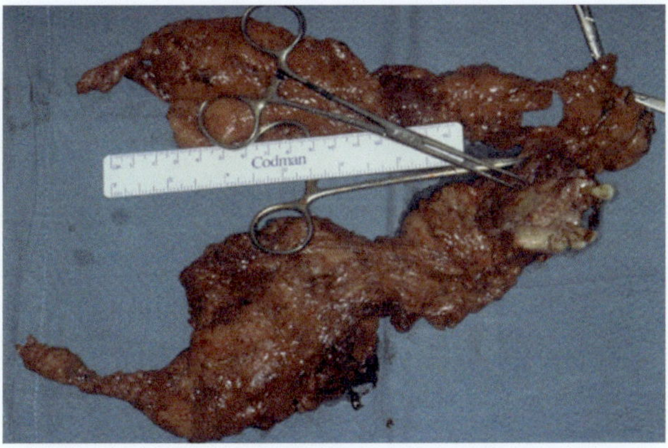

Fig. 1.32 Tumor dissection

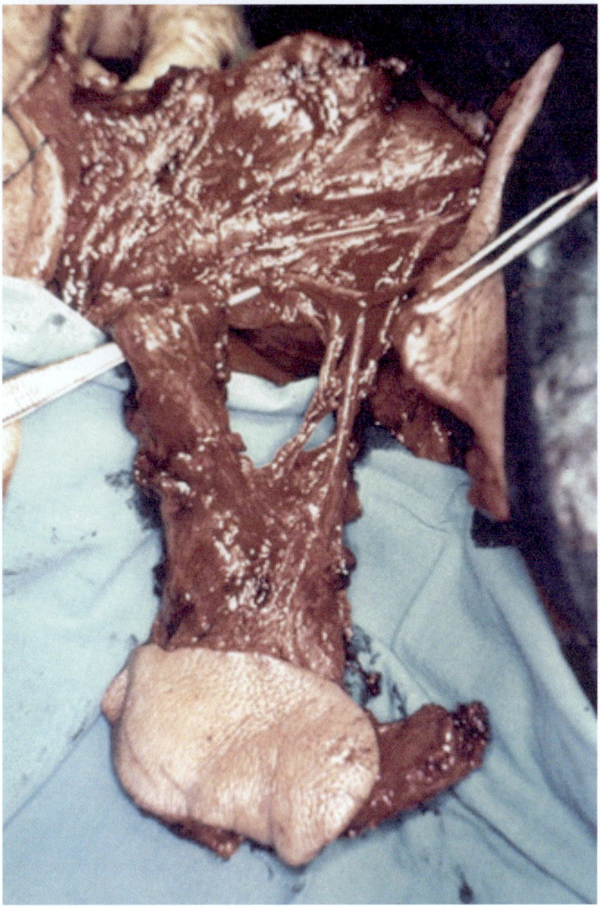

Fig. 1.33 Osteomyocutaneous trapezius flap isolated in its vascular pedicle

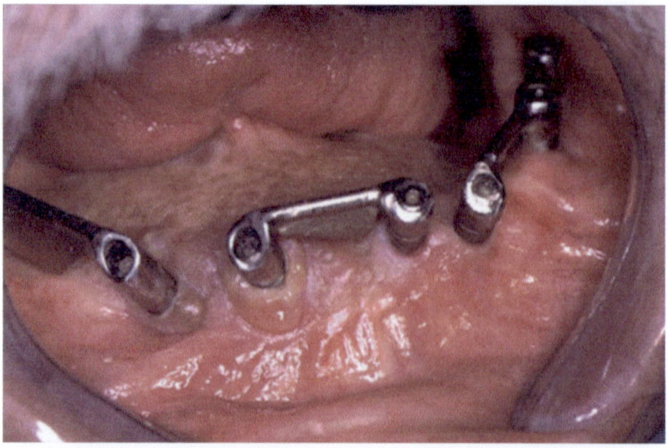

Fig. 1.34 Dental rehabilitation

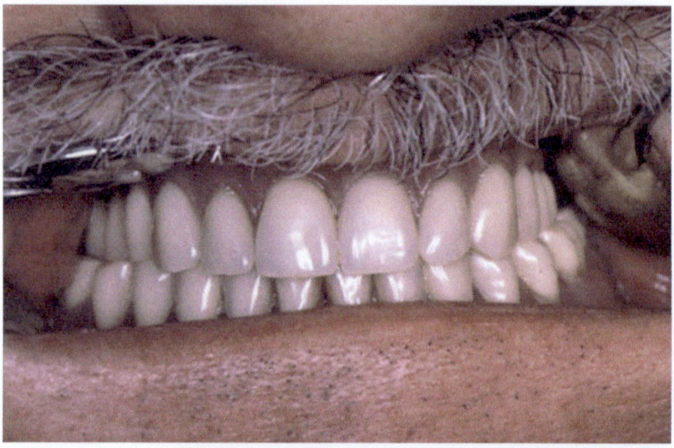

Fig. 1.35 Final occlusion

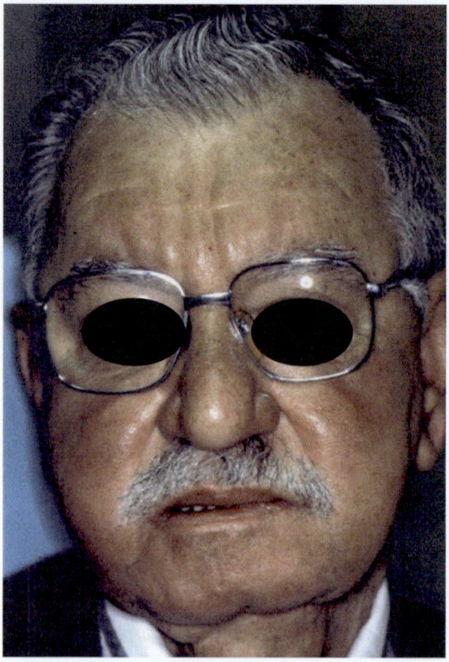

Fig. 1.36 Postoperative anteroposterior view of the patient

1.10 Reconstruction of the Condyle

The condyle is one of the main components of the temporomandibular joint (TMJ). Condylar defects are usually caused by tumors and often involve severe facial deformity and difficulty in mouth opening and mastication, thus significantly affecting quality of life.

Any discussion on the reconstruction of the TMJ necessarily [80] shows a significant difference between cases of a dysfunctional joint caused by a degenerative disease or ankylosis and cases in which reconstruction of a section of the mandible includes the TMJ. Advances in surgery to treat cancer of the head and neck have led to the creation of subtotal defects on an irradiated bed or and are that could be irradiated. These defects require a larger quantity of tissue and better vascularization; therefore, microvascular flaps tend to be used.

Condylar reconstruction techniques include costochondral grafts, vertical sliding osteotomy of the upper border of the ramus, sternoclavicular grafts, grafts of the second metatarsal, and prosthesis.

The system used by Kaban et al. [81, 82] to describe condylar defects can be applied to tumor resection, as follows:

- Class I defects, which only affect the condyle. The reconstruction articulates with the intact joint surface.
- Class II defects, in which condyle and articular disc are absent. The reconstruction articulates with the fibrous cartilage of the glenoid fossa and eminence of the temporal bone.
- Class III defects, in which the condyle, articular disc, and glenoid fossa are absent. Reconstruction of the middle cranial fossa and the joint is necessary.

Therefore, depending on the resected area, reconstruction must be adapted to anatomy and function. In unilateral openings, the objective is 35–40 mm; in bilateral openings, it is 30 mm. Potter and Dierks [80] report their reconstruction schedule according to the class of defect.

- Class I defects should have a good functional prognosis; therefore, the key to a successful procedure is careful remodeling of the proximal end of the fibula flap and its anatomical placement. A free condylar graft can also be added to the end of the fibula.
- Class II defects can be better restored with a contoured fibula and interposition of an auricular cartilage graft. This provides a stable bone reconstruction and the formation of pseudoarthrosis in the joint. The second metatarsal can also be used when only the structures of the TMJ are to be reconstructed.
- Class III defects that extend along the proximal mandible can be reconstructed by combining the fibula and the second metatarsal, or the fossa can be reconstructed with nonvascularized grafts, placement of an interposition flap, and mandibular reconstruction with a fibula flap.

In addition to the classic techniques described, it is also possible to use 2-step distraction osteogenesis for the reconstruction of the horizontal ramus and the ascending ramus, as described by Wang et al. [83], and to apply new technology to design double-barrel fibula flaps in which one fragment slides along the other for reconstruction of the condyle [84].

The promising results of Liu et al. [85] were based on three-dimensional porous titanium scaffold or allogenic bone scaffold combined with osteogenic and chondrogenic material and bone marrow stromal stem cells for repair of condylar defects in vivo using tissue engineering.

1.11 Application of Technology in Mandibular Reconstruction

Current advances in reconstruction in oral and maxillofacial surgery include navigation systems, 3D imaging, virtual planning, stereolithographic models, and custom prostheses.

Navigation systems enable the surgeon to know the position of surgical instruments in the patient's anatomy in real time. They were first described in the mid-1990s for stereotactic brain surgery. Taylor subsequently began to use them in our specialty this century.

Computer-assisted surgery is based on acquisition of preoperative images, which are processed to create three-dimensional models, plan surgery, and perform the intervention virtually.

Another important advantage of computer-assisted surgery is that it enables us to create stereolithographic models, cutting guides, and custom prostheses. The main benefit of this approach is that it can create mirror images of healthy areas for reconstruction of resected areas.

CAD/CAM enables us to improve surgical accuracy, improve rehabilitation prostheses, and reduce postoperative morbidity and surgical time.

When applying this technology in our practice, the necessary steps are as follows:

- Definition of the surgical problem.
- Analysis of all the options taking into account the diagnosis, prognosis, and patient preferences.
- Selection of the surgical strategy.
- Acquisition and processing of images to create three-dimensional images.
- Performance of virtual surgery on the images using specific software that enables us to make all three-dimensional movements.
- Creation of cutting guides, surgical models, and custom prostheses using CAD/CAM.
- Use of the material obtained during virtual surgery to guide surgical incisions. We can also use intraoperative surgery in order to perform guided resections and place custom prostheses.

Mandibular reconstructions that were unthinkable only 10 years ago are now being performed. Levine et al. [86] published a study of four complete mandibular reconstructions with prosthesis fitted during the same procedure, as did Wang et al. [84], who applied 3D technology for reconstruction of the mandible with the condyle using microsurgical double-barrel fibular flaps.

Thanks to these advances, we can perform complex reconstructive surgery while being sure of the outcome, since we know exactly where to make incisions in both ablative and reconstructive surgeries [89]. We will also be able to use mandibular reconstruction plates and previously modeled custom prostheses (Figs. 1.37, 1.38, 1.39, 1.40, 1.41, 1.42, 1.43, 1.44, 1.45, and 1.46).

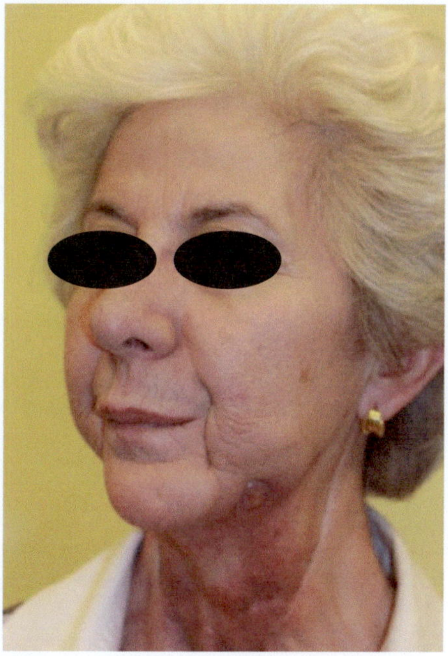

Fig. 1.37 Preoperative view

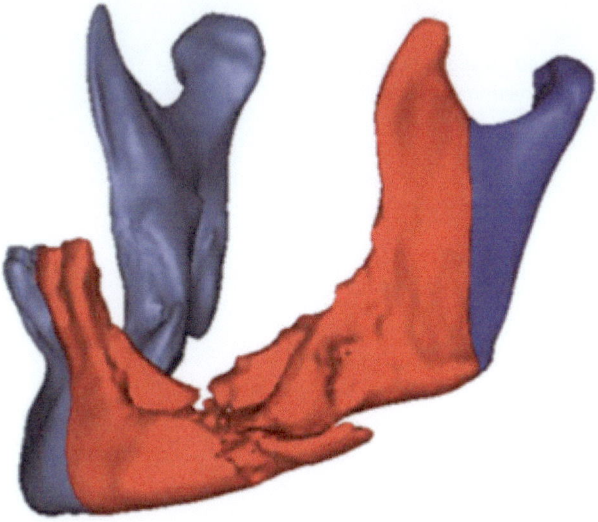

Fig. 1.38 Virtual planning resection

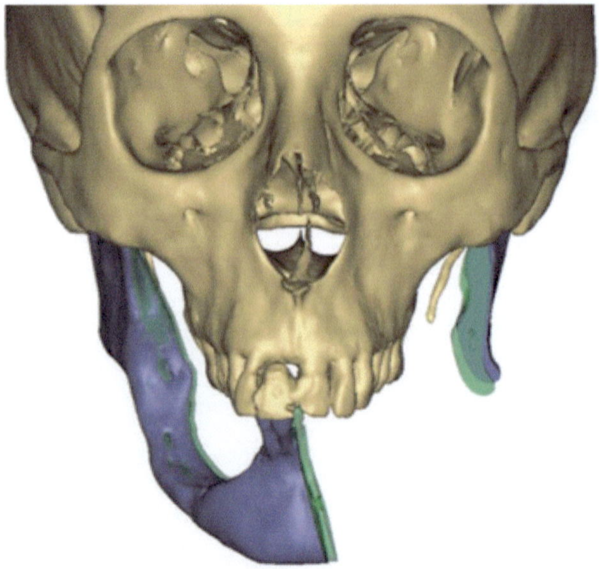

Fig. 1.39 Virtual planning defect

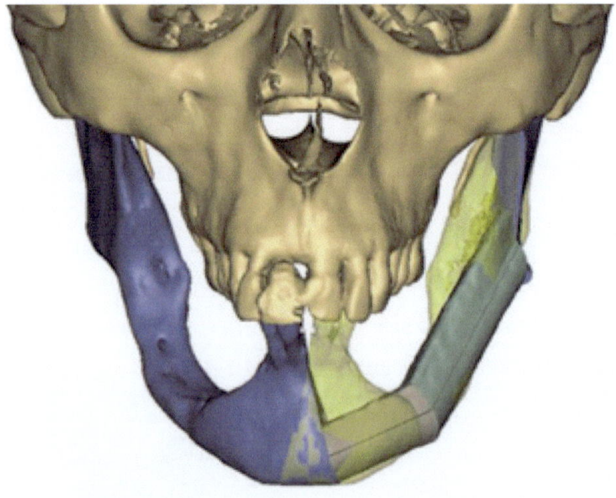

Fig. 1.40 Virtual planning reconstruction with fibula free flap

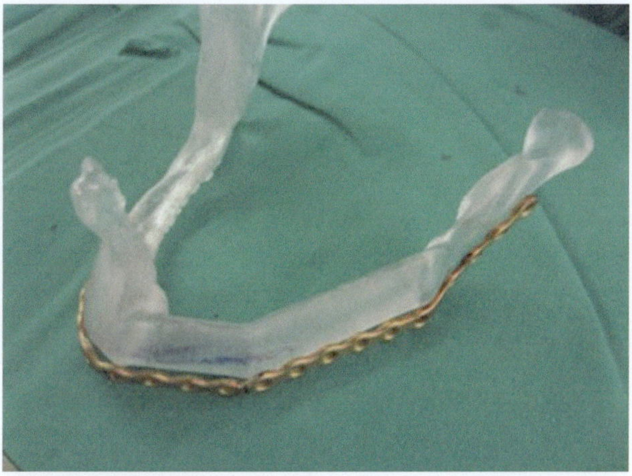

Fig. 1.41 Stereolithographic model with adapted plate

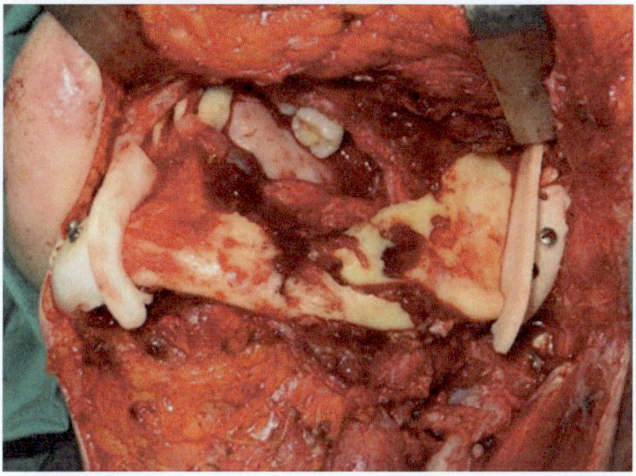

Fig. 1.42 Surgical guided resection at mandibular tumor

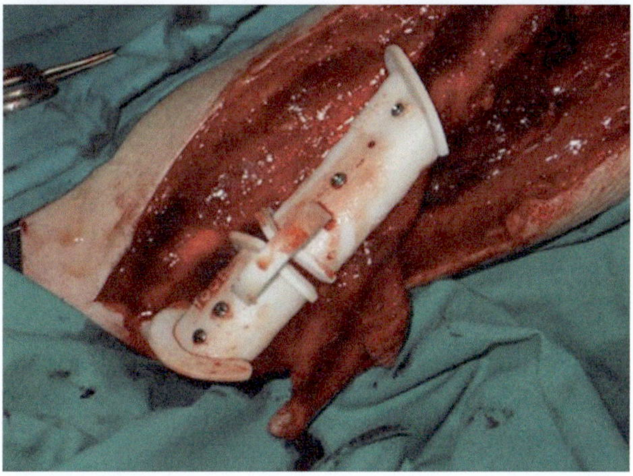

Fig. 1.43 Surgical guided resection of fibula flap

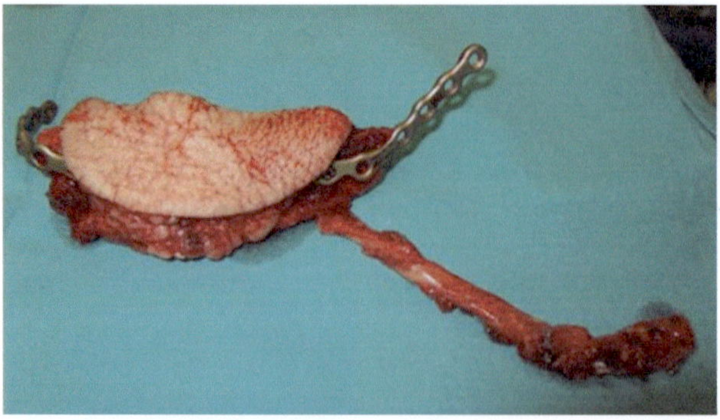

Fig. 1.44 Fibula free flap with reconstructed plate

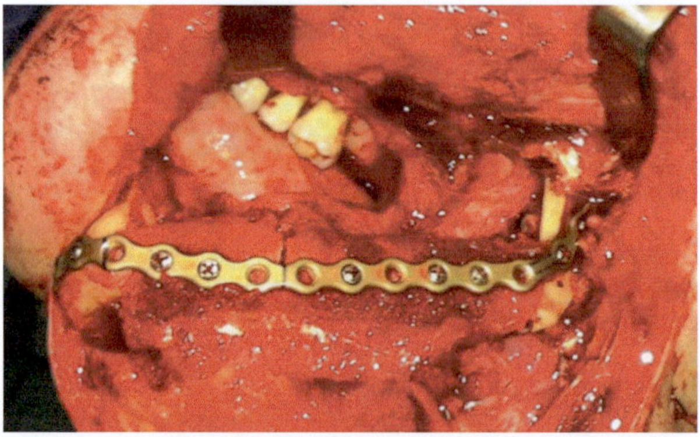

Fig. 1.45 Intraoperative reconstruction

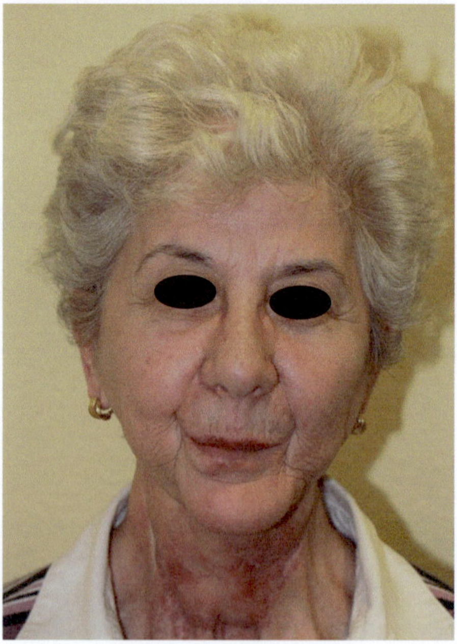

Fig. 1.46 Postoperative view

References

1. Bhishagratna KK. An English translation of the Sushruta Samhita based on original Sanskrit text. 3rd ed. Calcutta: Bose; 1916. p. 107.
2. Rogers BO. The historical evolution of plastic and reconstructive surgery. In: Wood-Smith D, Porowski PC, editors. Nursing care of the plastic surgery patient. St. Louis: C.V. Mosby; 1967. p. 4.
3. Taylor GI, Palmer JH. The vascular territories (angiosomes) of the body: experimental study and clinical applications. Br J Plast Surg. 1987;40(2):113.
4. Taylor GI, Palmer JH. Angiosome theory. Br J Plast Surg. 1992;45:327.
5. Wong RC, Tideman H, Kin L, Merkx MA. Biomechanics of mandibular reconstruction: a review. Int J Oral Maxillofac Surg. 2010;39:313–9.
6. Bardenheuer F. Verhandlung der Deutsch Gesellschaft Zentralbibliothek. Chirurgie. 1892;21:68.
7. Skyoff W. Frage der Knocken-plastik am Unterkiefer Zentralbibliothek. Chirurgie. 1900;35:881.
8. Ivy R, Epes BM. Bone grafting for defects of the mandible. Mil Surg. 1927;60:286–300.
9. Blocker TC, Stout RA. Mandibular reconstruction, World War II. Plast Reconstr Surg. 1949;4:153.
10. Brown RG, Vasquez LO, Jurkiewicz MJ. Reconstruction of the central mandible with a single block of iliac bone. Br J Plast Surg. 1976;29:191–5.
11. Millard RD, Deane M, Garst WP. Bending an iliac bone graft for anterior mandibular arch repair. Plast Reconstr Surg. 1976;48:600–1.
12. Wersal J, Bergsted H, Korlof B, Lind MG. Split rib graft for reconstruction of the mandible. Otolaryngol Head Neck Surg. 1984;92:270–5.
13. Hamaker R. Irradiated autogenous mandibular grafts in primary reconstruction. Laryngoscope. 1981;91:1031–51.
14. Hamaker R, Singer M, Schockley W. Irradiated mandibular autograft. Cancer. 1983;52:1017–21.
15. Cummings C, Leipzig B. Replacement of tumor involved mandible by cryosurgically devitalized autograft. Arch Otolaryngol. 1980;106:252–4.
16. DeFries HO, Marble HB, Sell KW. Reconstruction of the mandible: use of a homograft combined with autogenous bone and marrow. Arch Otolaryngol. 1971;93(4):426–32.
17. Akbay E, Aydogan F. Reconstruction of isolated mandibular bone defects with non-vascularized corticocancellous bone autograft and graft viability. Auris Nasus Larynx. 2014;41:56–62.
18. Luckey HA, Kubli F. Titanium alloys in surgical implants. ASTM ATP 796. Philadelphia: American Society for Testing and Materials; 1983.
19. Castermans A, Van Garse R, Vanwick R. Primary reconstruction of the mandible after resection for oral cancer. Acta Chir Belg. 1977;2:205–8.
20. Joyce LD, McQuarrie DG. Application of contemporary reconstructive techniques in head and neck for anterior oro-facial cancers. Surgery. 1976;80:373–8.
21. Bowerman JE. Noes on mandibular reconstruction. Proc R Soc Med. 1974;67:610–4.
22. Conley JJ. The use of vitallium prosthesis and implants in the reconstruction of the mandibular arch. Plast Reconstr Surg. 1951;8:150.
23. Cook HP. Immediate reconstruction of the mandible by metallic implant following resection for neoplasm. Ann R Coll Surg Engl. 1968;42:233–58.
24. Gullane PJ, Havas T, Holmes H. Mandibular reconstruction with metal plate and myocutaneous flap. Aust N Z J Surg. 1986;56:701–6.
25. Abbas AT. Reconstruction skeleton for the lower human jaw using CAD/CAM/CAE. J of King Saud Univ-Eng Sci. 2012;2:159–64.
26. Moulem R. Cancellous chip bone grafts. Lancet. 1944;2:146–748.
27. Boyne PJ, Zarem H. Osseous reconstruction of the resected mandible. Am J Surg. 1976;132: 49–53.
28. Lawson W, Loscalzo L, Baek SM. Experience with immediate and delayed mandibular reconstruction. Laryngoscope. 1982;92:5–10.
29. Albert TW, Smith JD, Everts E, Cook TA. Dacron mesh tray and cancellous bone in reconstruction of mandibular defects. Arch Otolaryngol Head Neck Surg. 1986;112:53–9.

30. Branemark PI, Lindstrom J, Hallen O. Reconstruction of the defective mandible. Scand J Plast Reconstr Surg. 1975;9:116–28.
31. Klotch DW, Prein J. Mandibular reconstruction using A-O plates. Am J Surg. 1987;154: 384–8.
32. Komisar A, Warman S, Danzinger E. A critical analysis of immediate and delayed mandibular reconstruction using A-O plates. Arch Otolaryngol Head Neck Surg. 1989;115(7):830–3.
33. Saunders JR, Hirata RM, Jaques DA. Definitive mandibular replacement using reconstruction plates. Am J Surg. 1990;160:387–9.
34. Gullane PJ. Primary mandibular reconstruction: analysis of 64 patients and evaluation of interface radiation dosimetry on bridging plates. Laryngoscope. 1991;101(54):1–24.
35. Zhou L, Zhao J, Shang H, Liu W, Feng Z, Liu G, Wang G, Liu Y. Reconstruction of mandibular defects using a custom-made titanium tray in combination with autologous cancellous bone. J Oral Maxillofac Surg. 2011;69:1508–18.
36. Yagihara K, Okabe S, Ishii J, Amagasa T, Yamashiro M, Yamaguchi S, Yokoya S, Yamazaki T, Kinoshita Y. Mandibular reconstruction using a poly(L-lactide) mesh combined with autogenous particulate cancellous bone and marrow: a prospective clinical study. Int J Oral Maxillofac Surg. 2013;42:962–9.
37. McCarthy JG, Williams JK, Grayson BH, Crombie JS. Controlled multiplanar distraction of the mandible: device development and clinical application. J Craniofac Surg. 1998;9(4):322–9.
38. Cuono C, Ariyan S. Immediate reconstruction of a composite mandibular defect with a regional osteomusculocutaneous flap. Plast Reconstr Surg. 1980;65:477.
39. Demergasso F, Piazza M. Trapezius myocutaneous flap in reconstructive surgery for head and neck cancer: an original technique. Am J Surg. 1979;138:533.
40. Panje W, Cutting C. Trapezius osteomyocutaneous island flap for reconstruction of the anterior floor of the mouth and the mandible. Head Neck Surg. 1980;3:66–71.
41. Panje WR. Mandible reconstruction with the trapezius osteomusculocutaneous flap. Arch Otolaryngol. 1985;111:223–9.
42. Little JW, McCulloch DT, Lyons JR. The lateral pectoral composite flap in one-stage reconstruction of the irradiated mandible. Plast Reconstr Surg. 1983;71:326–37.
43. Kudo K, Miyasawa M, Fujikoka Y, Sasaki J. Immediate repair of mandibular defects following surgery for carcinoma of the lower alveolus and gingiva using a pectoralis major osteomyocutaneous flap. J Maxillofac Surg. 1985;13:116–20.
44. Strauch B, Bloomberg AE, Lewin ML. An experimental approach to mandibular replacement: island vascular composite rib grafts. Br J Plast Surg. 1971;24:334–9.
45. Ostrup LT, Fredrickson JM. Reconstruction of mandibular defects after radiation using a free living bone graft transferred by microvascular anastomosis. Plast Reconstr Surg. 1975;55: 563–672.
46. Daniel RK. Mandibular reconstruction with free tissue transfer. Ann Plast Surg. 1978;1:346.
47. Taylor GI, Miller DH, Ham FJ. The free vascularized bone graft. A clinical extension of microvascular techniques. Plast Reconstr Surg. 1975;55:533–44.
48. Franklin JD, Shack BR, Stone J. Single stage reconstruction of mandible and soft tissue defects using a free osteocutaneous groin flap. Am J Surg. 1980;140:494–8.
49. MacLeod AM, Robinson DW. Reconstruction of defects involving the mandible and floor of the mouth by free osteocutaneous flaps derived from the foot. Br J Plast Surg. 1982;35:239–46.
50. Soutar DS, Widdowson WP. Immediate reconstruction of the mandible using a vascularized segment of radius. Head Neck Surg. 1986;8:232–46.
51. Cordeiro PG, Hidalgo DA. Soft tissue coverage of mandibular reconstruction plates. Head Neck. 1994;16(2):112–5.
52. Schusterman MA, Reece GP, Kroll SS, Weldon ME. Use of the A-O plate for immediate mandibular reconstruction in cancer patients. Plast Reconstr Surg. 1991;88(4):588–93.
53. Hoffmeister B, Fleiner B, Dunsche A. Significance of vascularization of jejunal transplants in secondary reconstruction of the mandible. Fortschr Kiefer Gesichtschir. 1994;39:111–4.
54. Hidalgo D. Fibula free flap: a new method of mandible reconstruction. Plast Reconstr Surg. 1989;84:71807.

55. Moscoso JF, Keller J, Geneden E, Weinberg H, Biller H, Buchbinder D, et al. Vascularized bone flaps in oromandibular reconstruction. Arch Otolaryngol Head Neck Surg. 1994;120:36–43.
56. Urken ML. Composite free flaps in oromandibular reconstruction. Review of the literature. Arch Otolaryngol Head Neck Surg. 1991;117:724–32.
57. Horiuchi K, Hattori A, Inada I, Kamibayashi T, Sagimura M, Yajima H, et al. Mandibular reconstruction using the double barrel fibular graft. Microsurgery. 1995;16:450–4.
58. Siciliano S, Lengele B, Reychler H. Distraction osteogenesis of a fibula free flap used for mandibular reconstruction: preliminary re- port. J Craniomaxillofac Surg. 1998;26:386–90.
59. Wei FC, Chen HC, Chuang CC, Noordhoff MS. Fibular osteosepto-cutaneous flap: anatomic study and clinical application. Plast Reconstr Surg. 1986;78:191–9.
60. Futran N, Stack BC, Payne LP. Use of color Doppler flow imaging for preoperative assessment in fibular osteoseptocutaneous free tissue transfer. Otolaryngol Head Neck Surg. 1997;117:660–3.
61. Futran N, Stack BC, Zaccardi MJ. Preoperative color flow Doppler imaging for fibula free tissue transfers. Ann Vasc Surg. 1998;12:445–50.
62. Wei F, Seah C, Tsai Y, Liu S, Tseu M. Hidalgo D. discussion "Fibula osteoseptocutaneous flap for reconstruction of composite mandibular defects". Plast Reconstr Surg. 1994;93:294–304.
63. Genden E, Buchbinder D, Chaplin JM, Lueg E, Funk GF, Urken ML. Reconstruction of the pediatric maxillae and mandible. Arch Otolaryngol Head Neck Surg. 2000;126:293–300.
64. Cuesta-Gil M, Ochandiano Caicoya S, Riba García F, Duarte Ruiz B, Navarro Cuéllar C, Navarro Vila C. Oral rehabilitation with osseointegrated implants in oncologic patients. J Oral Maxillofac Surg. 2009;67(11):2485–96.
65. Cuellar CN, Caicoya SJ, Sanz JJA, Cuéllar IN, Maza Muela C, Vila CN. Mandibular reconstruction with iliac crest free flap, nasolabial flap and osseointegrated implants. J Oral Maxillofac Surg. 2014;72(6):1226.e1–15.
66. Teot L, Bosse JP, Maffaregz R, et al. The scapular crest pedicled bone graft. Int J Micro surg. 1981;3:257–62.
67. Swartz WM, Banis JC, Newton ED, Ramasastry SS, Jones NF, Acland R. The osteocutaneous scapular flap for mandibular and maxillary reconstruction. Plast Reconstr Surg. 1986;77:530–45.
68. Baker SR, Sullivan MJ. Osteocutaneous free scapular flap for one stage mandibular reconstruction. Arch Otolaryngol Head Neck Surg. 1988;114:267.
69. Sullivan MJ, Carroll WR, Baker SR. The cutaneous scapular free flap in head and neck reconstruction. Arch Otolaryngol Head Neck Surg. 1990;116:600–3.
70. Kuriloff D, Sullivan M. Mandibular reconstruction using vascularized bone grafts. Otolaryngol Clin North Am. 1991;24:1391–418.
71. Neukam FW, Schmelzeisen R, Schliephake H. Oromandibular reconstruction with vascularized bone grafts in combination with implants. Oral and Maxill of Surg Clin N Am. 1994;7:717–38.
72. Deschler DG, Hayden RE. The optimum method for reconstruction of complex lateral oromandibular-cutaneous defects. Head Neck. 2000;22:674–9.
73. Demergasso F, Piazza M. Colgajo cutáneo aislado a pedículo muscular en cirugía reconstructiva por cáncer de cabeza y cuello. Téc-nica original. Actas de XLVII Congreso Argentino de Cirugía. Fórum de investigación. Buenos Aires; 1976.
74. Navarro-Vila C, Borja-Morant A, Cuesta M, López de Atalaya F, Salmerón JI, Barrios JM. Aesthetic and functional reconstruction with the trapezius osseomyocutaneous flap and dental implants in oral cavity cancer patients. J Craniomaxillofac Surg. 1996;24:322–9.
75. Navarro Vila C, Zárate Salazar J, Molini Dezotti D, Martínez Alegría J, Izaguirre Espinozo H, Suñer Machado M, et al. Reconstruction experience with myocutaneous and osteomyocutaneous skin flaps in oncological surgery of the head and neck. J Maxillofac Surg. 1984;12:107–13.
76. Netterville JL, Panje WR, Maves MD. The trapezius myocutaneous flap. Dependability and limitations. Arch Otolaryngol Head Neck Surg. 1987;113:271–81.
77. Cuesta Gil M, Navarro Vila C. Reconstrucción mandibular con el colgajo osteomiocutáneo trapecial. Estudio de 42 casos. Rev Esp Cirug Oral Maxil of. 1995;17:63–81.
78. Panje W, Morris M. Trapezius osteomusculocutaneous flap. In: Komisar A, editor. Mandibular reconstruction. New York: Thieme; 1997. p. 45–55.

79. Cuesta M, Ochandiano S, Barrios JM, Navarro Vila C. Rehabilitación oral con implantes osteointegrados en pacientes oncológicos. Rev Esp Cirug Oral Maxilof. 2001;23:171–82.
80. Potter JK, Dierks EJ. Vascularized options for reconstruction of the mandibular condyle. Semin Plast Surg. 2008;22(3):156–60.
81. Kaban LB, Moses MH, Mulliken JB. Surgical correction of hemifacial microsomia in the growing child. Plast Reconstr Surg. 1988;82:9–19.
82. Kaban LB, Moses MH, Mulliken JB. Correction of hemifacial microsomia in the growing child: a follow up study. Cleft Palate J. 1986;23 Suppl 1:50–2.
83. Wang JJ, Chen J, Ping FY, Yan FG. Double-step transport distraction osteogenesis in the reconstruction of unilateral large mandibular defects after tumour resection using internal distraction devices. Int J Oral Maxillofac Surg. 2012;41:587–95.
84. Wang WH, Zhu J, Deng JY, Xia B, Xu B. Three-dimensional virtual technology in reconstruction of mandibular defect including condyle using double-barrel vascularized fibula flap. J Craniomaxillofac Surg. 2013;41:417–22.
85. Liu CK, Jing CX, Tan XY, Xu J, Hu M. Using three-dimensional porous internal titanium scaffold or allogenic bone scaffold for tissue-engineering condyle as a novel reconstruction of mandibular condylar defects. J Med Hypotheses and Ideas. 2014;8:69–73.
86. Levine JP, Bae JS, Soares M, Brecht LE, Saadeh PB, Ceradini DJ, Hirsch DL. Jaw in a day: total maxillofacial reconstruction using digital technology. Plast Reconstr Surg. 2013;131(6): 1386–91.
87. López de Atalaya FJ. Utilización de los colgajos microquirúrgicos en cirugía maxilofacial [PhD thesis]. Madrid: Universidad Complutense; 1996.
88. Navarro-Vila C, Ochandiano S, López de Atalaya FJ, Cuesta M, Acero J, Barrios JM, et al. Reconstrucción mandibular: colgajos pediculados y microquirúrgicos. Cir Esp. 2002;72(5): 287–96.
89. Kontio R. Update on mandibular reconstruction: computer-aided design, imaging, stem cells and future applications. Curr Opin Otolaryngol Head Neck Surg. 2014;22(4):307–15.

Maxillary and Middle Face Reconstruction

2

Carlos Navarro Vila, Ana María López López, Cristina Maza Muela, and Carlos Navarro Cuellar

Abstract

Reconstruction of the maxilla is a challenge for the maxillofacial and oral surgeon. Defects caused by injury or tumor resection alter the stomatognathic system, leading to cosmetic and functional abnormalities.

Surgery for primary reconstruction of defects resulting from tumor resection is less complicated because no radiation therapy has been administered and fibrosis is not present. Consequently, the patient can return to work and regain a normal social and personal life.

Since there is no ideal surgical technique for reconstruction of the middle third, the type of defect, general status, and experience of the surgical team are key factors.

C. Navarro Vila, MD, DMD, PhD, FEBOMS (✉)
Full Professor Medical Faculty, Complutense University of Madrid, Madrid, Spain

Head of Oral and Maxillofacial Surgery Department, Gregorio Marañón General University Hospital, Madrid, Spain

Académico Correspondiente of the Royal National Academy of Medicine of Spain, Madrid, Spain
e-mail: cnavarro.vila@clinicanavarrovila.com

A.M. López López, MD, DDS, FEBOMS
Consultant at Oral and Maxillofacial Surgery Department, Miguel Servet University Hospital, Zaragoza, Spain
e-mail: anitalopez@gmail.com

C. Maza Muela, MD, DDS, FEBOMS
Consultant at Oral and Maxillofacial Surgery Department, Gregorio Marañón General University Hospital, Madrid, Spain
e-mail: crismazamuela@gmail.com

C. Navarro Cuellar, MD, DDS, PhD, FEBOMS

Associate Professor Medical Faculty, Complutense University of Madrid, Madrid, Spain

Consultant at Oral and Maxillofacial Surgery Department, Gregorio Marañón General University Hospital, Madrid, Spain
e-mail: cnavarrocuellar@gmail.com

C. Navarro Vila (ed.), *Reconstructive Oral and Maxillofacial Surgery*,
DOI 10.1007/978-3-319-20487-1_2

2.1 Introduction

The maxilla is the most important bone of the facial skeleton. It provides support to essential cosmetic structures and is involved in major functions such as chewing, speech, and swallowing.

Reconstruction of middle third defects is a challenge for the surgeon. According to Smolka et al. [1], ablative surgery, which is performed to treat tumors and injuries, necessarily implies a modification of the stomatognathic system.

Few patients undergo maxillectomy for maxillary cancer or gum cancer. Kreeft et al. [2] reported that the incidence of maxillary cancer in the United States was less than one case per 100,000 inhabitants. The different histologic types include adenocarcinoma, squamous cell carcinoma, adenoid cystic carcinoma, minor salivary gland carcinoma, and melanoma.

Many of these tumors, especially those located in the maxillary sinus, grow progressively to cause minor symptoms such as recurrent sinusitis, displacement of teeth, nasal respiratory insufficiency, and allergic processes. Therefore, at diagnosis, the tumors are considered advanced and invasive.

The treatment of choice for maxillary tumors is surgery, which involves resection with safety margins and immediate reconstruction. During the last few decades, a considerable percentage of maxillary tumors have been observed to metastasize to the cervical region, with the result that many authors recommend regional cervical treatment, mainly in stage III and IV maxillary sinus tumors and in undifferentiated tumors. Many such tumors subsequently require adjuvant approaches, such as radiation therapy and chemotherapy. In this chapter, we do not establish the indications for the different treatments; rather, we attempt to identify the most appropriate reconstruction technique for the postsurgical defect.

The first use of reconstructive surgery can be traced back to India before 2000 BC, when a nasal reconstruction procedure was performed using a frontal flap.

The maxilla enables us to chew, prevents the passage of solids and liquids to the nostrils and maxillary sinus, supports the eyeball, holds the teeth (which are involved in phonation, chewing, and physical appearance), ensures appropriate positioning of the eyeball, and enables the patient to speak. Therefore, all of these functions must be restored after maxillectomy. According to Okay et al. [3], the best cosmetic and functional results are obtained when the objective of surgery is oral rehabilitation and recovery of occlusion using dental prostheses. Cordeiro and Chen [4] state that maxillary reconstruction should achieve the following objectives:

1. Closure of the surgical wound
2. Elimination of the maxillary defect
3. Provision of support to the eyeball (if retained) or filling of the cavity after exenteration
4. Maintenance of the barrier between the paranasal sinuses and the anterior cranial fossa
5. Recovery of facial contour
6. Reconstruction of the palate
7. Provision of functional dentition

Since no single surgical technique can achieve all these objectives, maxillary reconstruction can vary depending on the extent of the resection (of both hard and soft tissue) and comorbidities.

Defects were traditionally repaired using obturators; however, the advances in the use of other tissues described by Futran and Mendez [5], particularly microvascular free flaps and pedicle flaps, have considerably increased the number of options for reconstruction.

Reconstruction of the maxilla and intraoral and/or extraoral soft tissue defects can be performed immediately (together with ablative surgery) or delayed (during a second procedure). Reconstruction performed during the initial procedure for head and neck defects was first proposed by Edgerton [6] in 1951.

According to Navarro Cuellar [7], the advantages of immediate reconstruction are as follows:

- Only one procedure required
- Greater simplicity: no fibrosis after surgery or radiation therapy
- More cost-effective
- Earlier return to work and a normal social and personal life
- Better recovery from the psychological problems caused by the deformity and by concern over the need for surgery in the future

Nevertheless, reconstructive procedures are long and require two teams working simultaneously.

The advantages of delayed reconstruction are as follows:

- Recurrences are detected more easily in patients who have not undergone a reconstructive procedure.
- Approximately 50 % of patients die within 3 years; therefore, it is better to wait and perform reconstruction surgery in patients in whom no recurrences are detected.

The disadvantages are higher costs, more complicated technique, and modification of vascular structures by radiation therapy. Finally, we cannot forget the psychological effects and severe functional restrictions associated with facial defects.

According to some authors, immediate reconstruction has the disadvantage that recurrences may be difficult to detect in 50 % of T3 and T4 tumors, although current imaging techniques (e.g., computed tomography, magnetic resonance, and endoscopy) make it easy to overcome this disadvantage, since even minute recurrences can be detected. Consequently, today, the possibility of early recurrence is no longer a contraindication for immediate reconstruction.

In summary, we are very much in favor of immediate reconstruction.

2.2 Classification of Maxillectomy Defects

Maxillectomy involves partial or total resection of the maxilla. Lizards [8] first described total maxillectomy in 1826. Two years later, Syme [9] performed the first maxillectomy combined with enucleation without a general anesthetic.

According to Eley and Watt-Smith [9], the indications for maxillectomy include benign and malignant tumors of the bone itself, as well as cancer of neighboring tissue.

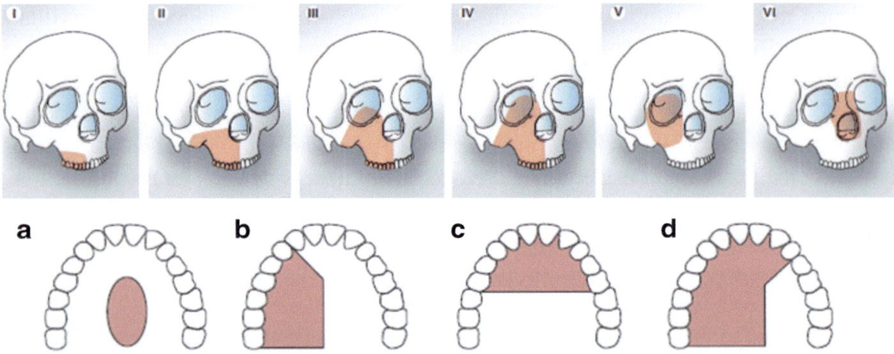

Fig. 2.1 Vertical and horizontal defects. Brown classification 2010

The objective of surgery is to ensure an adequate safety margin. In most cases, the procedure is performed to treat malignant tumors, mainly squamous cell carcinoma (80 %).

Given that there is no single internationally accepted classification for maxillectomy, the literature contains several options, such as the classifications of Wells and Luce [10], Spiro et al. [11], Davison et al. [12], Cordeiro and Santamaria [13], and Triana et al. [14], which are based on the nature of the procedure itself or on the resulting defect, as stated by Bidra et al. [15].

We use the classification proposed by Brown et al. [16, 17].

2.2.1 2010 Brown Classification

In 2000, Brown published a classification of maxillectomy defects [16] that was modified in 2010 [17]. Thus, defects are classified according to their vertical and horizontal components.

Vertical

I. Maxillectomy not causing an oroantral fistula
II. Maxillectomy not involving the orbit
III. Maxillectomy involving the orbital adnexa with orbital retention
IV. Maxillectomy with orbital enucleation or exenteration
V. Orbitomaxillary defect
VI. Nasomaxillary defect
VII. Maxillary defect not causing an oronasal fistula

Horizontal

(a) Palatal defect only, not involving the dental alveolus
(b) Defect less than or equal to one half unilateral
(c) Defect less than or equal to one half bilateral or transverse anterior
(d) Defect greater than one half maxillectomy (Fig. 2.1)

Poetker et al. [18] report complications arising from surgery, including cerebrospinal fluid leak, mucocele, trigeminal nerve pain, osteomyelitis, perforation of the nasal septum, oroantral and oronasal communications, loss of midface projection, nasal collapse, formation of synechiae, alar retraction, and ectropion.

2.3 Reconstructive Techniques

2.3.1 Obturators

An obturator is any dental prosthesis that prevents oroantral and oronasal communication while reestablishing dentition and speech. It is a simple, nonsurgical option. Pittman and Zender [19] favor performing a dental assessment before surgery so that the necessary extractions of infected teeth can be made and an impression can be taken for the obturator if reconstruction of resected tissue is not planned. However, it may be difficult for these prostheses to remain in place, as they are made before surgery. Park and Kwon [20] maintain that delayed surgical obturators can provide better functional results than immediate obturators.

We are against the use of obturators for the following disadvantages:

- Deficient aesthetic and functional reconstruction
- Rhinolalia
- Midface retrusion
- Inadequate prosthetic rehabilitation
- Difficult insertion in patients with trismus (Figs. 2.2 and 2.3)

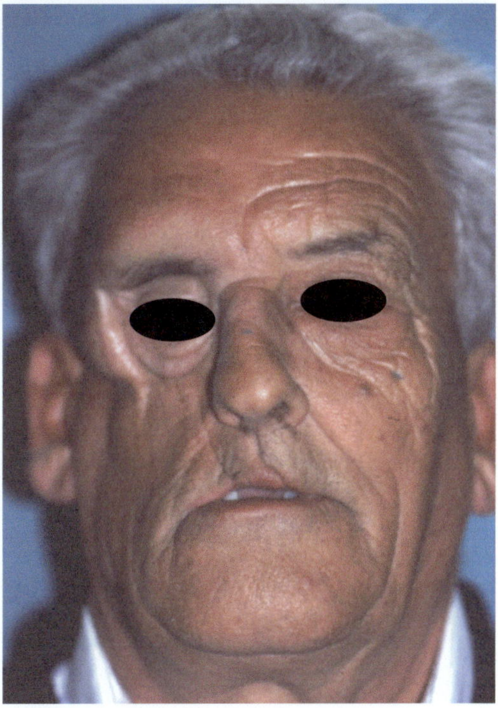

Fig. 2.2 Right maxillectomy. Reconstruction with an obturator

Fig. 2.3 Midface retraction

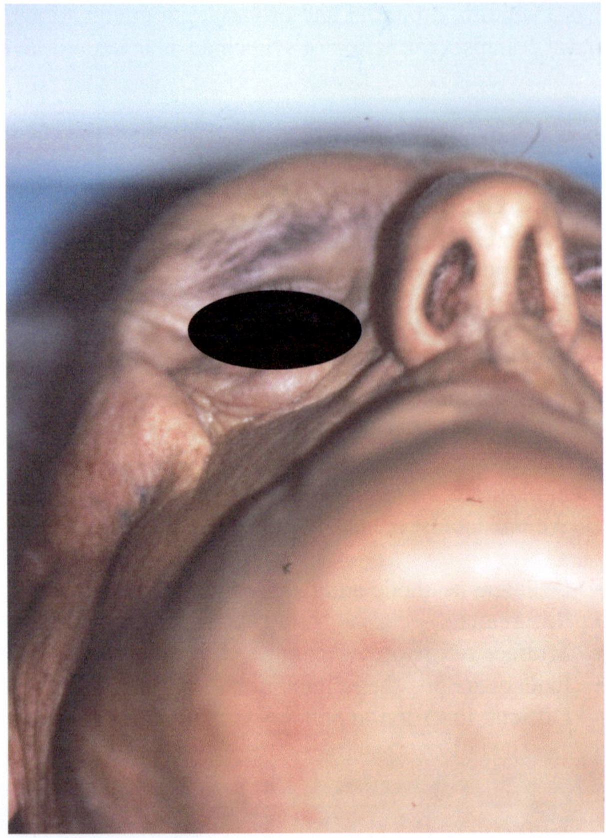

The nineteenth century saw the first descriptions of pedicle flaps, which were an alternative in the management of maxillectomy defects. Other surgical techniques became available over time, including nonvascularized grafts, free flaps, and distraction osteogenesis. The size of the soft or hard tissue defect is crucial when deciding on a reconstruction technique. Nevertheless, there is no consensus on the ideal approach for each type of defect [1].

2.3.2 Local Flaps

Local and regional flaps are the first choice for small defects such as those affecting the palate, maxillary tuberosity, and oroantral communications.

2.3.2.1 Bichat Fat Pad

This structure was reported by Bichat in 1802, although it had already been described by Heister in 1732 and Winslow in 1753. Egyedi was first to use it for reconstruction of the oral cavity in 1977 [21–25].

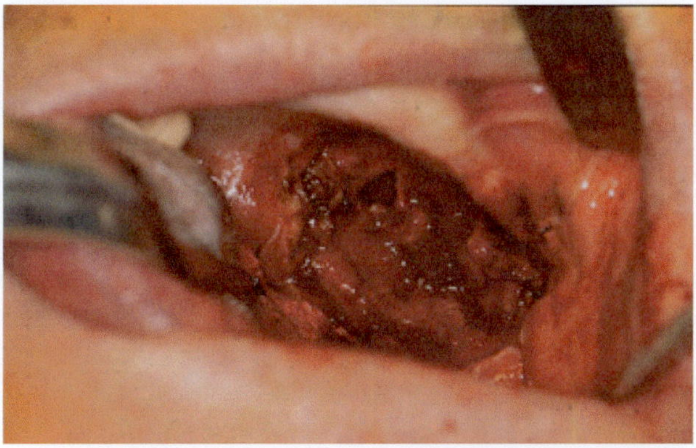

Fig. 2.4 Reconstruction of the maxillary tuberosity with Bichat fat pad

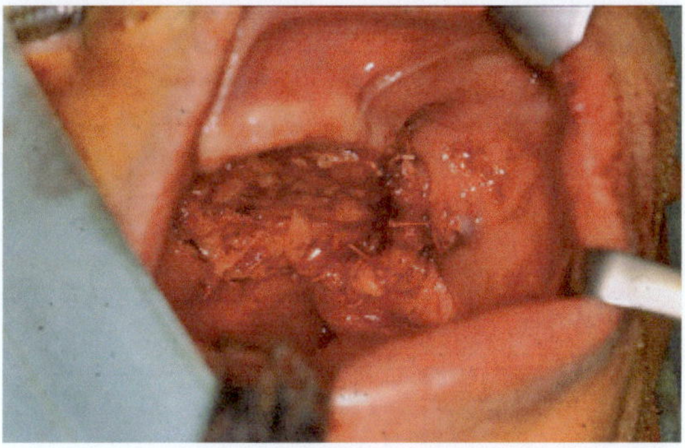

Fig. 2.5 Intraoperative result

Vascularization depends on three arteries: the buccal branch and the deep temporal branch, both of which are branches of the internal maxillary artery, and the transverse facial artery, which is a branch of the superficial temporal artery. Blood supply is also provided by small branches of the facial artery. Such diversity of supply ensures the safety of this option.

The Bichat fat pad can be used to close fistulas of the palate (post-extraction, post-maxillectomy) and small mucosal defects (Figs. 2.4 and 2.5).

2.3.3 Regional Pedicle Flaps

Regional pedicle flaps were first used in the nineteenth century. Flap survival always depends on integrity and appropriate vascularization once the flap has been surgically designed.

According to Muzaffar et al. [26], the first flaps used for reconstruction of the midface were the deltopectoral flap, pectoralis major flap, latissimus dorsi flap, temporalis flap, sternocleidomastoid flap, and trapezius flap. The pectoralis, latissimus dorsi, and trapezius are too bulky and difficult to adapt for most defects.

Pedicle flaps are used for larger defects. Carstens et al. [27] stated that pedicle flaps were limited by the length of the vascular pedicle and the lack of sufficient tissue to fill the defect. Their intrinsic characteristics make these flaps ideal for elderly patients with a high cardiovascular risk.

2.3.3.1 Buccinator Flap

The buccinator is made of flexible, thin tissue, and, according to Zhao et al. [28], its properties are satisfactory. It is covered medially by mucosa and laterally by the masseter, the ascending mandibular branch, the Bichat fat pad, and the buccopharyngeal fascia. Anteriorly, it is intertwined with the orbicularis oculi; posteriorly, it inserts into the pterygomandibular ligament.

Kaplan [29] first used the buccal mucosa in 1975, followed by Maeda et al. [30], who incorporated fibers from the buccinator. Bozola et al. [31] reported that the buccal artery and facial artery [27, 32] provided the main supply to the flap. Venous drainage is by the pterygoid plexus and the facial vein.

The buccinator can be used for posterior-based flaps. It can be tunneled below the pterygomandibular ligament to close defects of the palatine and pharyngeal mucosa, dental alveolus, and floor of the mouth. Its design can also be anterior based to close defects of the anterior hard palate, dental alveolus, maxillary sinus, floor of the nasal cavity, lip, and orbit.

Nowadays, we do not use this flap for any maxillary defects.

2.3.3.2 Temporalis Muscle Flap

The temporalis muscle flap was first described in 1898 by Golovine [33] for reconstruction of an orbital defect after exenteration.

In a study with rhesus monkeys in 1981, Bradley and Brockbank [34] reported the possibility of rotating the temporalis muscle toward the mouth after division of the zygomatic arch and base of the coronoid.

Cheung [35] described the rich microvascular network of the temporalis muscle, which depends on three main arteries: the anterior deep temporal artery, the posterior deep temporal artery, and the middle temporal artery. The first two arteries are branches of the internal maxillary artery, whereas the third arises from the superficial temporal artery. Such extensive vascularization makes the temporalis flap a very safe reconstructive technique for intraoral defects, with relatively few complications during recovery. Survival of this flap is based on preservation of the deep temporal artery.

Ahmed Djae et al. [36] report the following advantages for the temporalis muscle flap:

- Both the flap and the area to be reconstructed are found in the same surgical field.
- The muscle is quite bulky.
- Adequate vascularization.
- The flap comprises muscle and fascia.
- Minimal morbidity.
- The cosmetic defect in the temporal fossa can be corrected with a prosthesis.

We use this flap for Brown type IA and IIA defects [17]. In the case of type IIIA defects, we use it to reconstruct the palate in combination with other flaps.

Functional rehabilitation is done with a mixed prosthesis based on the contralateral teeth and a removable partial denture with attachments or implants in the contralateral maxilla. In our experience, we place Mozo Grau implants (MG osseous) in the contralateral maxilla with excellent results.

Although Cheung [35] describes submucosal neovascularization during the first weeks after muscle transfer, the approach does permit subsequent surgery for reconstruction with cortical-cancellous chips and titanium mesh before dental rehabilitation with implants. We do not use this technique.

Complications are often associated with the size of the defect and the location of the structure to be replaced. They include the following:

- Oroantral communications
- Partial/total flap loss
- Difficulties with chewing and/or mouth opening
- Paresis/paralysis of the frontal branch of the facial nerve
- Hematoma, superinfection, and cosmetic defects at the donor site (Figs. 2.6, 2.7, 2.8, 2.9, 2.10, 2.11, and 2.12)

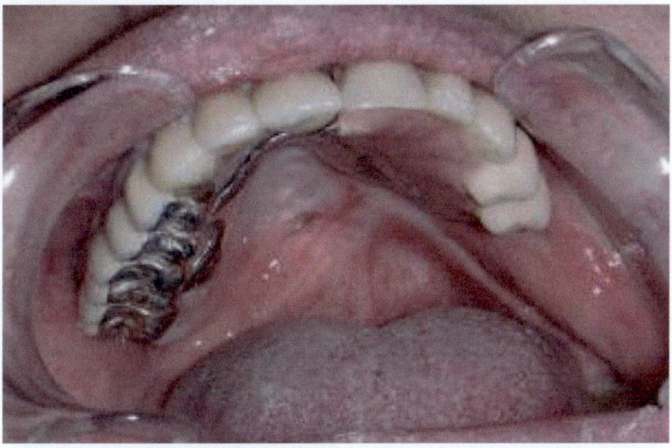

Fig. 2.6 Palatal reconstruction after IA maxillectomy

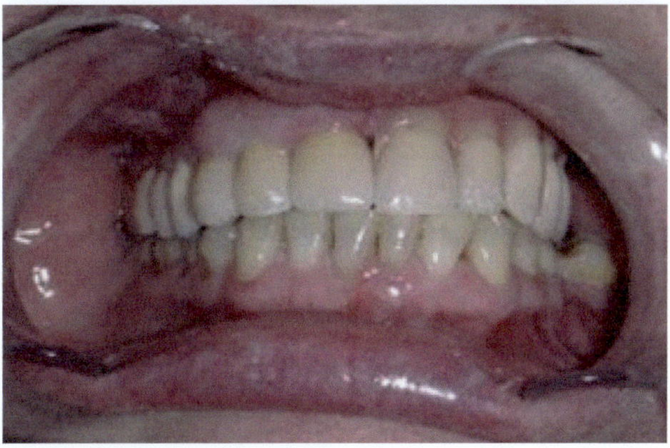

Fig 2.7 Definitive occlusion

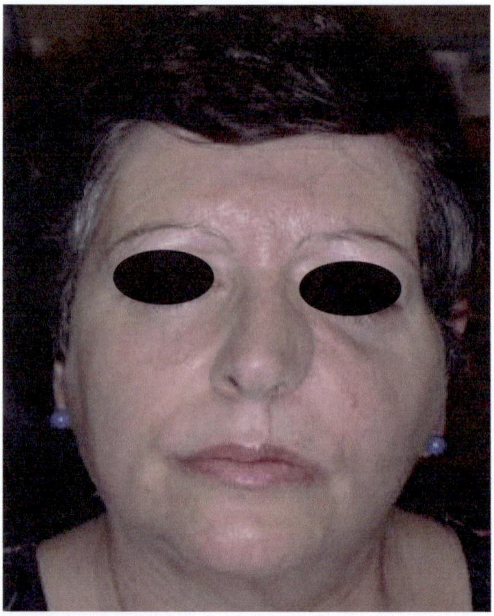

Fig. 2.8 Postoperative view

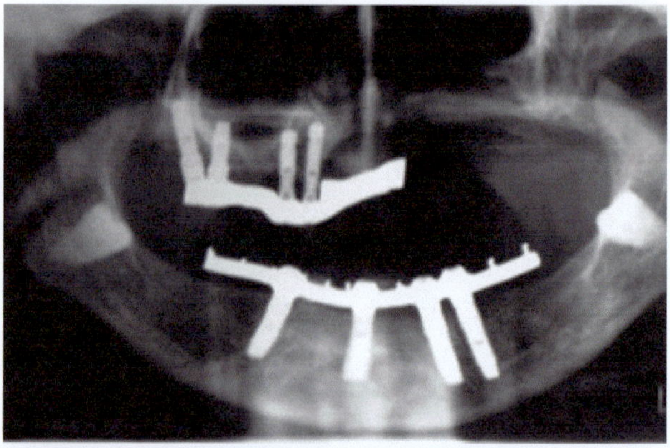

Fig. 2.9 Prosthetic rehabilitation with dental implants on the contralateral hemimaxilla

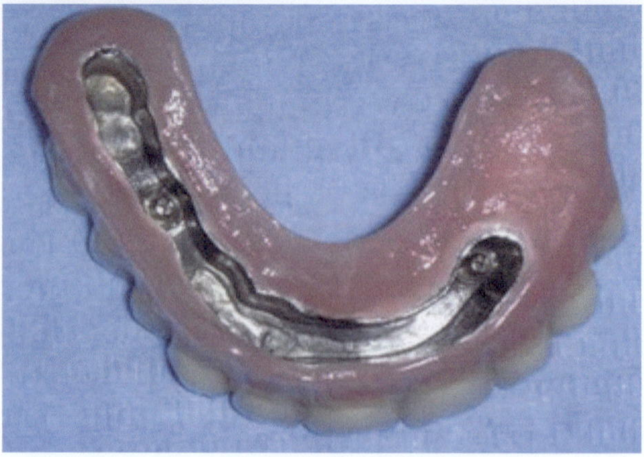

Fig. 2.10 Prosthesis

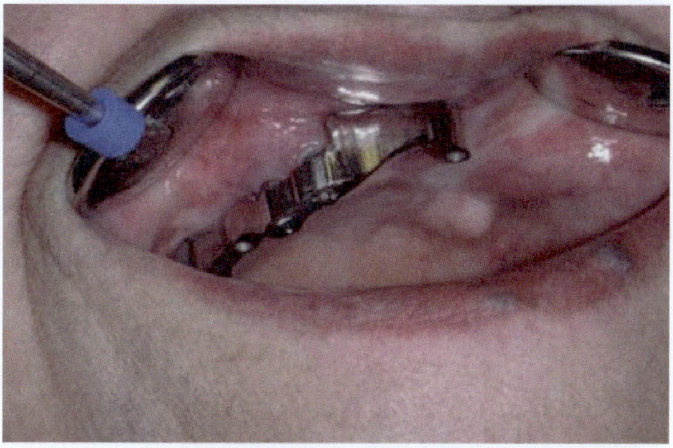

Fig. 2.11 Postoperative intraoral view

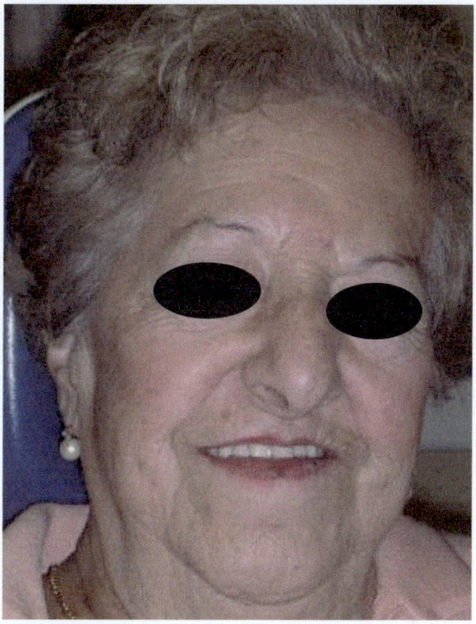

Fig. 2.12 Postoperative view

2.3.3.3 Temporoparietal Fascial Flap with Parietal Bone Flap

In 1898, Brown [37] and Monks [38] first reported using this flap to reconstruct the external ear and upper eyelid.

The temporoparietal fascial flap has a very long axis of rotation, which, according to Roy et al. [39], enables high mobility. Furthermore, Lam and Carlson [40] report that the anatomy of the temporal artery system is very constant, with blood supply to the flap provided by the superficial temporal vein and artery.

Mokal et al. [41] state that this reconstruction technique can be jeopardized by local traumatic injuries, previous surgery, radiation therapy, and carotid artery occlusion.

Its advantages include the following:

- Large area (approximately 14 × 17 cm)
- Thinness (2–4 mm)
- Inclusion of parietal bone

Its complications include the following:

- Possible lesion of the frontal branch of the facial nerve
- Unsightly scars
- Alopecia on scar tissue

We rarely use this flap; sometimes we apply it to maxillectomy IIIA in combination with temporalis muscle flap. The parietal bone supports the eye in the right position, and the temporalis myofascial flap reconstructs the palate.

It can include parietal bone for reconstruction of malar bone defects.

Therefore, we use it in type IIA defects, where it holds the eyeball in place (Figs. 2.13, 2.14, 2.15, and 2.16).

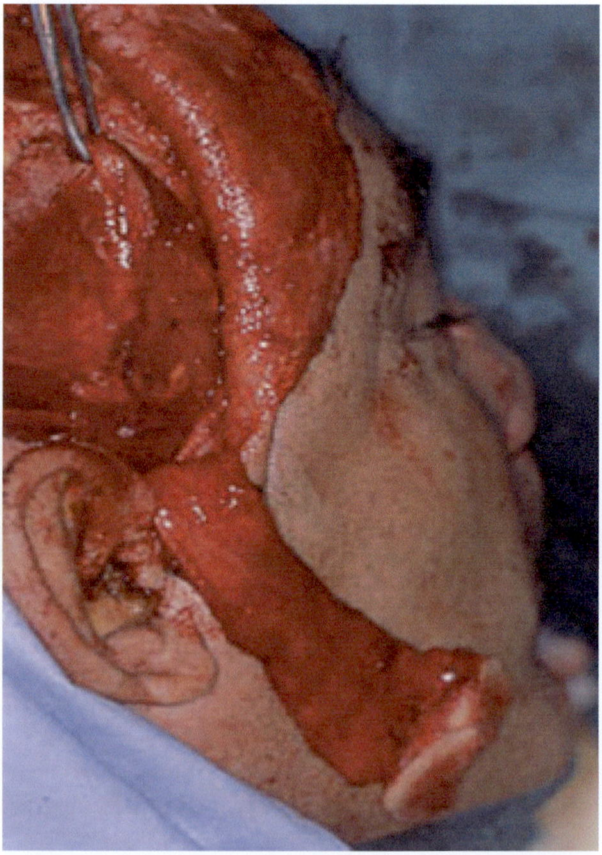

Fig. 2.13 Harvesting myofascial temporalis flap and temporoparietal flap

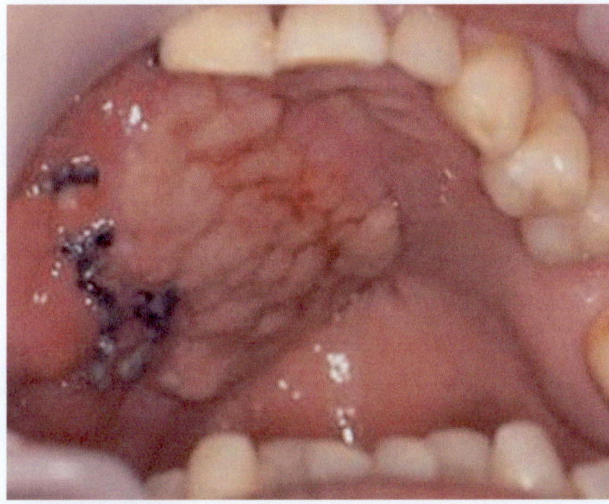

Fig. 2.14 Early postoperative intraoral view

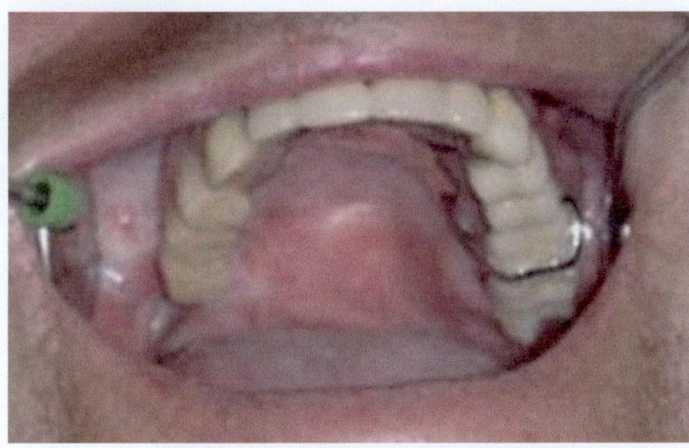

Fig. 2.15 Mucosalization of the myofascial flap after 6 months

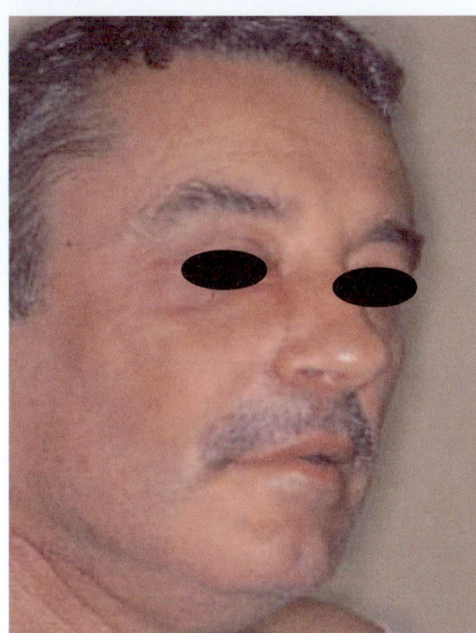

Fig. 2.16 Postoperative view

2.3.3.4 Cervicopectoral Flap

For maxillary defects that require large reconstructions of facial skin, Sakellariou and Salama [42] consider the cervicoparietal flap an excellent alternative that provides an adequate cosmetic appearance and prevents the patchy effect of other techniques. In addition, morbidity of the donor site is minimal, as reported by Shestak et al. [43]. According to Soler-Presas et al. [44], dissection is quick, easy, and safe.

The cervicopectoral flap can be used in combination with other flaps such as the rectus abdominis and temporal myofascial flaps, which provide bulk (Figs. 2.17, 2.18, 2.19, 2.20, 2.21, 2.22, and 2.23).

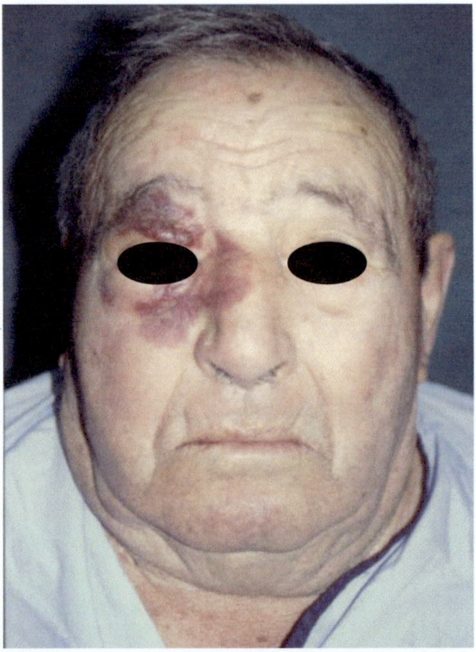

Fig. 2.17 Preoperative view

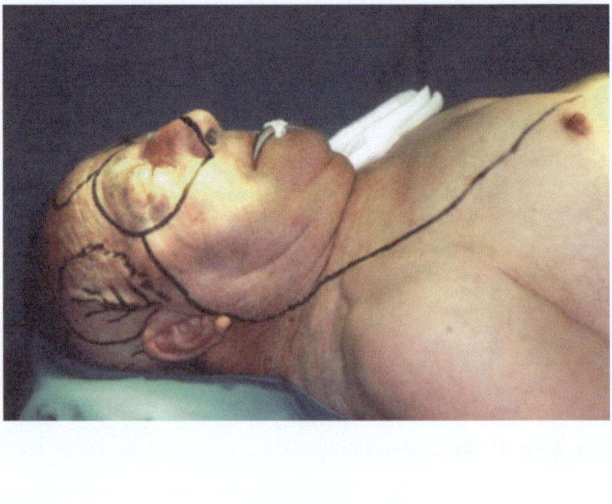

Fig. 2.18 Intraoperative resection and reconstruction design

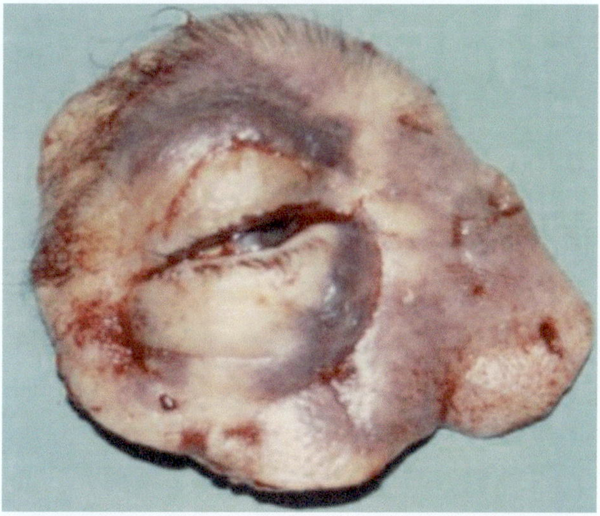

Fig. 2.19 Tumor resection

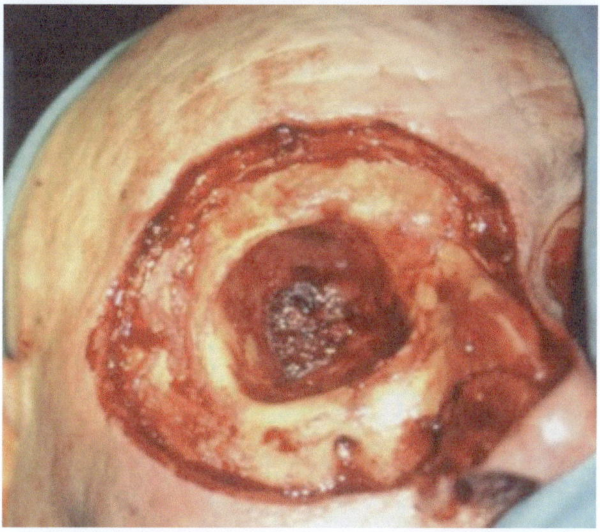

Fig. 2.20 Intraoperative defect

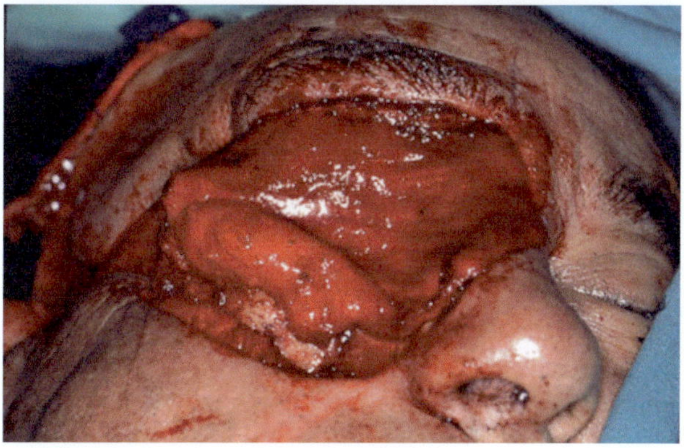

Fig. 2.21 Filling of the orbital cavity with myofascial temporalis flap

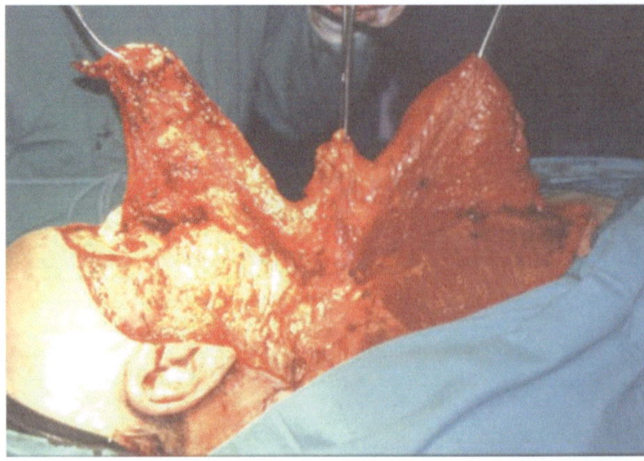

Fig. 2.22 Cervicopectoral flap dissection

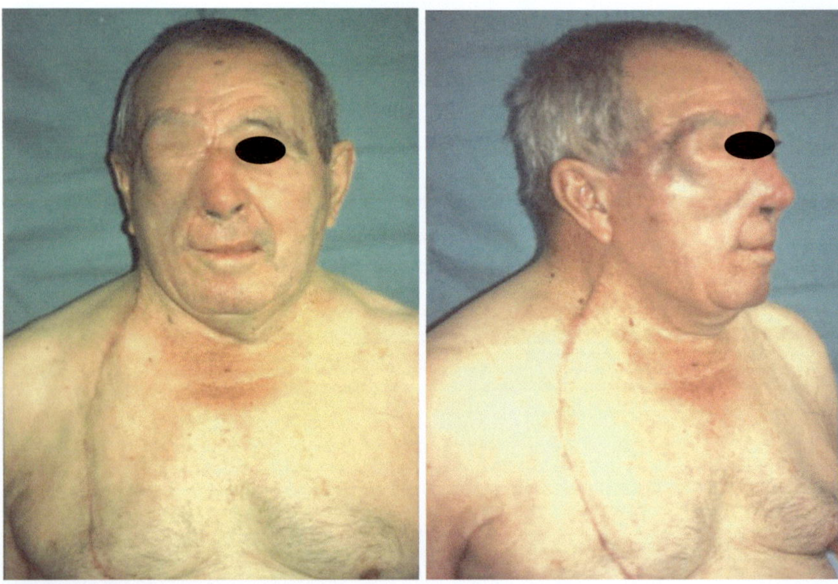

Fig. 2.23 Postoperative view

2.3.4 Microvascular Free Flaps

In cases where the defect is extensive and involves the palate, with few teeth remaining, Brida et al. [15] recommend surgical reconstruction aimed at a more favorable outcome of prosthodontic treatment in order to guarantee that the patient can speak and swallow again. Therefore, in our hands, free bone flaps are the approach of choice, since they make it possible to fit osseointegrated MG osseous implants and manufacture a prosthesis for dental-alveolar rehabilitation.

During the last 25 years, microvascular free flaps have been a unique alternative for the reconstructive surgeon. Many options are available, depending on the need for soft and bony tissue.

This alternative prevents the length of the vascular pedicle from being a limitation to reconstruction. In addition, it enables the flap to be directed in such a way that it can adapt more accurately to the defect.

Futran [45] proposed the use of microvascular flaps, although no benefit has been shown with a single flap.

Nevertheless, as reported by Kajikawa et al. [46], the main problems are the resulting scar, the variation in the color of the flap, and the difference in texture with respect to the rest of the facial tissue.

Reconstruction of extensive composite defects involving bone, oral mucosa, skin, and soft tissue sometimes requires a combination of flaps, as reported by Wei et al. [47]. Schliephake [48] recommends reconstructing the alveolar process, buttresses, orbital walls, and zygomatic bone using bony components to achieve a satisfactory outcome in the long term.

Kokemueller et al. [49] reported on computer-assisted primary reconstruction of bone contour with tailored titanium implants combined with soft tissue free flaps to fill defects.

2.3.4.1 Rectus Abdominis Flap

The rectus abdominis flap is an easily designed musculocutaneous flap with a large pedicle (inferior epigastric vessels).

Brown type IVA defects are the ideal indication for this flap, which provides the bulk of the missing soft tissue.

We use the rectus abdominis flap in combination with the temporalis myofascial flap: the rectus abdominis provides bulk, and the temporalis muscle is used to reconstruct the soft and/or hard palate defect. It is an excellent alternative to the iliac crest microsurgical flap.

We also use it to provide bulk in type IIIA defects (Figs. 2.24, 2.25, 2.26, 2.27, 2.28, 2.29, and 2.30).

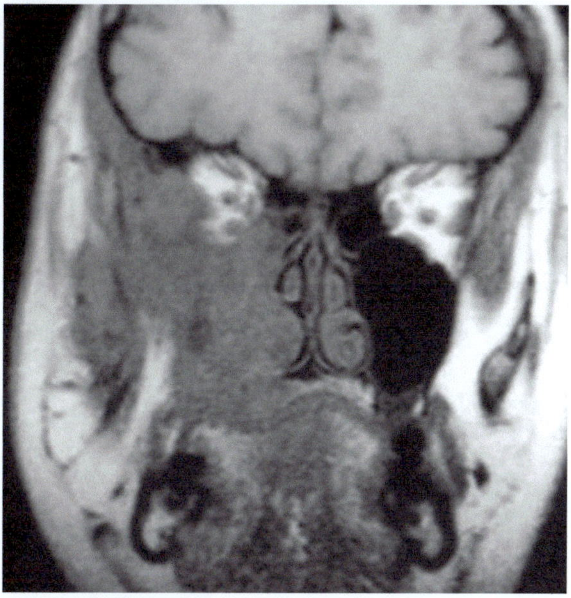

Fig. 2.24 MRI image of the tumor

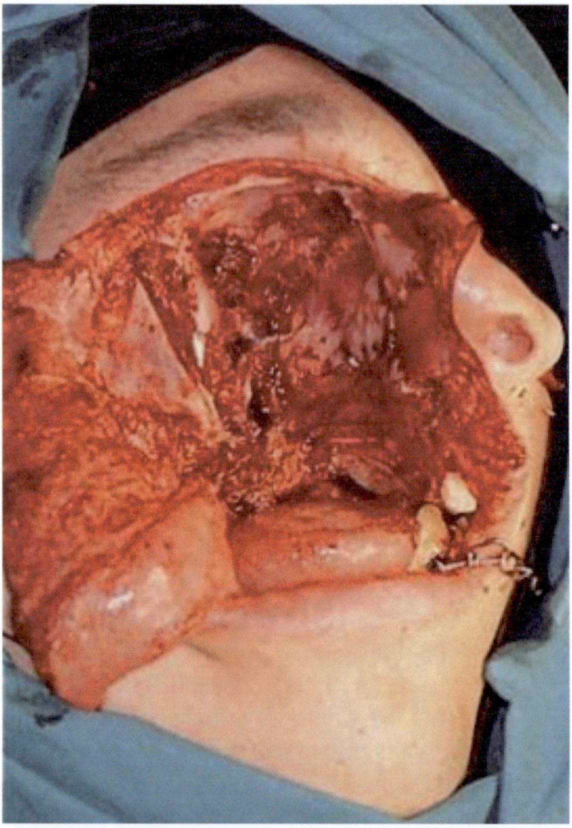

Fig. 2.25 Surgical defect

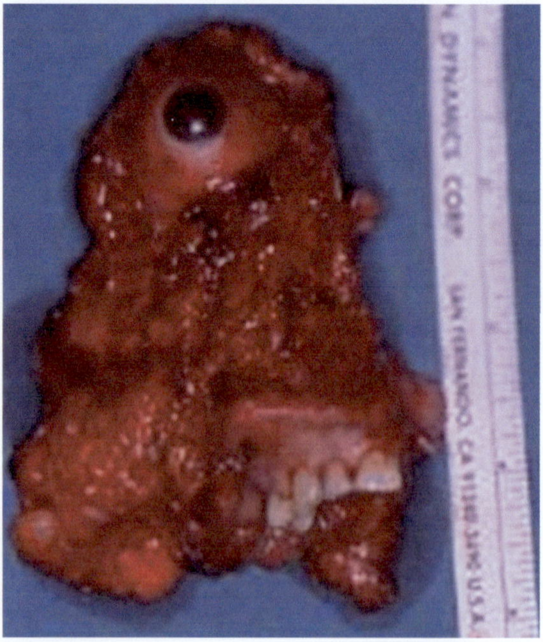

Fig. 2.26 Specimen

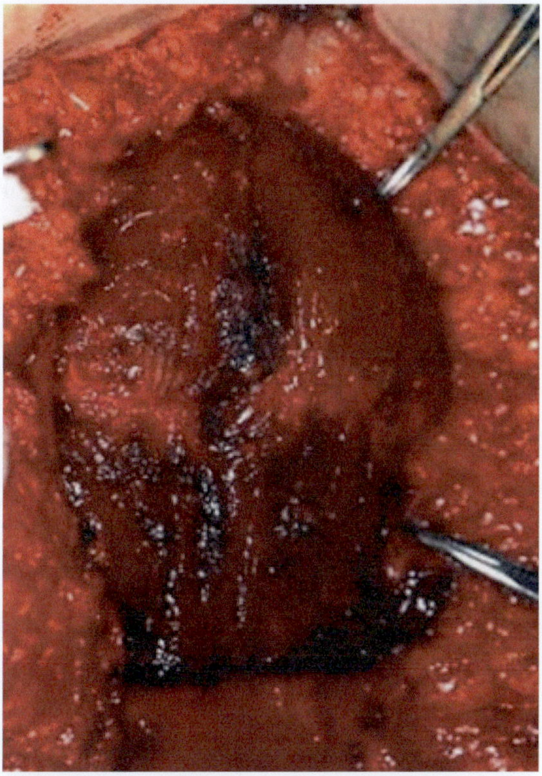

Fig. 2.27 Harvesting of the rectus abdominis free flap

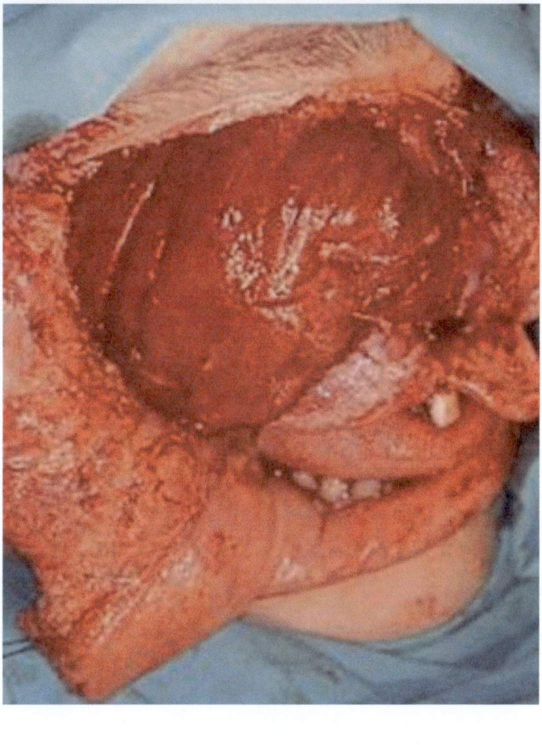

Fig. 2.28 Position of the flap at the face

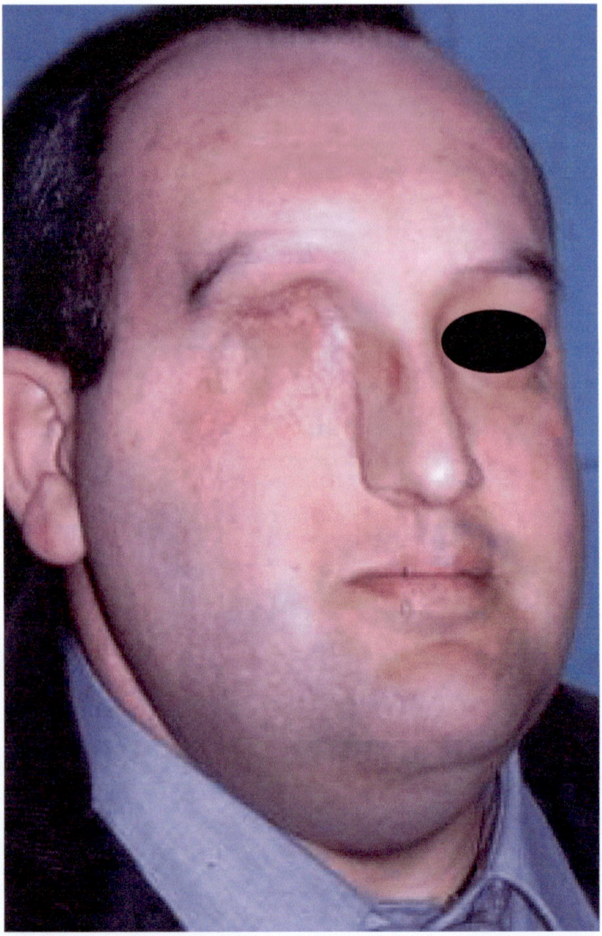

Fig. 2.29 Postoperative view

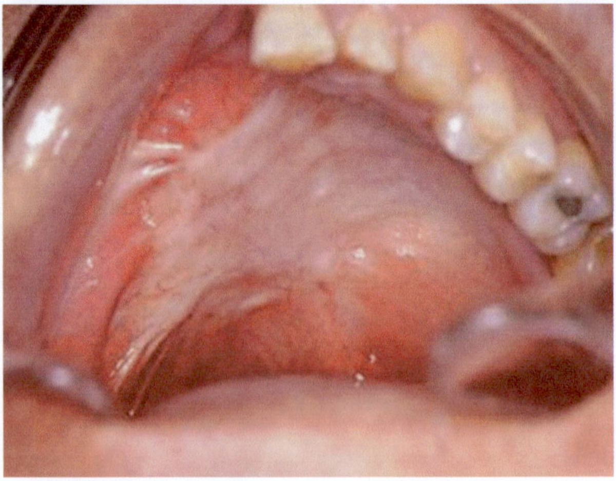

Fig. 2.30 Intraoral aspect of the reconstruction

2.3.4.2 Osteofasciocutaneous Fibula Flap

The first microvascular flap with bone was used by Taylor et al. [50] to treat a post-traumatic tibial defect in 1975. In 1979, Gilbert [51] reported a lateral approach for dissecting the flap. In 1983, Chen and Yan [52] became the first authors to incorporate a skin paddle. However, it was not until 6 years later that Hidalgo [53] used the flap for reconstruction of the mandible.

The constant caliber of the pedicle enabled Wei et al. [54] to the distal end of the fibular vessels as an anastomosis site for a second free flap.

Periosteal supply from the peroneal artery and endosteal blood supply from the nutrient artery, a branch of the peroneal artery, as reported by Pototschnig et al. [55], make it possible to perform multiple osteotomies providing that no damage has been done to the periosteum.

This technique is useful for type Ic and Id defects and is an alternative in Brown type II defects [17]. Reconstruction of soft tissue defects can be achieved using the skin paddle reported by Navarro Vila et al. [56].

Advantages

- The large quantity of bone available (4 cm up to 25 cm) makes the osteofasciocutaneous fibula flap the largest bone flap, as described by Navarro Cuellar et al. [57].
- The associated skin paddle can be molded.
- Two surgical teams can work simultaneously.
- Minimum donor morbidity.
- Long pedicle with considerable vascular caliber that favors microsurgical anastomosis.
- Possibility of rehabilitation with implants owing to the primary stability resulting from the thickness of the cortex.
- The approach of choice in obese patients who need a bone flap.
- Abundant vascularization facilitates osteotomy and adaptation of the flap to the resulting maxillary defect.

Complications

- Vestibuloplasty is necessary in order to place the prosthesis on the implants.
- Placement of the implants must be delayed owing to the large amount of osteosynthesis material necessary for shaping the reconstruction.
- Implants should be placed 12–18 months after radiation therapy, once the osteosynthesis material has been removed (Figs. 2.31, 2.32, 2.33, 2.34, 2.35, 2.36, 2.37, 2.38, 2.39, 2.40, 2.41, 2.42, 2.43, 2.44, and 2.45).

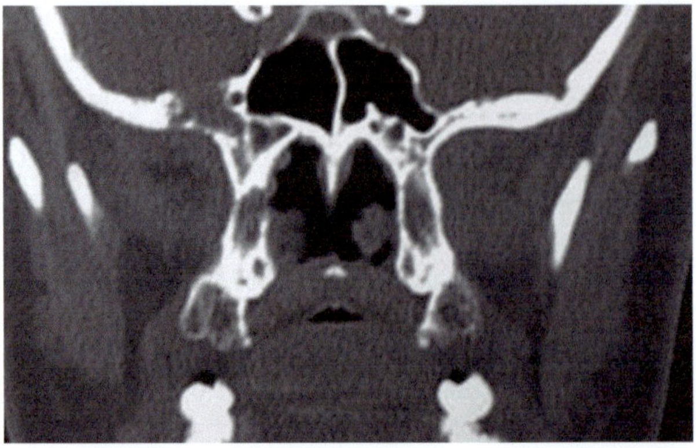

Fig. 2.31 Preoperative CT

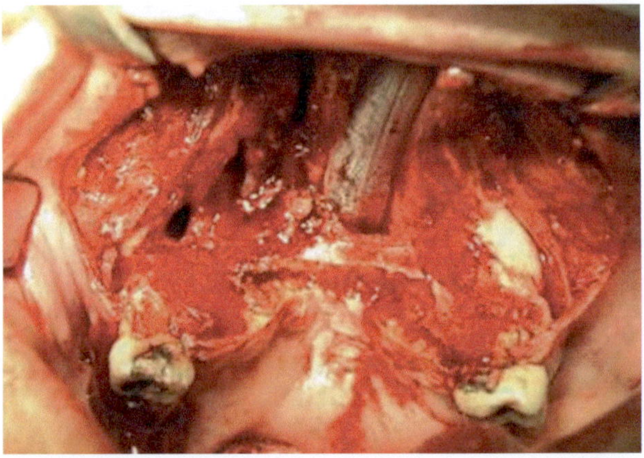

Fig. 2.32 Surgical defect

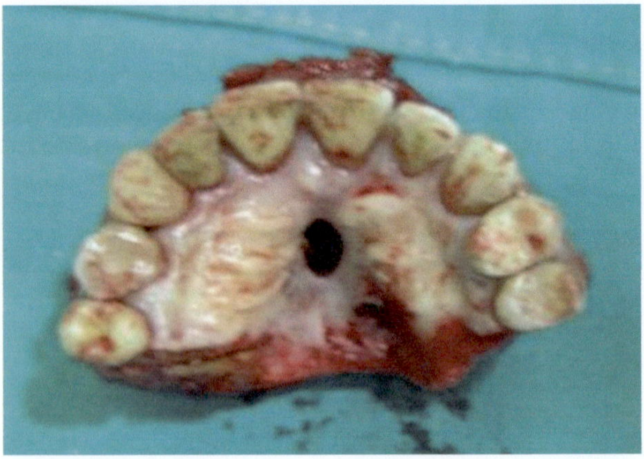

Fig. 2.33 Surgical specimen

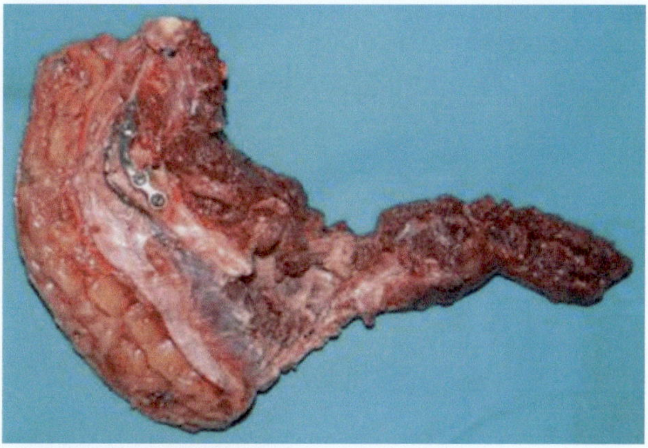

Fig. 2.34 Fibula free flap

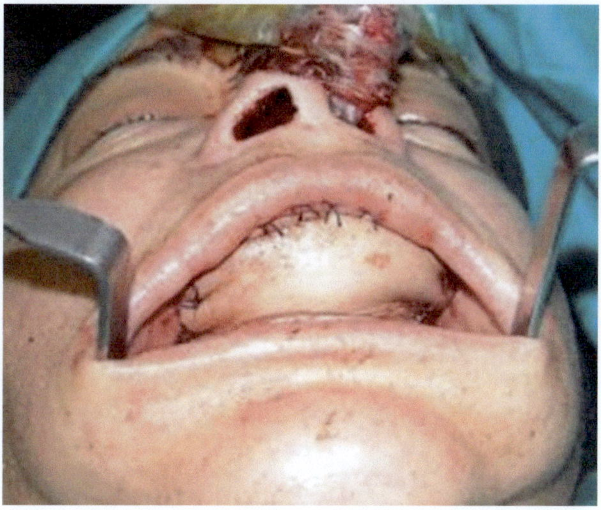

Fig. 2.35 Early postoperative image

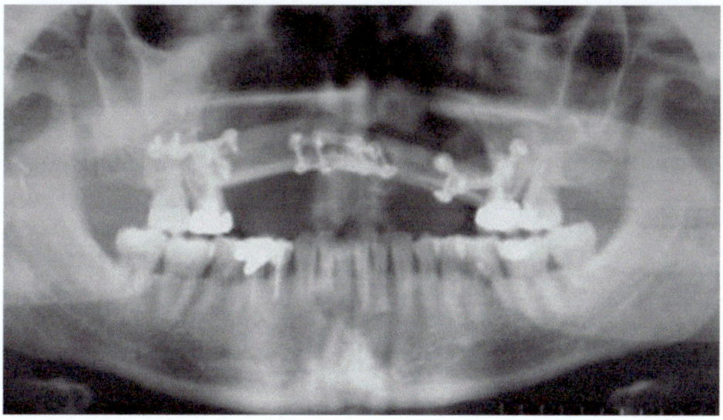

Fig. 2.36 OPT control

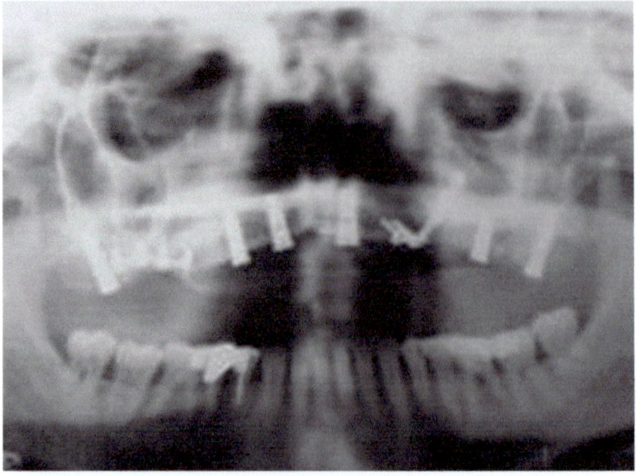

Fig. 2.37 OPT with MG osseous implants

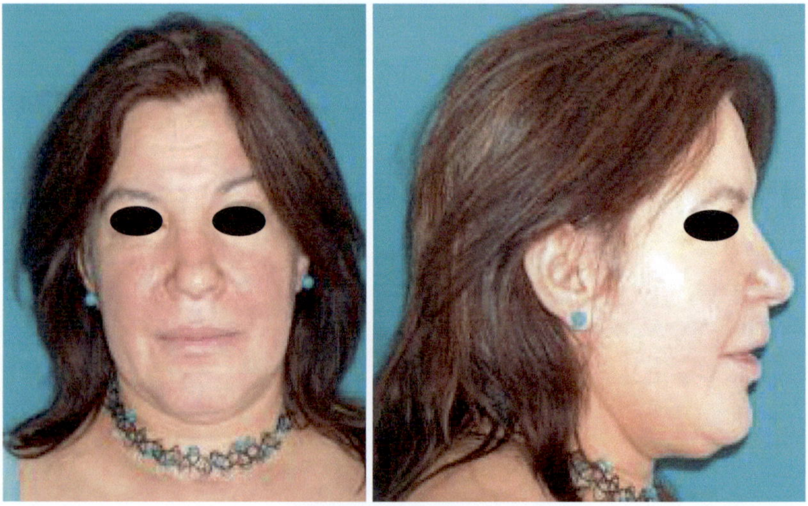

Fig. 2.38 Six months after dental rehabilitation

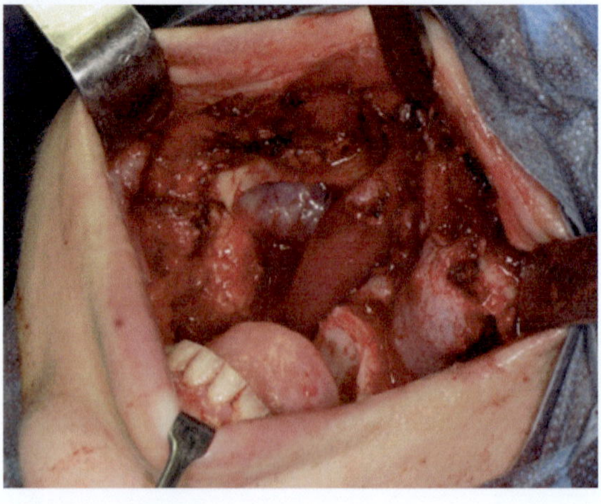

Fig. 2.39 Surgical defect

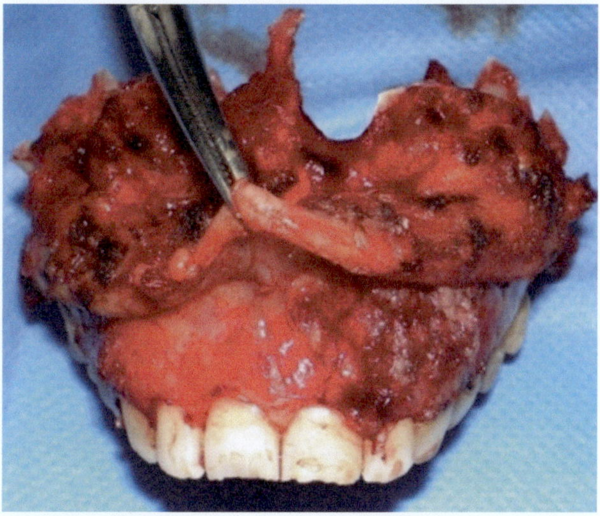

Fig. 2.40 Bilateral maxillectomy

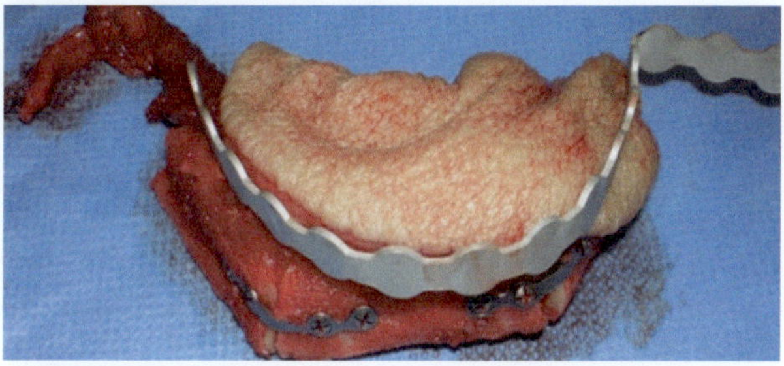

Fig. 2.41 Contouring free fibula flap

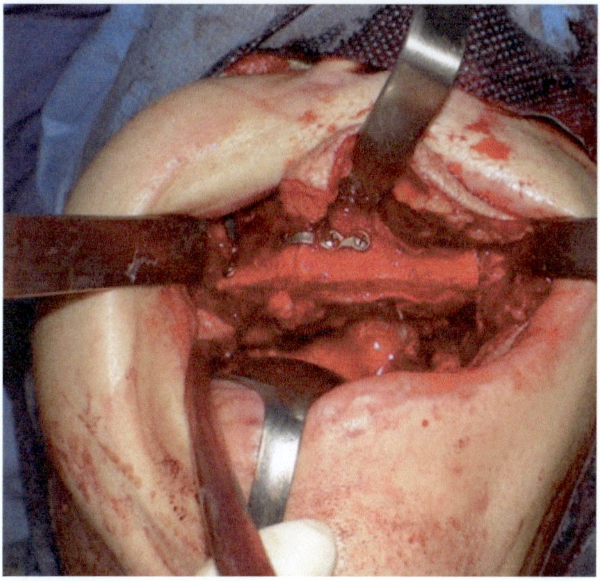

Fig. 2.42 Fibula flap reconstruction

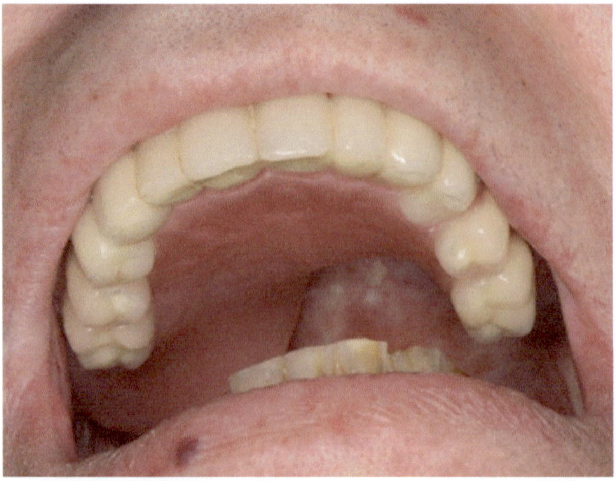

Fig. 2.43 Dental prosthesis

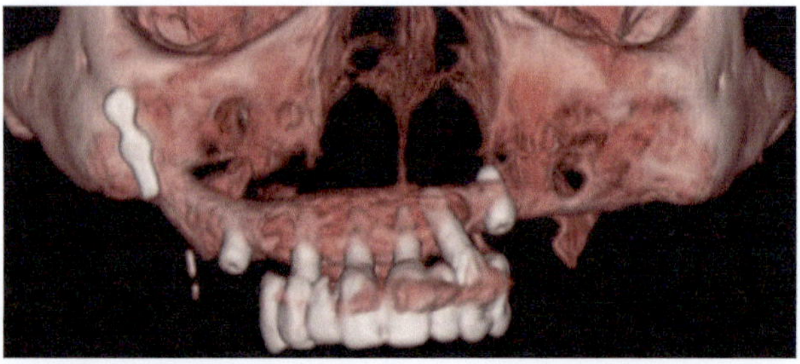

Fig. 2.44 CT with free fibula flap and MG osseous implants reconstruction

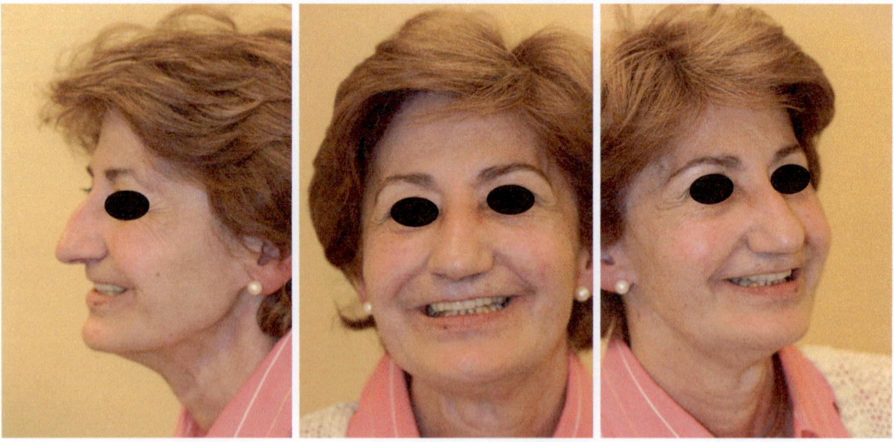

Fig. 2.45 Postoperative views

2.3.4.3 Radial Forearm Fasciocutaneous Flap

Also known as the Chinese flap, the radial forearm fasciocutaneous flap was first reported in 1981 by Yang et al. [58] and they used it to treat burns of the head and neck.

Its vascular pedicle is based on the radial artery, which is accompanied by two veins of the same length and half the diameter that drain into the ulnar vein. A superficial vein, the cephalic vein, is also present.

Futran [45] reported that the radial flap can be dissected with bone, although the length and width of the available bone restricts its use to small anterior defects that do not require implants. Furthermore, in patients requiring reconstruction of a bone defect, our first option is always the osteofasciocutaneous fibula flap.

For Duflo et al. [59], this is an ideal flap for the reconstruction of mucosal defects and defects of the soft tissue of the oral cavity and soft palate. It is ideal for extensive surfaces and small volumes.

In our daily practice, we never use the radial forearm osteofasciocutaneous flap for maxillary reconstruction for these reasons:

- The amount of bone that we can obtain is limited because it is necessary to maintain the continuity of the remnant radial bone and bone availability is limited to 40 % of the radius circumference.
- Great morbidity of the donor site with up to 25 % of pathological fractures.
- The dental implants we can use are very short, so they are not useful for prosthetic rehabilitation.

2.3.4.4 Iliac Crest Flap

In 1979, Taylor et al. [60] reported the usefulness of the deep circumflex iliac artery, which supplies the iliac bone. Five years later, Ramasastry et al. [61] identified the ascending branch of the deep circumflex iliac artery as the main artery of the internal oblique muscle.

The iliac crest flap is indicated for type II and IIIA defects. In type IIIA defects, orbital volume can be restored by placing the bony component in a vertical position. If the internal oblique muscle is incorporated as described by Duflo et al. [59], the maxillectomy defect can be safely reconstructed, since the fistula is obliterated with the muscle, which reepithelializes without providing excessive bulk.

Baliarsing et al. [62] report the use of this bone flap for maxillary reconstruction. It enables the alveolar ridge to be restored for dental rehabilitation, provides soft tissue for separating oral and nasal defects, supports the orbit, and ensures appropriate malar projection.

Advantages

- The flap can be used to shape the alveolar ridge, the infraorbital ridge, and the zygomatic process of the maxilla.
- Immediate placement of osseointegrated implants.

- The internal oblique muscle can be used to reconstruct intraoral soft tissue.
- The skin paddle can be used to reconstruct extraoral defect that is present.
- The bone is short, up to7–9 cm.
- The flap cannot be used for bilateral defects.
- Limited mobility of soft tissue with respect to bone.
- Donor site morbidity.
- Relatively short pedicle. In some cases, venous grafts are necessary, and it can increase the risk of thrombosis, as reported by Brown et al. [63] (Figs. 2.46, 2.47, 2.48, 2.49, and 2.50).

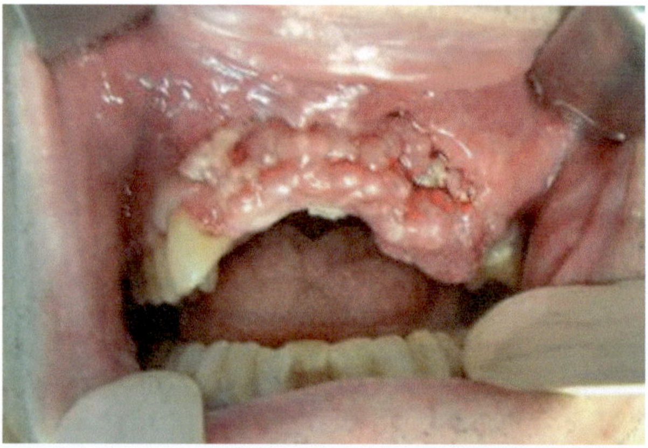

Fig. 2.46 Maxillary squamous cell carcinoma

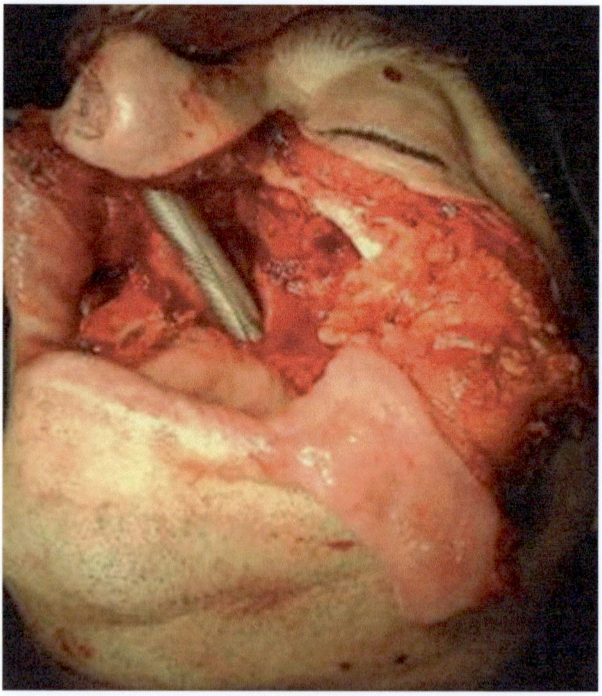

Fig. 2.47 Surgical defect

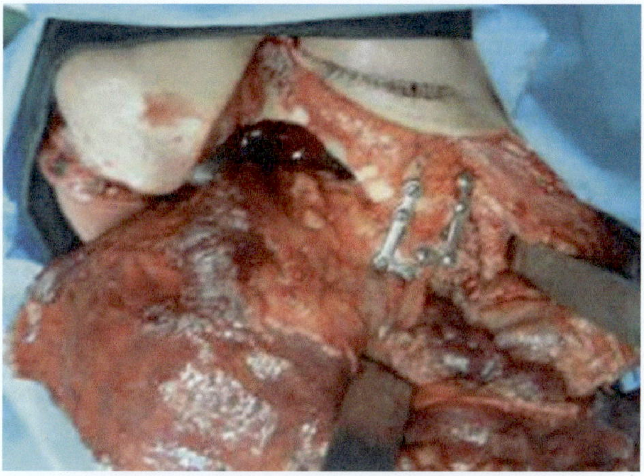

Fig. 2.48 Intraoperative view of the reconstruction

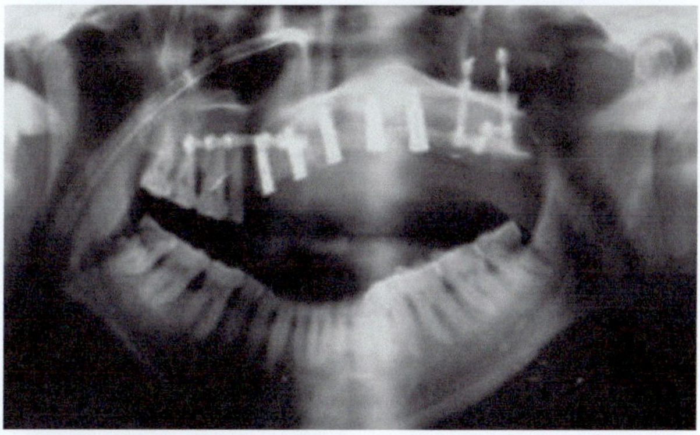

Fig. 2.49 OPT postoperative control

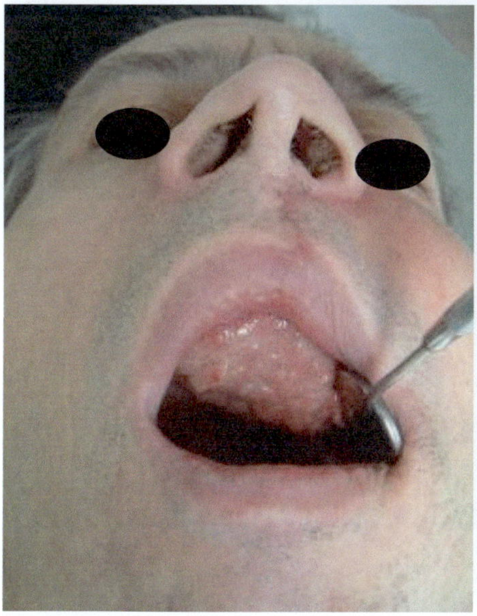

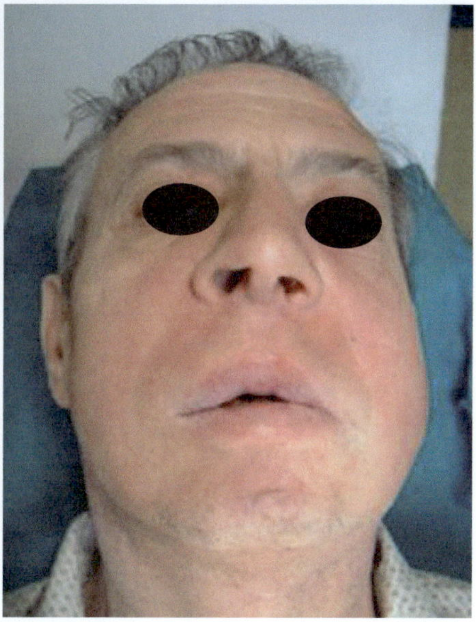

Fig. 2.50 Early and 6 months postoperative views

2.3.4.5 Scapular Flap

According to Duflo et al. [59], the scapular flap has the advantage that soft tissue can be rotated and placed in many different ways, thus making it more versatile than other microsurgical flaps. If the angular branch of the thoracodorsal artery is included in the design, as proposed by Triana et al. [14], then both the tip and the most lateral area of the bone can be included in the flap. Similarly, several flaps from the subscapular system have been described.

Their surgical indications are similar to those of the osteofasciocutaneous fibula flap.

Advantages

- Greater mobility of soft tissue than with other flaps

Disadvantages

- The scapular flap cannot be harvested simultaneously with another flap because of the need to vary the patient's position.
- Complex bone orientation.
- Relatively short pedicle.
- Possible lower volume in women (Figs. 2.51, 2.52, 2.53, 2.54, and 2.55).

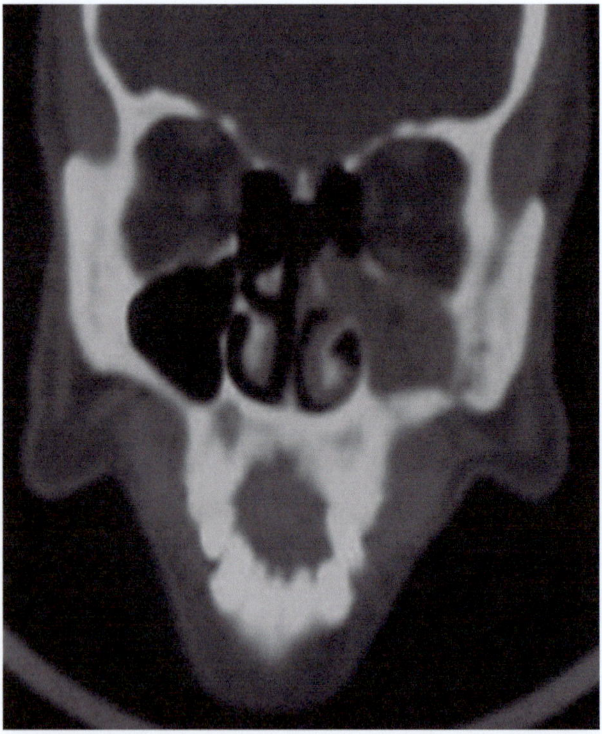

Fig. 2.51 Preoperative CT

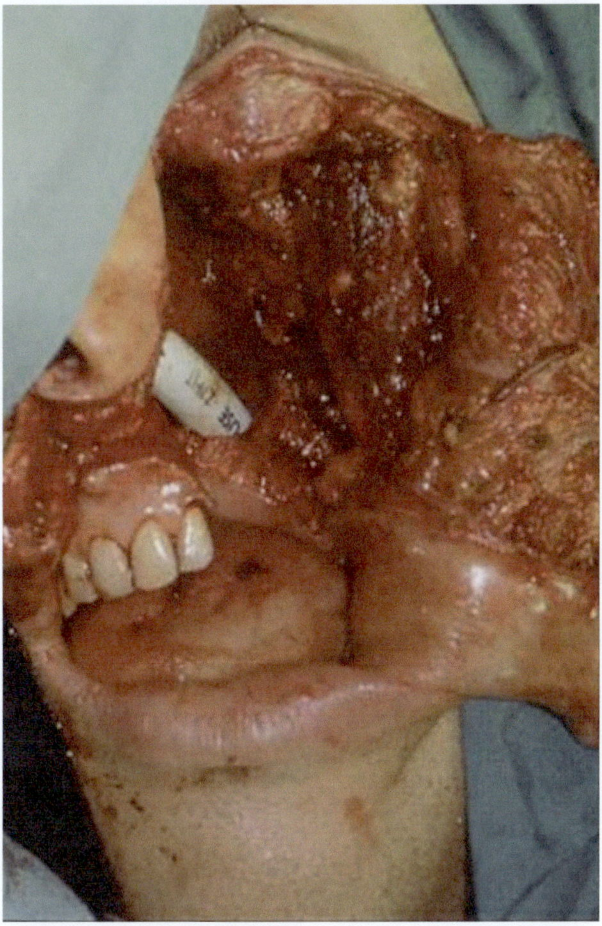

Fig. 2.52 Surgical defect

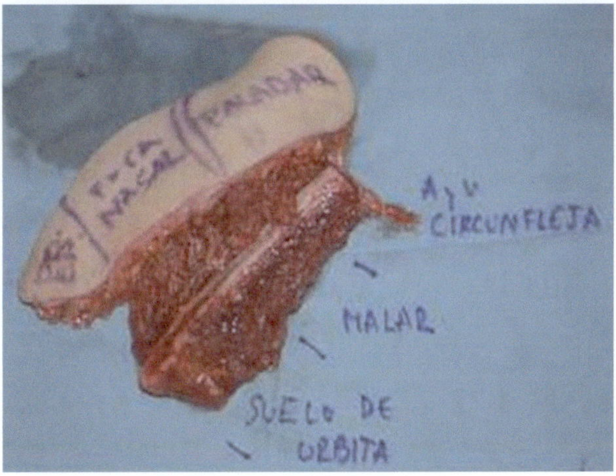

Fig. 2.53 Scapular flap design

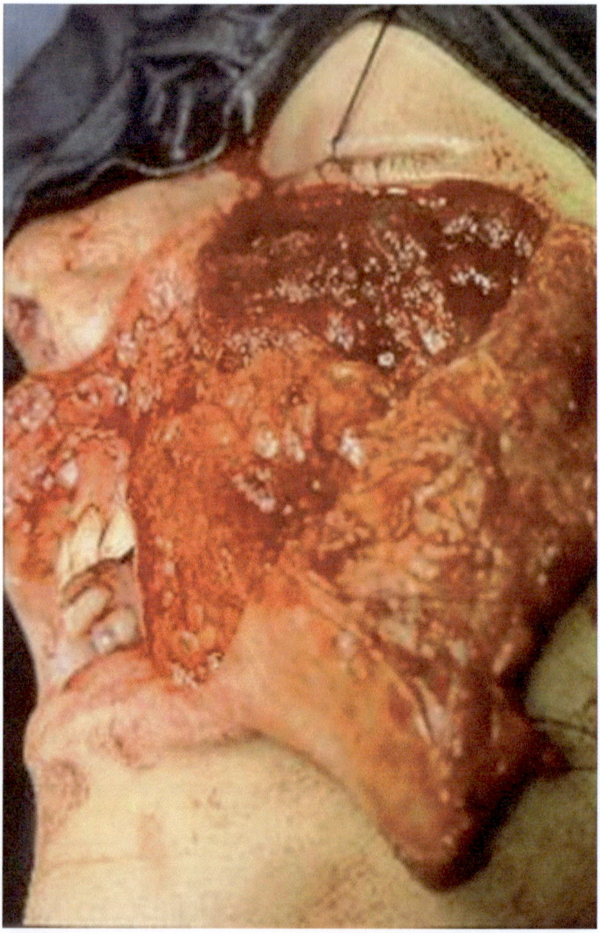

Fig. 2.54 Intraoperative view of the placement of the flap

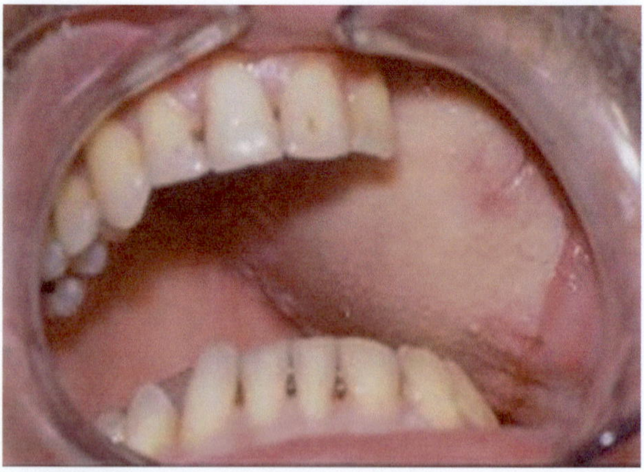

Fig. 2.55 Intraoral postoperative view

2.3.5 Distraction Osteogenesis

Initially used to lengthen long bones, distraction osteogenesis is another option for reconstructing maxillary defects. In 1905, Codivilla [64] first used the technique to lengthen a femur and thus correct differences in leg length.

In 1988, Ilizarov and Soybelman [65] began a series of investigations and applications for distraction osteogenesis in the facial bones.

The surgical procedure is followed by different periods:

- Latency period: 5–7 days
- Distraction (lengthening) period: approximately 1 mm per day
- Consolidation period: 8–12 weeks
- Withdrawal of the distraction device once ossification has been confirmed

The complications of this technique are as follows:

- Incorrect distraction vector
- Dehiscence and exposure of the fragment to be transferred
- Fracture of the transferred element during surgery or difficulty performing the osteotomy
- Defects of bone formation

Niu et al. [66] state that distraction osteogenesis can reestablish the lost architecture of the maxilla by providing a natural facial appearance with normal speech and swallowing. Furthermore, Bengi et al. [67] report that it enables the soft tissue profile to be improved.

We use distraction for defects of the alveolar crest in the cases of very low tumors and very well-differentiated ones and in patients with very high maxilla (Figs. 2.56, 2.57, 2.58, 2.59, 2.60, and 2.61).

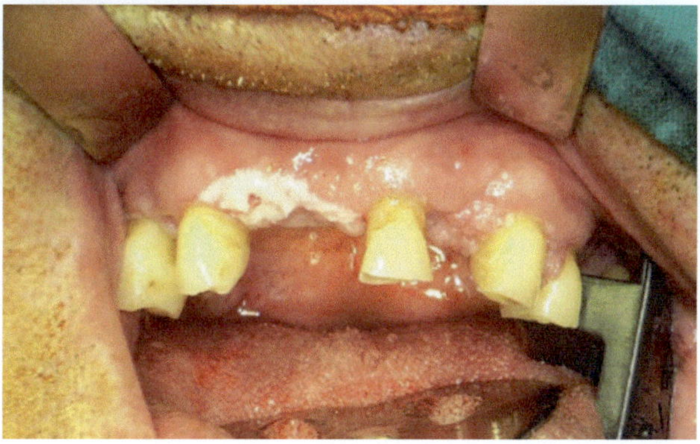

Fig. 2.56 Epidermoid carcinoma arising from a previous lichen planus

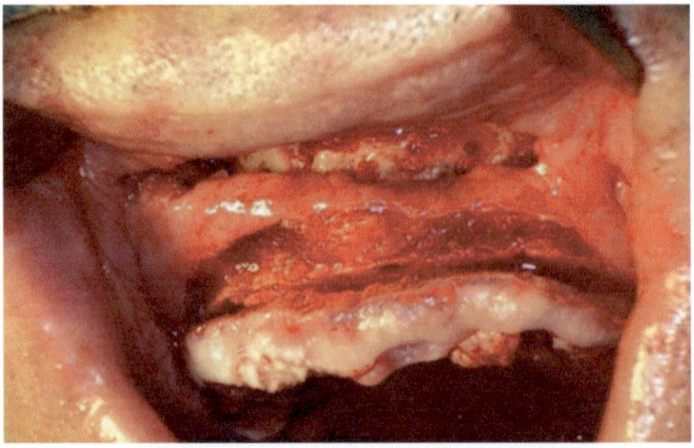

Fig. 2.57 Resection

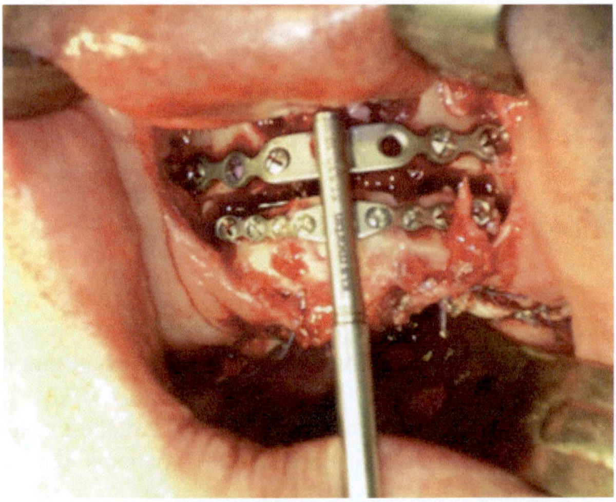

Fig. 2.58 Starting distraction

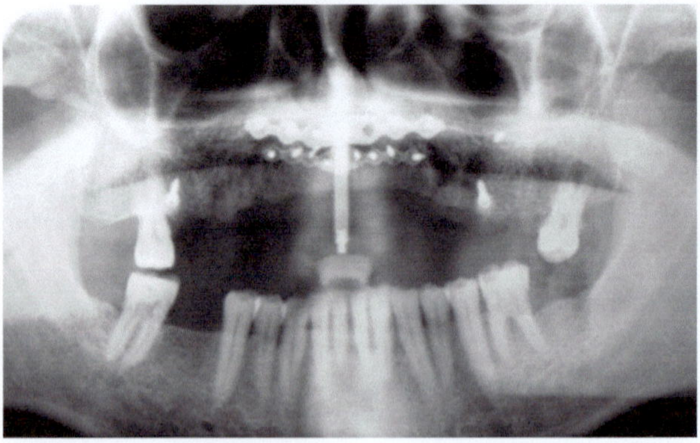

Fig. 2.59 OPT during the latency period

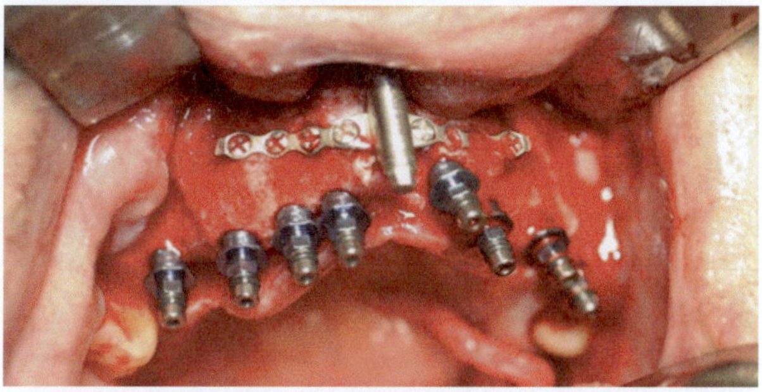

Fig. 2.60 Eight MG osseous implants placed in the distracted bone before we remove the distractor

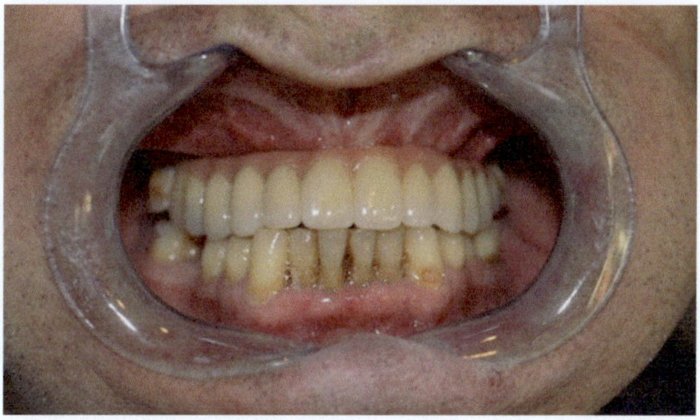

Fig. 2.61 Final occlusion

References

1. Smolka W, Iizuka T. Surgical reconstruction of maxilla and midface: clinical outcome and factors relating to postoperative complications. J Craniomaxillofac Surg. 2005;33(1):1–7.
2. Kreeft AM, Krap M, Wismeijer D, Speksnijder CM, Smeele LE, Bosch SD. Oral function after maxillectomy and reconstruction with an obturator. Int J Oral Maxillofac Surg. 2012;41(11): 1387–92.
3. Okay DJ, Genden E, Buchbinder D, Urken M. Prosthodontic guidelines for surgical reconstruction of the maxilla: a classification system of defects. J Prosthet Dent. 2001;86(4): 352–63.
4. Cordeiro PG, Chen CM. A 15-year review of midface reconstruction after total and subtotal maxillectomy: part I. Algorithm and outcomes. Plast Reconstr Surg. 2012;129(1):124–36.
5. Futran ND, Mendez E. Developments in reconstruction of midface and maxilla. Lancet Oncol. 2006;7(3):249–58.
6. Edgerton Jr MT. Replacement of lining to oral cavity following surgery. Cancer. 1951;4(1):110–9.
7. Navarro Cuellar C. Reconstrucción mandibular: colgajos libres vs colgajos pediculados (PhD thesis). Madrid; 2005
8. Willemot J, Michel J. Naissance et développement de l'Oto-rhino-laryngologie dans l'histoire de la médicine. Acta Oto-Rhino-Laryngologica. 1981;35:654–70.
9. Eley KA, Watt-Smith SR. The nasolabial approach: a potential alternative to the lip-splitting incision for maxillectomy. Br J Oral Maxillofac Surg. 2012;50(1):e6–8.
10. Wells MD, Luce EA. Reconstruction of midfacial defects after surgical resection of malignancies. Clin Plast Surg. 1995;22(1):79–89.

11. Spiro RH, Strong EW, Shah JP. Maxillectomy and its classification. Head Neck. 1997;19(4): 309–14.
12. Davison SP, Sherris DA, Meland NB. An algorithm for maxillectomy defect reconstruction. Laryngoscope. 1998;108(2):215–9.
13. Cordeiro PG, Santamaria E. A classification system and algorithm for reconstruction of maxillectomy and midfacial defects. Plast Reconstr Surg. 2000;105(7):2331–46; discussion 47–8.
14. Triana Jr RJ, Uglesic V, Virag M, Varga SG, Knezevic P, Milenovic A, et al. Microvascular free flap reconstructive options in patients with partial and total maxillectomy defects. Arch Facial Plast Surg. 2000;2(2):91–101.
15. Bidra AS, Jacob RF, Taylor TD. Classification of maxillectomy defects: a systematic review and criteria necessary for a universal description. J Prosthet Dent. 2012;107(4):261–70.
16. Brown JS, Rogers SN, McNally DN, Boyle M. A modified classification for the maxillectomy defect. Head Neck. 2000;22(1):17–26.
17. Brown JS, Shaw RJ. Reconstruction of the maxilla and midface: introducing a new classification. Lancet Oncol. 2010;11(10):1001–8.
18. Poetker DM, Loehrl TA, Toohill RJ. External medial maxillectomy. Oper Tech Otolaryngol-Head Neck Surg. 2010;21(2):107–10.
19. Pittman AL, Zender CA. Total maxillectomy. Oper Tech Otolaryngol-Head Neck Surg. 2010; 21(3):166–70.
20. Park KT, Kwon HB. The evaluation of the use of a delayed surgical obturator in dentate maxillectomy patients by considering days elapsed prior to commencement of postoperative oral feeding. J Prosthet Dent. 2006;96(6):449–53.
21. Yasuo H, Kohsuke I, Toshinori M, Kenichi S. Closure of oroantral communications using a pedicled buccal fat pad graft. J Oral Maxillofac Surg. 1995;53:771–5.
22. Wallace JH, Greg A, Russel R, Chambers K. Use of pedicled fat pad graft as an adjunct in the reconstruction of palatal cleft defects. Oral Surg Oral Med Oral Pathol Oral Radiol Endod. 1995;80:24–7.
23. Khouw YLN, Van Der Wal KGH. Bilateral palatal reconstruction using 2 pedicled buccal fat pads in rhinolalea aperta after extensive necrotizing tonsillitis: a case report. J Oral Maxillofac Surg. 2004;62:749–51.
24. Kim Y-K. The use of a pedicled buccal fat pad graft for coverage in primary palatorrhaphy: a case report. J Oral Maxillofac Surg. 2001;59:1499–501.
25. Matarasso A. Managing the buccal fat pad. Aesthet Surg J. 2006;26:330–6.
26. Muzaffar AR, Adams Jr WP, Hartog JM, Rohrich RJ, Byrd HS. Maxillary reconstruction: functional and aesthetic considerations. Plast Reconstr Surg. 1999;104(7):2172–83; quiz 84.
27. Carstens MH, Stofman GM, Hurwitz DJ, Futrell JW, Patterson GT, Sotereanos GC. The buccinator myomucosal island pedicle flap: anatomic study and case report. Plast Reconstr Surg. 1991;88(1):39–50; discussion 1–2.
28. Zhao Z, Zhang Z, Li Y, Li S, Xiao S, Fan X, et al. The buccinator musculomucosal island flap for partial tongue reconstruction. J Am Coll Surg. 2003;196(5):753–60.
29. Kaplan EN. Soft palate repair by levator muscle reconstruction and a buccal mucosal flap. Plast Reconstr Surg. 1975;56:129.
30. Maeda K, Ojimi H, Utsugi R, Ando S. A T-shaped musculomucosal buccal flap method for cleft palate surgery. Plast Reconstr Surg. 1987;79(6):888–96.
31. Bozola AR, Gasques JA, Carriquiry CE, Cardoso de Oliveira M. The buccinator musculomucosal flap: anatomic study and clinical application. Plast Reconstr Surg. 1989;84(2):250–7.
32. Zhao Z, Li S, Yan Y, Li Y, Yang M, Mu L, et al. New buccinator myomucosal island flap: anatomic study and clinical application. Plast Reconstr Surg. 1999;104(1):55–64.
33. Golovine SS. Procédé de cloture plastique de l'orbite aprés l'exentération. Arch Ophthalmol. 1898;18:679–80.
34. Bradley P, Brockbank J. The temporalis muscle flap in oral reconstruction. A cadaveric, animal and clinical study. J Maxillofac Surg. 1981;9(3):139–45.

35. Cheung LK. Microvascular network of the healing surface over the temporalis flap in maxillary reconstruction. Int J Oral Maxillofac Surg. 1999;28(6):469–74.
36. Ahmed Djae K, Li Z, Li ZB. Temporalis muscle flap for immediate reconstruction of maxillary defects: review of 39 cases. Int J Oral Maxillofac Surg. 2011;40(7):715–21.
37. Brown WJ. Extraordinary case of horse bite: the external ear completely bitten off and successfully replaced. Lancet. 1898;1:1533.
38. Monks GH. The restoration of a lower lid by a new method. N Engl J Med. 1898;139:385.
39. Roy C, Bandyopadhyay M, Dubey S, Gupta AK. Temporoparietal fascia flap in intra-oral reconstruction without split thickness skin graft cover: a case report. J Indian Med Assoc. 2013;111(12):852, 4.
40. Lam D, Carlson ER. The temporalis muscle flap and temporoparietal fascial flap. Oral Maxillofac Surg Clin North Am. 2014;26(3):359–69.
41. Mokal NJ, Ghalme AN, Kothari DS, Desai M. The use of the temporoparietal fascia flap in various clinical scenarios: a review of 71 cases. Indian J Plast Surg. 2013;46(3):493–501.
42. Sakellariou A, Salama A. The use of cervicofacial flap in maxillofacial reconstruction. Oral Maxillofac Surg Clin North Am. 2014;26(3):389–400.
43. Shestak KC, Roth AG, Jones NF, Myers EN. The cervicopectoral rotation flap–a valuable technique for facial reconstruction. Br J Plast Surg. 1993;46(5):375–7.
44. Soler-Presas F, Cuesta-Gil M, Borja-Morant A, Concejo-Cutoli C, Acero-Sanz J, Navarro-Vila C. Midface soft tissue reconstruction with the facio-cervico-pectoral flap. J Craniomaxillofac Surg. 1997;25(1):39–45.
45. Futran ND. Primary reconstruction of the maxilla following maxillectomy with or without sacrifice of the orbit. J Oral Maxillofac Surg. 2005;63(12):1765–9.
46. Kajikawa A, Ueda K, Katsuragi Y, Hirose T, Asai E. Three-step orbitofacial reconstruction after extended total maxillectomy using free RAM flap and expanded cervicofacial flap with cartilage grafts. J Plast Reconstr Aesthet Surg. 2010;63(10):1608–14.
47. Wei FC, Demirkan F, Chen HC, Chen IH. Double free flaps in reconstruction of extensive composite mandibular defects in head and neck cancer. Plast Reconstr Surg. 1999;103(1): 39–47.
48. Schliephake H. Revascularized tissue transfer for the repair of complex midfacial defects in oncologic patients. J Oral Maxillofac Surg. 2000;58(11):1212–8.
49. Kokemueller H, Tavassol F, Rucker M, Gellrich NC. Complex midfacial reconstruction: a combined technique of computer-assisted surgery and microvascular tissue transfer. J Oral Maxillofac Surg. 2008;66(11):2398–406.
50. Taylor GL, Miller G, Ham F. The free vascularized bone graft. A clinical extension of microvascular techniques. Plast Reconstr Surg. 1975;55:533–44.
51. Gilbert A. Vascularized transfer of the fibular shaft. Int J Microsurg. 1979;1:100.
52. Chen Z, Yan W. The study and clinical application of the osteocutaneous flap of fibula. Microsurgery. 1983;4:11–6.
53. Hidalgo DA. Fibula free flap: a new method of mandible reconstruction. Plast Reconstr Surg. 1989;84(1):71–9.
54. Wei FC, Seah CS, Tsai YC, Liu SJ, Tsai MS. Fibula osteoseptocutaneous flap for reconstruction of composite mandibular defects. Plast Reconstr Surg. 1994;93(2):294–304; discussion 5–6.
55. Pototschnig H, Schaff J, Kovacs L, Biemer E, Papadopulos NA. The free osteofasciocutaneous fibula flap: clinical applications and surgical considerations. Injury. 2013;44(3):366–9.
56. Navarro Vila C, Ochandiano Cacioya S, García Marín F. Tratado de Cirugía Oral y Maxilofacial. 2nd ed. Madrid: St. Louis; 2009.
57. Navarro Cuéllar C, Ochandiano Caicoya S, Riba Garcia F, Lopez de Atalaya FJ, Acero Sanz J, Cuesta Gil M, et al. Rehabilitación implantosoportada en el colgajo libre de peroné. Revista Española de Cirugía Oral y Maxilofacial. 2006;28:263–75.
58. Yang G, Chen B, Gao Y, et al. Forearm free skin flap transplantation. Natl Med J China. 1981;61:39.

59. Duflo S, Lief F, Paris J, Giovanni A, Thibeault S, Zanaret M. Microvascular radial forearm fasciocutaneous free flap in hard palate reconstruction. Eur J Surg Oncol. 2005;31(7):784–91.
60. Taylor GI, Townsend P, Corlett M. Superiority of the deep circumflex iliac vessels as the supply for free groin free flaps: experimental work. Plast Reconstr Surg. 1979;64:595–604.
61. Ramasastry SS, Granick MS, Futrell JW. Clinical anatomy of the internal oblique muscle. J Reconstr Microsurg. 1986;2(2):117–22.
62. Baliarsing AS, Kumar VV, Malik NA, B DK. Reconstruction of maxillectomy defects using deep circumflex iliac artery-based composite free flap. Oral Surg Oral Med Oral Pathol Oral Radiol Endod. 2010;109(3):e8–13. doi:10.1016/j.tripleo.2009.10.055.
63. Brown JS, Jones DC, Summerwill A, Rogers SN, Howell RA, Cawood JI, et al. Vascularized iliac crest with internal oblique muscle for immediate reconstruction after maxillectomy. Br J Oral Maxillofac Surg. 2002;40(3):183–90.
64. Codivilla A. On the means of lengthening in the lower limbs, the muscles, and tissues which are shortened through deformity. Am J Orthop Surg. 1905;2:353–69.
65. Ilizarov GA, Soybelman LM. Some clinical and experimental data concerning lengthening of lower extremities. Eksp Khir Anesteziol. 1969;14:27.
66. Niu XG, Zhao YM, Han XX. Multiplanar and combined distraction osteogenesis for three-dimensional and functional reconstruction of unilateral large maxillary defects. Br J Oral Maxillofac Surg. 2009;47(2):106–10.
67. Bengi O, Karacay S, Akin E, Okcu KM, Olmez H, Mermut S. Cephalometric evaluation of patients treated by maxillary anterior segmental distraction: a preliminary report. J Craniomaxillofac Surg. 2007;35(6–7):302–10.

Reconstruction of the Cranio-Orbital Region

3

Julio Acero Sanz, Cristina Maza Muela,
José Ignacio Salmerón Escobar,
and Santiago José Ochanciano Caicoya

Abstract

Treatment of tumors of the cranio-orbital region is a challenge for the surgeon. It requires appropriate presurgical evaluation and planning of the reconstructive approach in order to ensure a favorable cosmetic and functional outcome and prevent potentially fatal complications. One of the main objectives of reconstruction of defects of the cranio-orbital region is that of ensuring complete closure of the dura mater using well-vascularized tissue that separates endocranial structures from the upper aerodigestive tract. The incorporation of microvascular flaps has made it possible to reach this objective with a low complication rate. In the case of bone resection that alters facial harmony, restoration should be based on bone grafts or biomaterial implants. Virtual planning techniques and surgical navigation constitute a major advance in the reconstruction of craniofacial skeletal defects.

J. Acero Sanz, MD, DDS, PhD, FEBOMS (✉)
Head of Oral and Maxillofacial Surgery Department, Ramón y Cajal University Hospital, Madrid, Spain

Associate Professor of Alcalá University, Madrid, Spain
e-mail: j-acero@telefonica.net

C. Maza Muela, MD, DDS, FEBOMS • S.J. Ochanciano Caicoya, MD, DDS, FEBOMS
Consultant at Oral and Maxillofacial Surgery Department, Gregorio Marañón General University Hospital, Madrid, Spain
e-mail: crismazamuela@gmail.com; sochandiano@hotmail.com

J.I. Salmerón Escobar, MD, PhD, FEBOMS
Associate Professor Medical Faculty, Complutense University, Madrid, Spain

Consultant at Oral and Maxillofacial Surgery Department, Gregorio Marañón General University Hospital, Madrid, Spain
e-mail: jisalmeron@telefonica.net

C. Navarro Vila (ed.), *Reconstructive Oral and Maxillofacial Surgery*,
DOI 10.1007/978-3-319-20487-1_3

3.1 Introduction

The cranio-orbital region is a complex anatomical region situated in the upper and middle thirds of the face. It includes the anterior cranial base. This region can be affected by a wide variety of benign and malignant tumors originating in any of its component structures and by inflammatory or traumatic processes leading to defects with major cosmetic and functional repercussions that require reconstruction. In this chapter, we focus on the reconstruction of defects resulting from resection of tumors, which are the most frequent defects in this region. Advances in surgical approaches and reconstruction techniques have considerably extended the indications for surgical treatment of tumors affecting the cranial base. Appropriate reconstruction of defects in this region is critical if severe complications are to be prevented [1].

3.2 Anatomy

The orbits are complex cavities formed by the mesenchymal tissue adjacent to the optic vesicle. They are situated on each side of the sagittal plane between the upper and middle third of the face. Each orbit has the form of a 4-sided pyramid whose function is to house and protect the eyeball and its adnexa. It is therefore essential for vision [2] (Fig. 3.1).

The structure of the orbit comprises an anterior base and four walls that converge on a posterior apex situated at the level of the optic foramen. The anterior base lacks a bony wall, although it has a sphincter muscle (orbicularis oculi) located in the tissue of the eyelids, which comprise mobile vertical skinfolds that protect the eyeball from light and foreign bodies. Structural stability is provided by the bony walls shaped around the orbital ridge thanks to seven facial bones: the upper portion of the maxilla, zygomatic bone, lacrimal bone, sphenoid bone, ethmoid bone, frontal bone, and palatine bone.

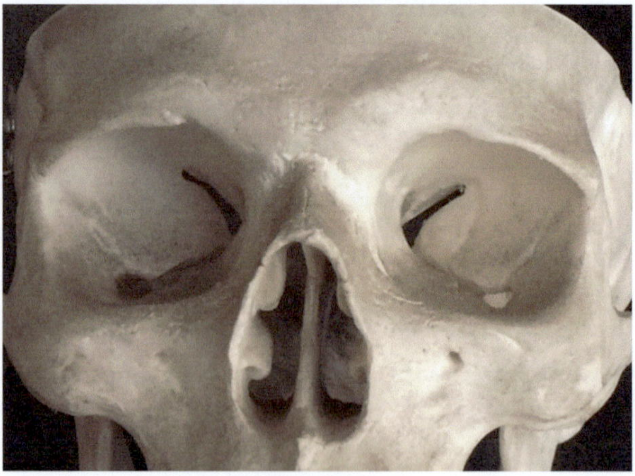

Fig. 3.1 Frontal view of orbital cavities

The orbital floor is formed medially by the orbital process of the maxilla, anteriorly and laterally by the zygomatic bone, and posteriorly by the orbital process of the palatine bone. It is concave, rests directly on the maxillary sinus, and is composed of a thin plate, making it prone to fracture. The infraorbital nerve courses across the orbital floor—first in a fissure and then in a canal 1.5 cm from the orbital ridge—from its entry via the infraorbital foramen. The medial orbital wall comprises the frontal process of the maxilla anteriorly, as well as the lacrimal bone and the lamina papyracea of the ethmoid bone. In the anterior portion, we find the anterior and posterior lacrimal crests, which form the lacrimal fossa, a key element in the insertion of the medial orbital canthus. The orbital floor is the weakest of the 4 walls and connects with the corresponding nostril. The lateral wall is formed by the frontal process of the zygomatic bone and the greater wing of the sphenoid. It is the most solid wall of the 4 and separates the orbit from the infratemporal fossa. The orbital roof is formed by the horizontal portion of the frontal bone and the lesser sphenoid wing. It sits directly between the orbit and the frontal sinus and communicates with the anterior cranial fossa at its most posterior part. Together with the lateral wall, the roof forms a solid structure. Given its closeness to the cranial cavity, the surgical approach to treat conditions affecting this area (both trauma and tumors) must be made from the anterior cranial fossa.

The apex of the orbit is limited inferiorly by the greater sphenoid wing and superiorly by the lesser sphenoid wing. Towards the external portion, a small part of the frontal bone fills the space between both wings at this level to create the superior and inferior orbital fissures. Deep within the structure and medially, we find the optic foramen, through which the optic nerve and ophthalmic artery enter the orbital cavity. The superior orbital fissure also serves as a conduit for the third, fourth, and fifth cranial nerves, the ophthalmic branch of the fifth nerve, the ophthalmic vein, and a branch of the middle meningeal artery. This is also the point of insertion of the orbital muscles, which provide mobility to the eyeball. The orbital muscles are surrounded by periorbital fat and periosteum as the last barrier attached to the bone.

The cranial floor separates the brain from the structures of the face. This complex region can be divided into the anterior, middle, and posterior cranial fossae. The anterior cranial fossa communicates with the viscerocranium. It is also the roof of the viscerocranium, including the orbital roof laterally and the upper aerodigestive tract in the central area. The region is interesting in surgical terms because it is close to the orbits and the frontal, sphenoid, and ethmoid sinuses. Therefore, knowledge of its anatomy is important when planning the reconstruction of defects caused by trauma, tumor, or infection. Repair must be followed by complete postsurgical closure to prevent cerebrospinal fluid leak to the facial region (Fig. 3.2).

The anterior cranial fossa is limited posteriorly by an imaginary horizontal line that is perpendicular to the major axis of the cranium, between the sella turcica and the horizontal portion of the lesser sphenoid wing. It is concave and courses anteriorly over the cribriform plate and crista galli on the midline that symmetrically divides the horizontal portion of the frontal bone, which in turn ascends to form the vertical portion of the frontal bone and thus create the anterior wall of the

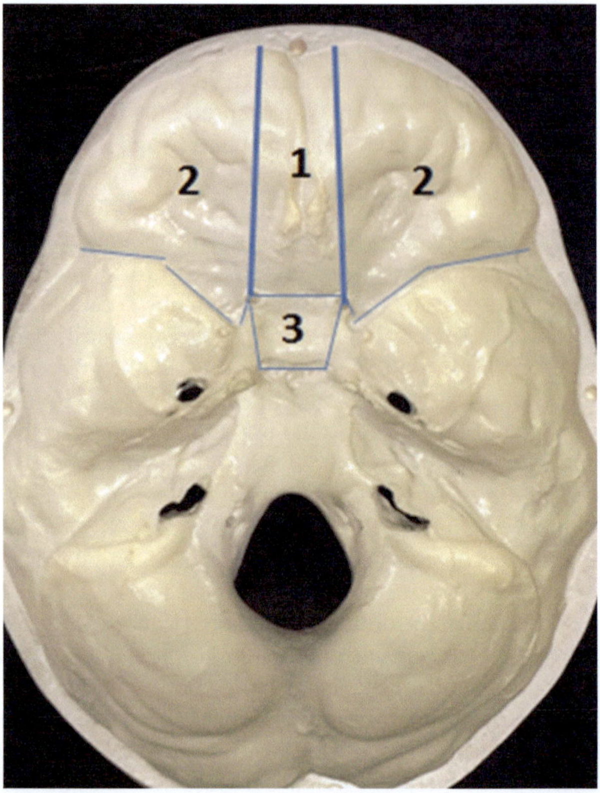

Fig. 3.2 Anterior cranial fossa: *1* medial area, *2* lateral area, *3* suprasellar area

cranial cavity. Laterally, the anterior cranial fossa is limited by the joint between the frontal and parietal bones (coronal suture). This area also contains the frontal lobes of the brain.

Exposure of the anterior cranial floor facilitates access to several facial structures. Laterally, access is gained to both orbits and, in the midzone, via the cribriform plate, to the roof of the nostrils and ethmoid air cells, which can contain tumors that are difficult to reach. Caution must be exercised with several major structures; for example, the anterior portion of the circle of Willis, lateral to the sphenoidal sinus, gives off the middle cerebral arteries (which in turn give off the ophthalmic arteries) and the anterior cerebral arteries, which are situated in the horizontal portion of the lesser sphenoid wing. Other major structures include the following: the optic canal, which arises at the prechiasmatic sulcus and runs across the sphenoid to the orbit; the posterior ethmoidal foramen, which is situated where the lesser sphenoid wing meets the cribriform plate of the ethmoid bone and is a conduit for the posterior ethmoidal nerve, vein, and artery; and the cribriform plate, which is perforated by several openings for the passage of olfactory nerve filaments. Damage to this plate could lead to anosmia. In the anterior portion, we find the anterior ethmoidal foramen (for the anterior ethmoidal nerve, vein, and artery), and at the midline, between the ethmoid and frontal bones, we find the foramen cecum, through which the emissary vein courses to the sagittal sinus.

3.3 Principles of Treatment of Tumors of the Cranio-Orbital Region

Tumors affecting the anterior cranial base and associated structures can originate in the orbit, lacrimal gland, paranasal septa, nasal cavity, skin, and intracranial structures. Given the large variety of possible origins, tumors in this region are also histologically varied. The most frequent are squamous cell carcinoma, adenocarcinoma, sarcoma, esthesioneuroblastoma, meningioma, and osteoma, as well as fibrous dysplasia, which is a tumorlike lesion. The treatment objectives in this region are control of the tumor and functional and anatomical reconstruction, as is the case in other tumors of the head and neck. A multidisciplinary approach is necessary.

According to Shah et al. [1], the first reports of a transfacial–transcranial approach to treat orbital tumors were by Cushing in 1938 and Dandy in 1941. The first resection using a combined cranial and facial approach was reported by Smith et al. in 1954 in a patient with a malignant tumor in the frontal sinus [3]. In 1963, Ketcham et al. reported a series of patients treated using anterior craniofacial resection for tumors in the ethmoidal sinuses [4]. Treatment of tumors in this region has improved thanks to the development of diagnostic methods such as 3D imaging, intraoperative imaging, neuronavigation, and intraoperative monitoring, as well as new surgical techniques (approach and reconstruction), especially the introduction of microvascular reconstruction techniques, which have fewer severe complications. Careful planning and in-depth knowledge of the local anatomy are essential.

The basic principles of anterior craniofacial resection are appropriate resection of the tumor according to its histologic type and extension. Malignant tumors should be addressed using en bloc resection covering major structures such as the ethmoidal sinuses, the anterior cranial fossa, or the roof of the nasal cavity (anterior craniofacial resection) or lateral structures such as the orbit and its contents (anterolateral craniofacial resection). If en bloc resection is impossible or the margin is too wide because of vital structures in the region (e.g., cavernous sinus, brain), the widest resection possible should be performed in combination with radiation therapy.

3.4 Diagnosis and Presurgical Planning

Before treatment, it is important to make a careful diagnosis based on the clinical history and the results of complementary tests [1]. The patient's age, general status, and comorbid conditions should be taken into account, as should the location, type, and extension of the lesion using imaging techniques such as magnetic resonance and computed tomography (CT). If necessary, vascular status should be explored using angio-CT or magnetic resonance angiography. Imaging data can be included in a navigation system to facilitate guided resection of the tumor. If possible, the histologic diagnosis should be made by means of biopsy or,

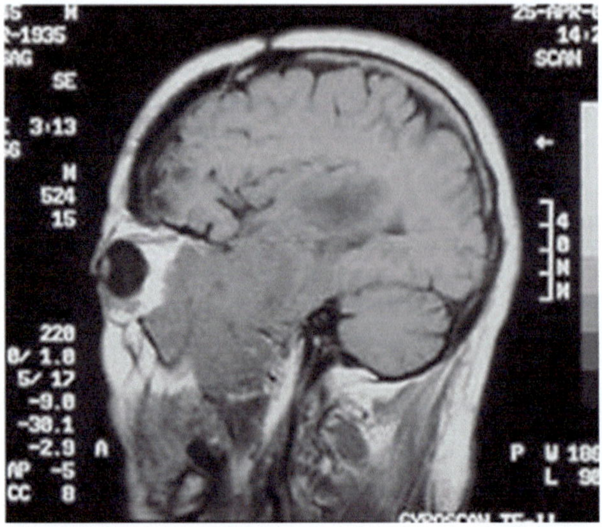

Fig. 3.3 RMI of a gigant meningioma

occasionally, endoscopy, although this may be impossible before surgery in tumors located at inaccessible sites. Knowledge of the nature of the tumor, the location and extension of the tumor, and its relationship with structures such as the carotid or vertebral vessels, the dura mater, brain, cranial nerves, or periorbital area is the basis for planning the surgical approach, resection of the tumor, and reconstruction [5] (Fig. 3.3).

3.5 Surgical Approaches

Access to the lesion can be gained using various approaches depending on the region as follows:

- Endoscopic techniques. The recent development of endoscopic techniques has enabled minimally invasive removal of selected tumors [6]. Although these techniques represent a clear advance, their indication remains controversial, especially in the case of advanced malignant tumors.
- Medial labiomandibulotomy: The approach is anterior to the cervical spine. The procedure can be combined with other craniofacial approaches.
- Le Fort I osteotomy. Le Fort I osteotomy provides good access to tumors affecting the cranial base and the central nasopharynx. Morbidity is low. This approach is not suitable for very extensive lesions, especially in the case of malignant tumors.
- Translocation of the facial middle third (pedicled maxillectomy). This group of approaches is based on freeing vascularized units of the middle third to enable broad access to the cranial base and deep facial regions. Reconstruction is safe once the units of the middle third are returned to their original location [5, 7–9].

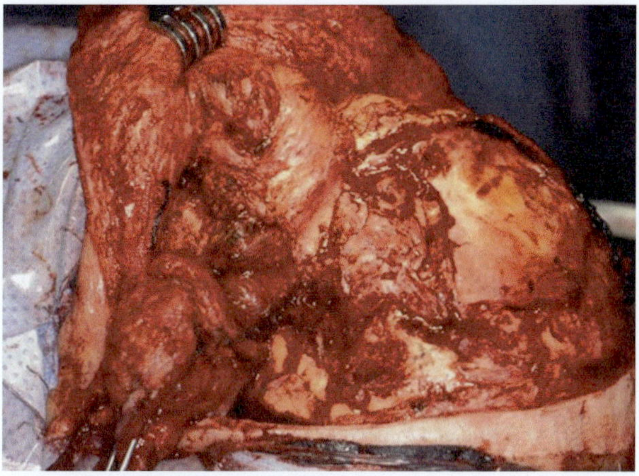

Fig. 3.4 Coronal approach extending preauricular regions

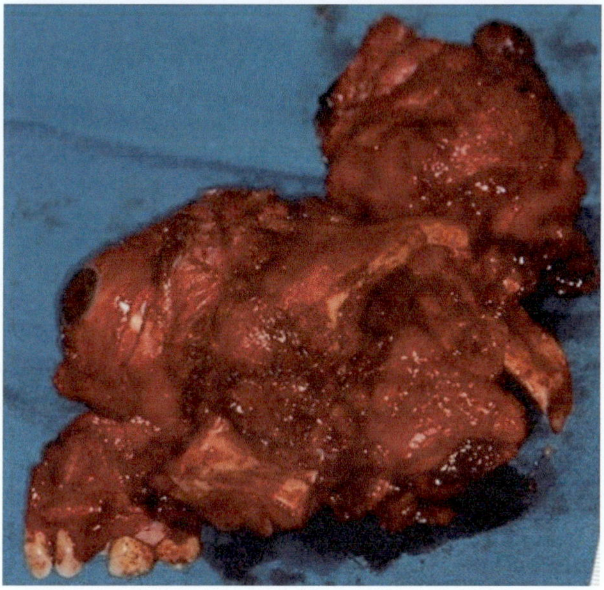

Fig. 3.5 Surgical specimen

This type of maxillectomy is an excellent alternative in extensive tumors affecting the central cranial base and deep anatomical regions such as the pterygomaxillary and infratemporal fossae and the orbit.

- Subfrontal approach to the anterior cranial fossa (unilateral or bilateral). This approach requires a coronal incision and more or less extensive frontal craniotomy [10].
- Combined approaches: In the anterolateral approach, it may be necessary to combine a subfrontal approach with any of the other approaches cited (Figs. 3.4 and 3.5).

3.6 Reconstruction of Defects of the Cranio-Orbital Region

3.6.1 Objectives

After tumor resection in this area and after defects caused by injury, the objectives of reconstruction are as follows:

- Complete sealing of the cranium
- Restoration of volume and craniofacial harmony
- Conservation of functions

In order to reach these objectives, a series of steps must be systematically completed [1, 11, 12] as follows:

- Repair of defects of the dura mater
- Placement of a well-vascularized tissue barrier between the cranial cavity and the upper aerodigestive tract
- Reconstruction of bone architecture if it is necessary to restore facial cosmesis
- Restoration of soft tissue bulk
- Reconstruction of skin defects, preferably with skin of similar quality, color, and texture

3.6.1.1 Surgical Techniques

Before the introduction of microvascular flaps, isolation of the cranial cavity and coverage of defects in this region were based on free grafts such as fragments of fascia, muscle, or fat in order to eliminate naso-ethmoidal defects, or local flaps, with a high rate of complications in large defects, especially in patients who had received radiation therapy [1, 12]. At present, the possibility of using microvascular free tissue and introducing new digital techniques in the diagnosis and planning of resection and reconstruction of cranio-orbital tumors has considerably improved outcomes and reduced the number of complications associated with this type of surgery.

3.7 Local and Regional Flaps

Local and regional flaps include flaps of the pericranium, epicranial aponeurosis, and the combination of both (galeal–pericranial flap), as well as the temporalis muscle flap. These flaps are simple and safe, although in extreme defects of the floor of the cranium and orbitofacial region, they cannot guarantee appropriate isolation and repair of intracranial structures. Local scalp flaps can be used to cover minor skin defects or major resections when it is impossible to perform more complex reconstructions or as a rescue approach when these fail.

- Mucosal flaps. Recently developed endoscopic approaches have increased the importance of mucoperiosteal and mucoperichondrial flaps. These flaps are based on the vessels of the nasal septum and are an alternative to nonvascularized

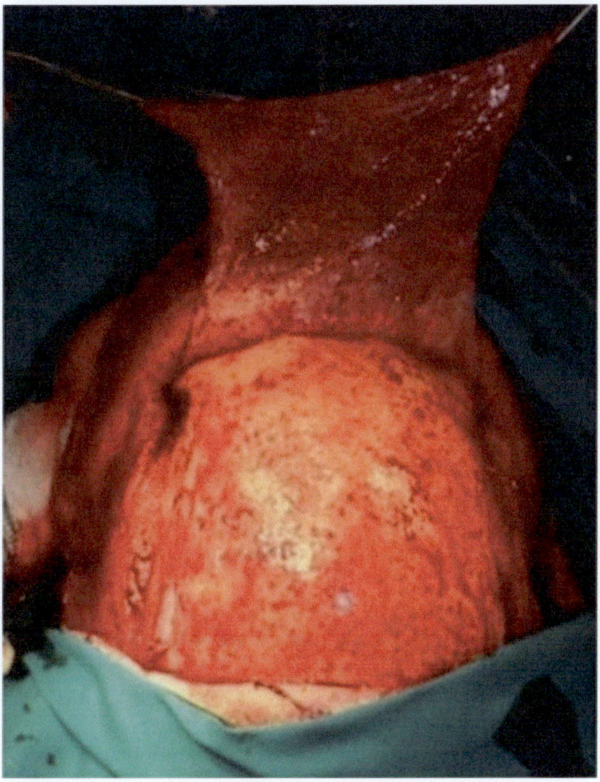

Fig. 3.6 Coronal approach and pericranial flap

fascial or mucous tissue free flaps to close small defects in the naso-ethmoidal region and thus prevent cerebrospinal fluid rhinorrhea [6, 12]

- Pericranial flaps or combined flaps (galeal–pericranial) can be used to repair defects of the dura mater and small defects of the anterior cranial fossa, especially for obturation at the nasofrontal duct and ethmoid–orbital area. This obturation should be accompanied by preparation of the frontal sinus through curettage of the mucosa and cranialization or obliteration [11]. Pericranial flaps are very adaptable and well vascularized. When a thicker flap is necessary, they can be combined with the epicranial aponeurosis, a subdermal layer of tissue that continues laterally with the superficial temporal fascia. If the design of the resection allows, these flaps should be prepared during surgery, with an anterior pedicle (supplied by the supratrochlear vessels), a lateral pedicle (supplied by the superficial temporal vessels), or a combined anterolateral pedicle [12] (Figs. 3.6, 3.7, and 3.8).
- Temporalis muscle flap. The temporalis muscle flap, which is supplied by the deep temporal branches of the internal maxillary artery, was first described by Golovine for obliteration of the orbital cavity after exenteration [13]. The temporalis flap is a good option for covering small to medium anterolateral defects of the cranial base. However, it is not useful in large defects that require a bulky flap or extensively affect the cranial base towards the midline, since its arc of rotation

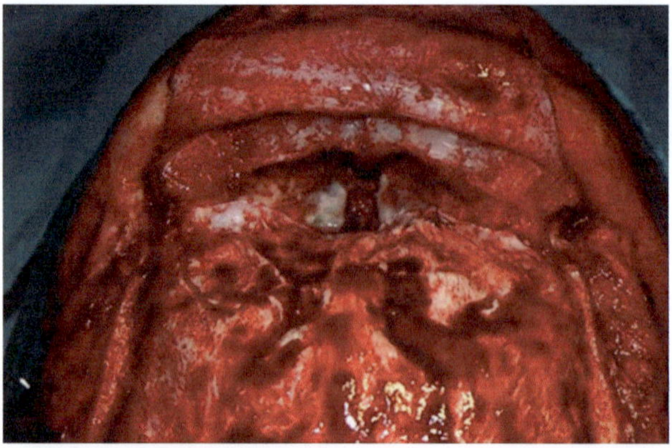

Fig. 3.7 Anterior skull base surgical defect

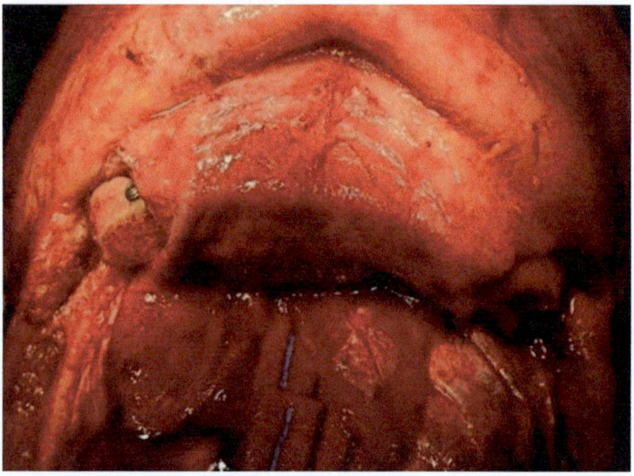

Fig. 3.8 Pericranial flap covering the defect

is limited, although it can be widened by cutting the coronoid process. This flap has the drawback of leaving a secondary cosmetic defect in the temporal fossa. In lesser reconstructions, the anterior portion of the muscle can be used, and the defect can be covered by sliding the posterior part of the muscle towards the retro-orbital area. In cases where the whole temporalis muscle must be used, the defect in the fossa can be significant, although it can be filled using prosthetic material (methyl methacrylate or polyethylene). However, this increases the risk of postsurgical infection, especially in patients who have undergone radiation therapy (Figs. 3.9, 3.10, 3.11, 3.12, 3.13, and 3.14).

- Distant pedicle flaps. Flaps such as the pectoralis major myocutaneous flap, the inferior or lateral inferior trapezius flap, and the latissimus dorsi pedicle flap are not the first choice in the reconstruction of major defects of the cranio-orbital area, especially at the level of the cranial floor, owing to the limited arc of rotation, which prevents the flap from reaching this region. In addition, the quality of reconstruction is poor, and complications, especially wound dehiscence, are

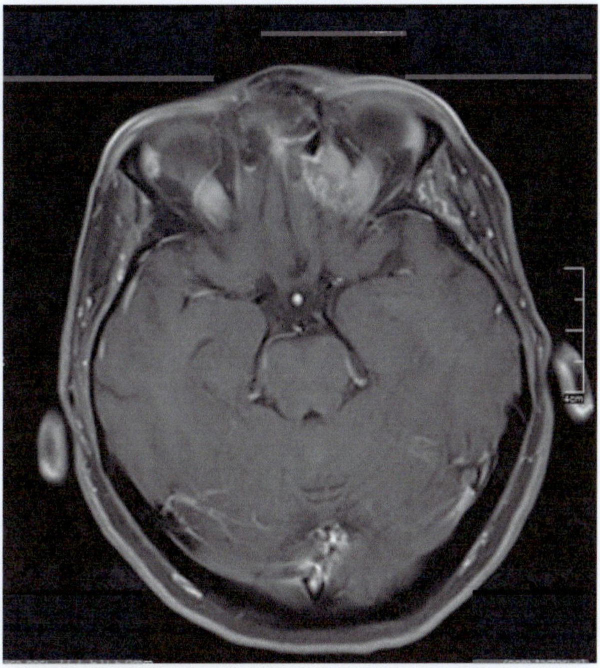

Fig. 3.9 Preoperative. MRI. Squamous cell carcinoma of the left orbitary region

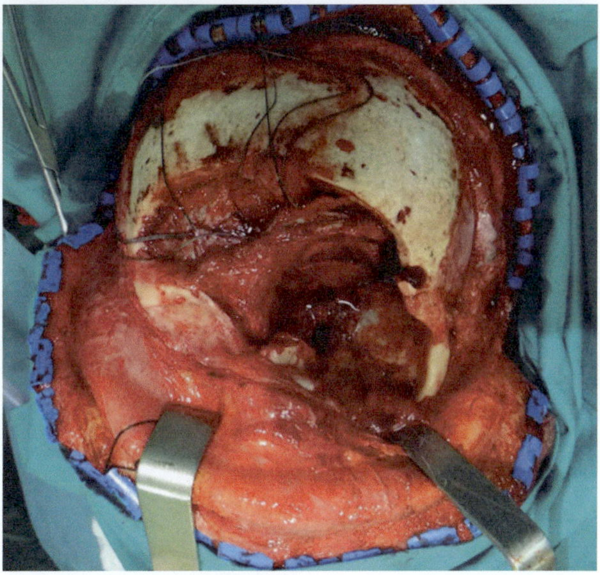

Fig. 3.10 Surgical defect

frequent. Pedicle flaps from other regions may be a second-choice alternative in patients with a poor general status, major vascular disorders, or failure of a more complex microvascular reconstruction [12].

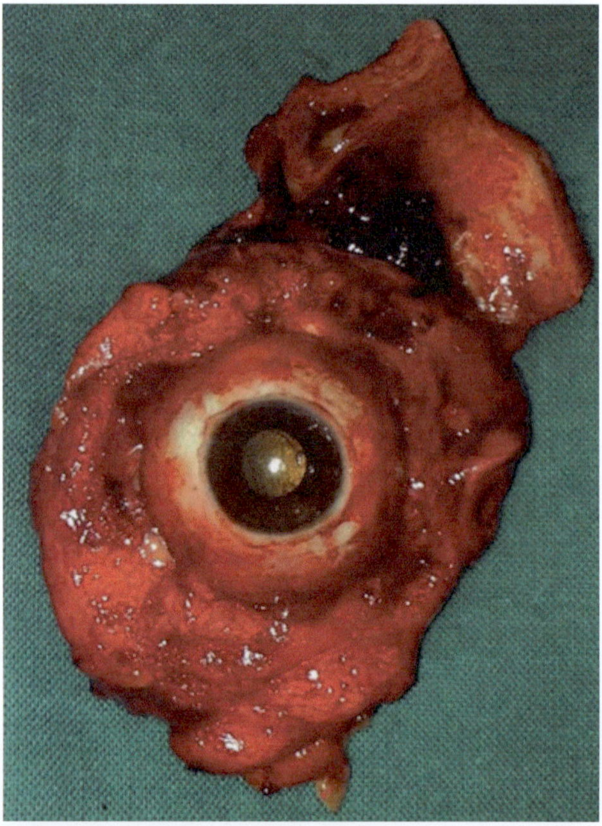

Fig. 3.11 Surgical specimen

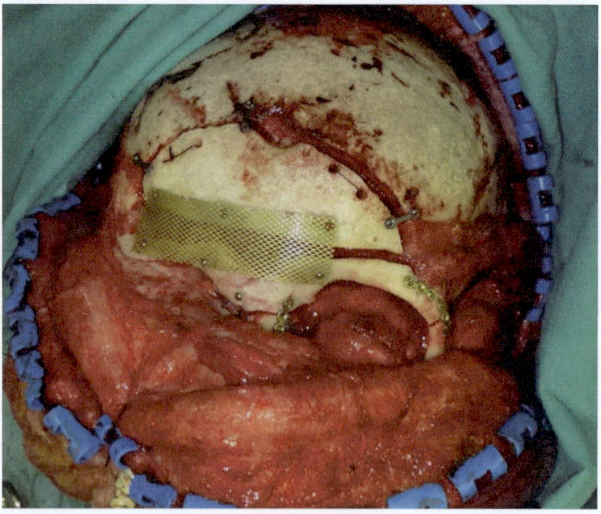

Fig. 3.12 Intraoperative view of the reconstruction

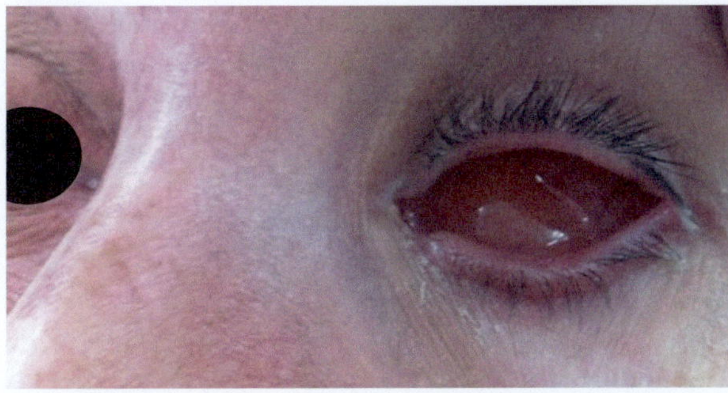

Fig. 3.13 Temporalis muscle flap filling the orbital cavity

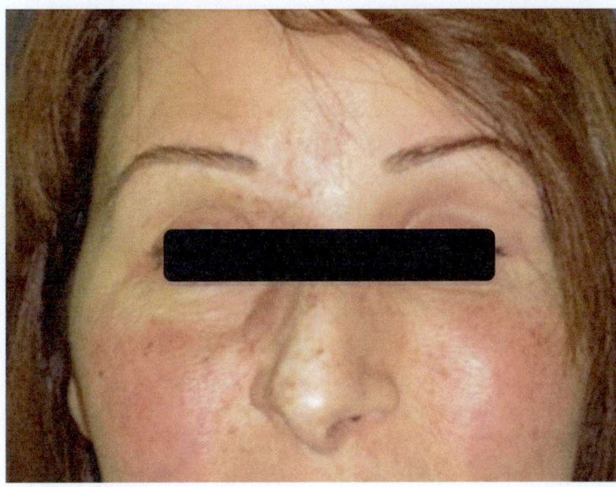

Fig. 3.14 Anteroposterior postoperative view

3.8 Microvascular Flaps

Transfer of free tissue using microvascular anastomosis is currently the method of choice for reconstructing complex defects of the craniofacial region, including the cranial base and the orbit [11, 14]. Its principal advantages include the 3-dimensional versatility of the reconstruction, which is limited only by the location of the receptor vessels, and the possibility of transferring a large volume of well-vascularized tissue to seal the intracranial contents, obliterate dead space, and provide skin cover. Microvascular flaps can include various tissues in compound flaps (muscle, dermis, skin, and bone), have reduced associated morbidity at donor sites, and enable 2 teams to work simultaneously in most cases. In addition, the reconstruction is highly reliable, with success rates of 95–98 %, although in cases of failure, the complications due to flap loss can be very severe. Reconstruction in the cranio-orbital region is limited by the reduced availability of receptor vessels near the defect to be repaired. The temporal vessels are used where possible and must be preserved during the preparation of a coronal flap. In cases where it is impossible to use the superficial temporalis pedicle flap, the alternatives include cervical vessels such as the facial vein and artery, the external carotid artery, and the external or internal jugular veins. The internal jugular vein is used with end-to-side anastomosis. Such circumstances will necessitate the use of very long vascular pedicle flaps, the most common being the radial fasciocutaneous flap, the anterolateral thigh flap, and musculocutaneous flaps of the rectus abdominis or latissimus dorsi. Flaps with a bone component are uncommon in craniofacial reconstruction, in which bone reconstruction is usually by nonvascularized free bone grafts or by implanting biomaterial (see below). An interesting indication of the fibular flap and iliac crest flap (albeit less frequently, owing to the shortness of its pedicle) is the reconstruction of posttraumatic defects in the orbit, as proposed by Rodriguez et al. [15].

- Radial fasciocutaneous forearm flap (radial flap). The radial forearm flap is supplied by the radial artery and its venae comitantes (deep system) and by the radial vein (superficial system). This long flap makes it possible to reach the receptor vessels in the neck. The radial forearm flap provides a very adaptable island of thin fasciocutaneous tissue. It can be used to cover thin defects of medium extension (maximum 15 × 15 cm) [12], such as defects of the pharyngeal mucosa and skin defects, and as a dermal flap at the level of the cranial base–orbit.
- Anterolateral thigh flap. The anterolateral thigh flap is based on the perforators of the descending branch of the lateral femoral circumflex artery and its venae comitantes. It has a long pedicle, although this could be limited by the various ways in which the perforators emerge. The anterolateral thigh flap is suitable for coverage of extensive defects of the craniofacial region (up to 15 × 30 cm) and can be used to fill dead space by de-epithelializing and folding the flap. Donor-site morbidity is very infrequent.
- Rectus abdominis flap. The rectus abdominis flap is based on the deep epigastric artery and its venae comitantes. It is widely used for reconstruction of the cranial base and orbit because of its good vascularization and the versatility of its design, which provides the option of using muscle tissue with sufficient bulk to fill large defects. The rectus abdominis flap can also be combined with fascia and a skin island to cover large defects with a long vascular pedicle (10–12 cm), thus making makes it possible to reach the cervical receptor vessels in cases where the temporal vessels cannot be used (Figs. 3.15, 3.16, 3.17, 3.18, 3.19, and 3.20).
- Latissimus dorsi flap. The latissimus dorsi flap is based on the thoracodorsal pedicle, which depends on the subscapular system. As with the rectus abdominis flap, the latissimus dorsi flap is often used to repair large cranio-orbital and facial defects, since it provides a large well-vascularized muscle or musculocutaneous flap (40 × 30 cm) and has a large caliber and long pedicle. The latissimus dorsi flap can also be prepared as a chimeric flap combined with other components of the subscapular system, such as the serratus muscle or the scapula osteofasciocutaneous flap when required for the repair of very complex defects.
- Omentum flap. The omentum is a double layer of peritoneum that inserts in the major curvature of the stomach and transverse colon. The omentum flap is supplied by the gastroepiploic vessels. Since it is a well-vascularized flap that can

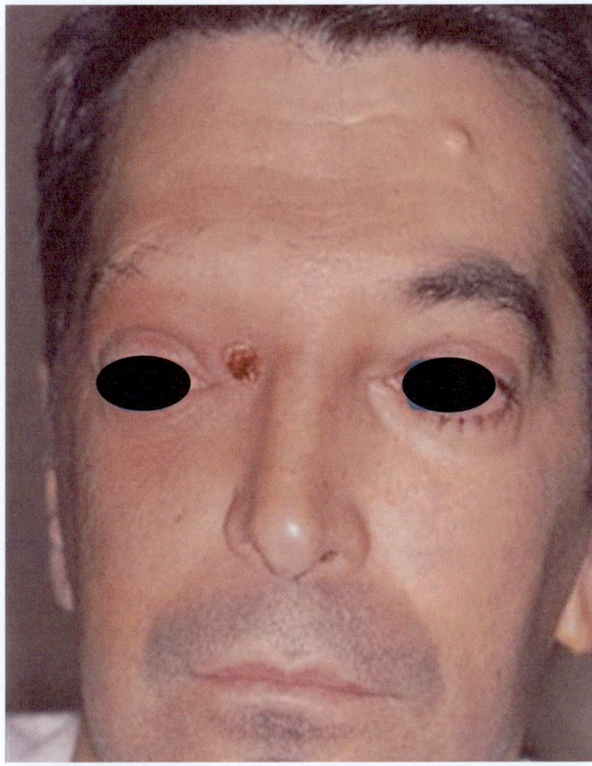

Fig. 3.15 Orbito-ethmoidal right tumor

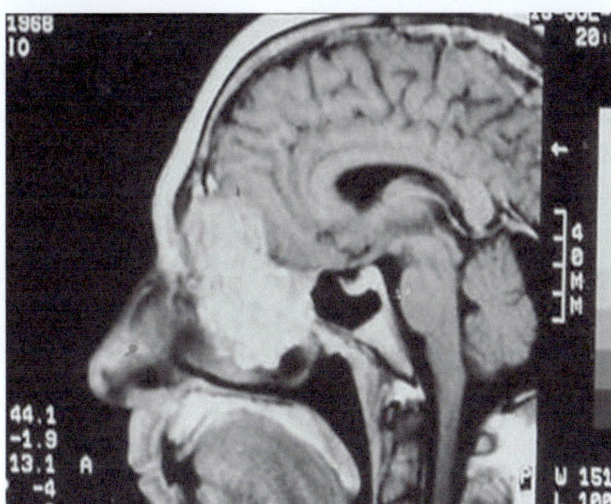

Fig. 3.16 Preoperative MRI. Invasion of anterior fossa and frontal bone

cover broad surfaces, it can be combined with a free skin graft to cover wider cranial defects. The main drawback of the omentum flap is the morbidity associated with the abdominal surgery needed to harvest the flap [16].

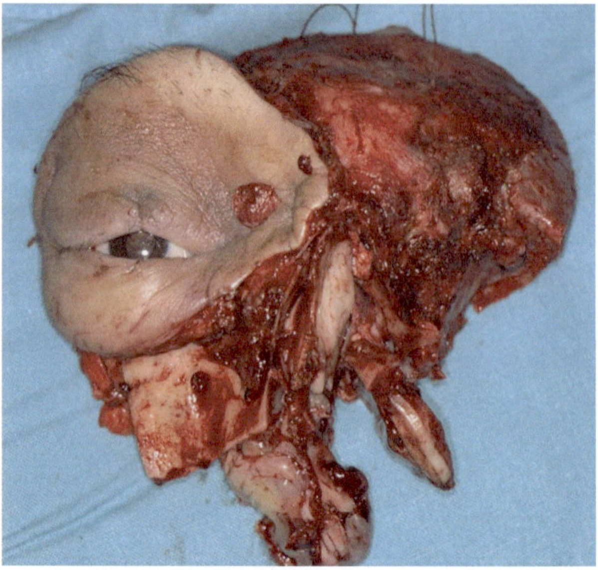

Fig. 3.17 Surgical specimen

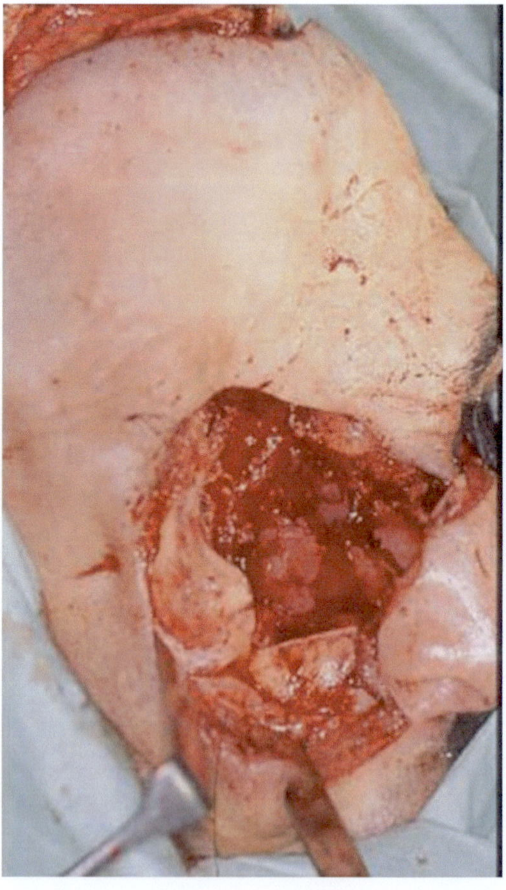

Fig. 3.18 Surgical defect

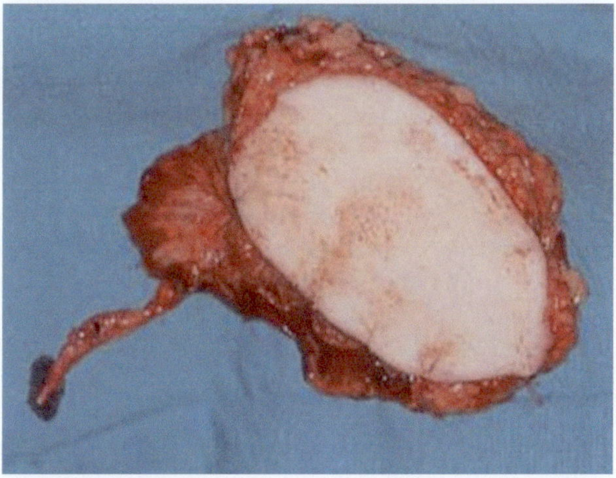

Fig. 3.19 Rectus abdominis flap

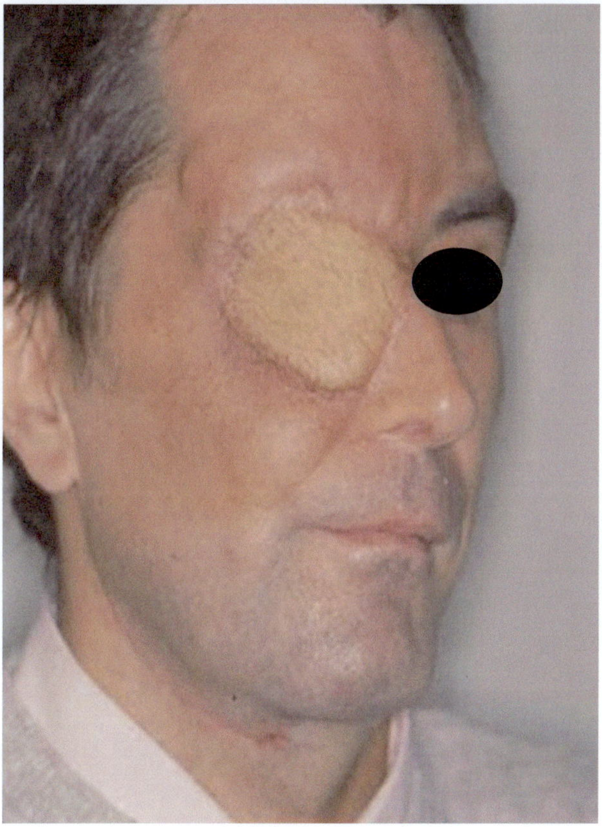

Fig. 3.20 Postoperative view

3.9 Bone Reconstruction

Reconstruction of bone defects after resection in the cranio-orbital region is indicated only if the defect of the craniofacial architecture causes a clear alteration of cosmesis or of the position of the eyeball, which can occur after resections of the frontal–malar or frontal–nasal skeleton or in wide wall resection, especially of the roof, medial wall, or floor. Bone reconstruction is generally not necessary after resections of the central region of the anterior cranial base (cribriform plate) or after resections in the temporal region, since coverage with soft tissue flaps (whether local, regional, or microvascular) enables the defect to be repaired. In the remaining cases, bone defects can be repaired using nonvascularized bone grafts or biomaterials prepared before or during surgery (custom prosthesis).

- Bone grafts. Restoration of cranial bone defects can be carried out using free bone grafts taken from the internal cortex of the bone flap removed during the craniotomy, generally at the frontoparietal level. Other sources of bone grafts include the iliac bone or ribs when large quantities of bone tissue are required, although taking tissue from these areas implies morbidity at an additional donor site. It is very important to cover the graft with well-vascularized soft tissue and anchor it with miniplates and screws to reduce resorption of the graft. Resorption is another disadvantage of bone grafts, especially in patients who have received radiation therapy. In selected cases involving microvascular reconstruction, the bone fragment of a compound flap can be used for reconstruction of the associated bone defect, as reported by Rodriguez et al. [15] (Figs. 3.21 and 3.22).

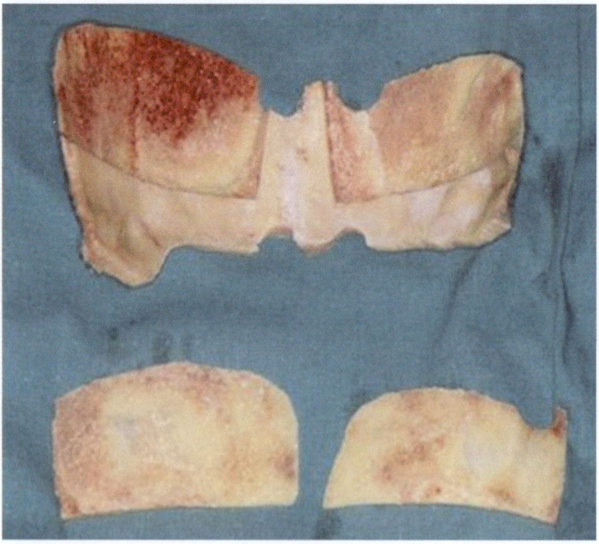

Fig. 3.21 Calvarian bone

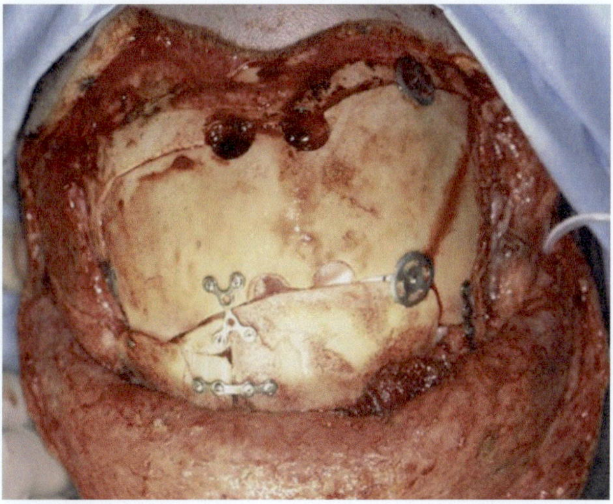

Fig. 3.22 Calvarian bone repositioned

- Alloplastic material. Several materials have been proposed as substitutes for bone grafts in order to shorten the duration of surgery, reduce morbidity (no donor site), and improve cosmetic outcome (no reabsorption). The materials used include several bone cements, hydroxyapatite, acrylic prostheses, titanium mesh, and polyether ether ketone. Titanium mesh has been used to cover complex cranial defects, although in this indication, it can lead to problems arising from heat conductivity. In addition, titanium mesh is expensive. The most common indication in the cranio-orbital region is repair of the orbital walls. The advent of digital technology has made it possible to customize prostheses to an existing craniofacial defect or even to perform virtual resection of the tumor and prepare the prosthesis before resection using a stable material such as polyether ether ketone. Planning data are downloaded to the navigation system for transfer to the operative field. Once the resection has been performed as planned, the previously prepared prosthesis can be inserted, thus reducing operative time and preventing donor-site morbidity [17]. The main risk in repair of cranio-orbital defects using alloplastic materials is the possibility of infection and exposure of the materials. Every attempt must be made to prevent this from happening by ensuring appropriate coverage with soft tissue (Figs. 3.23, 3.24, 3.25, 3.26, 3.27, 3.28, 3.29, 3.30, and 3.31).

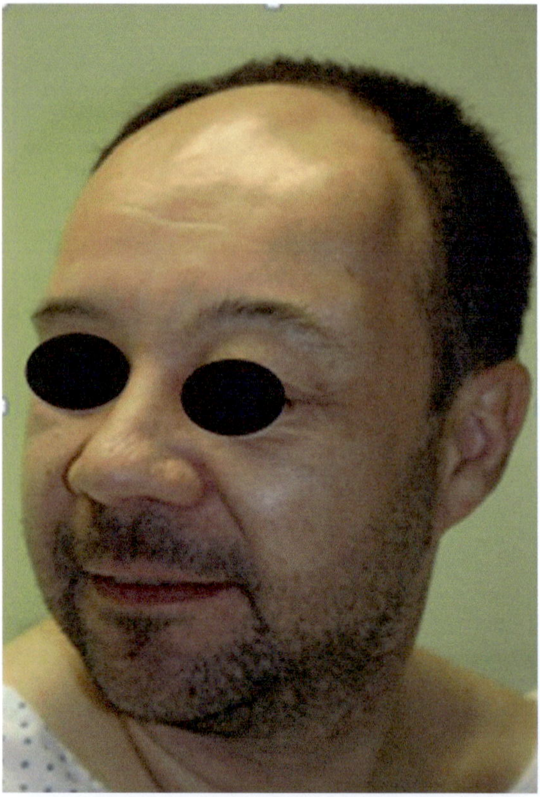

Fig. 3.23 Left fronto-orbital meningioma

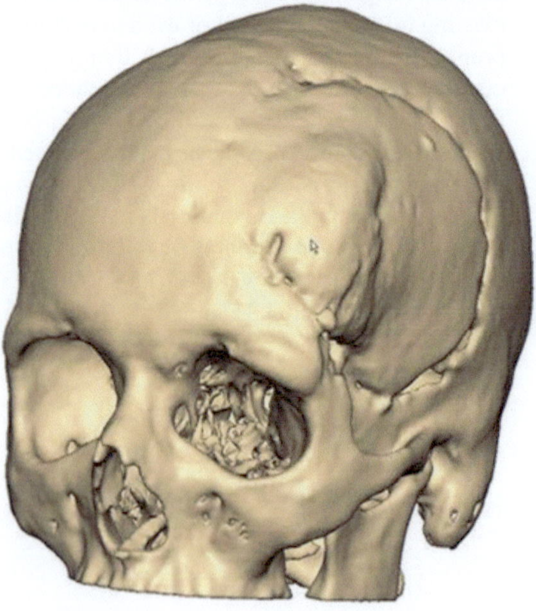

Fig. 3.24 3D CT reconstruction of the tumor

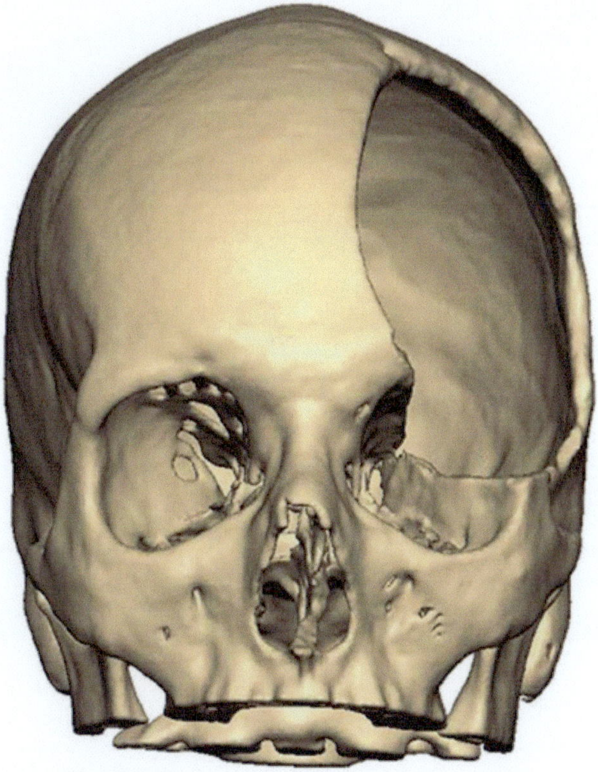

Fig. 3.25 Virtual surgical planning defect

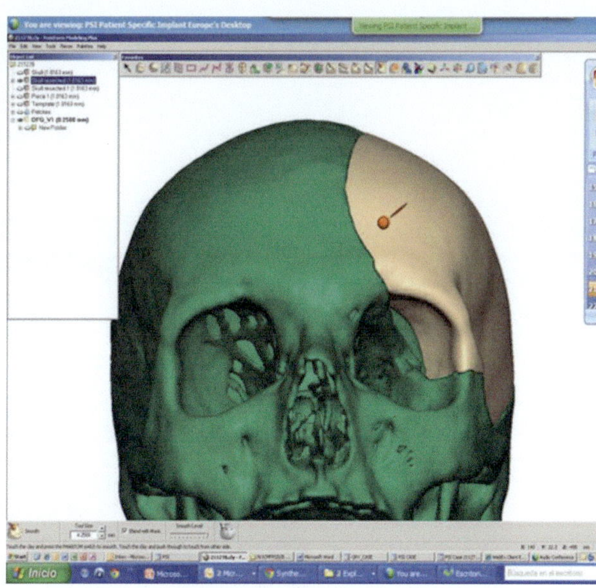

Fig. 3.26 Virtual reconstruction

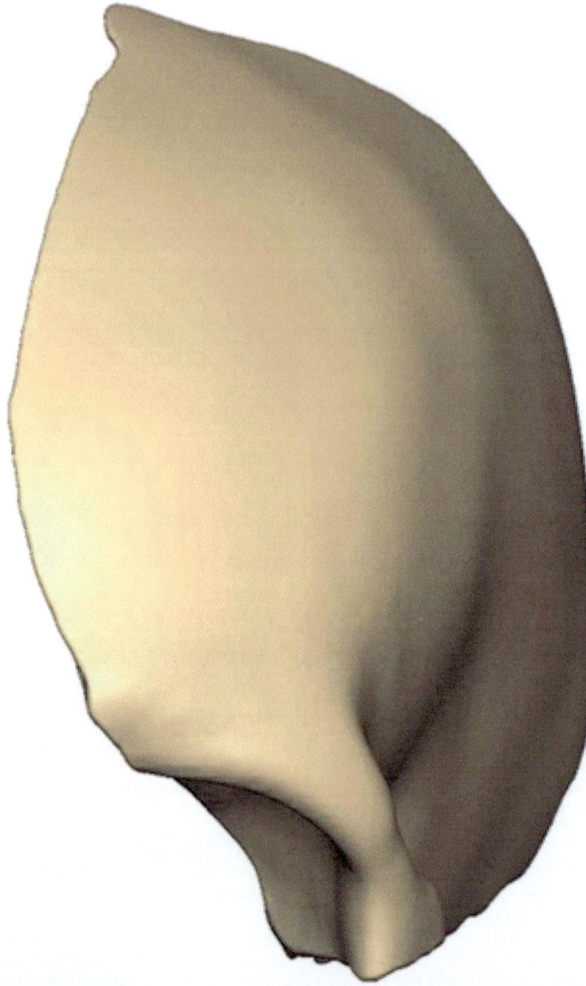

Fig. 3.27 PEEK prosthesis design

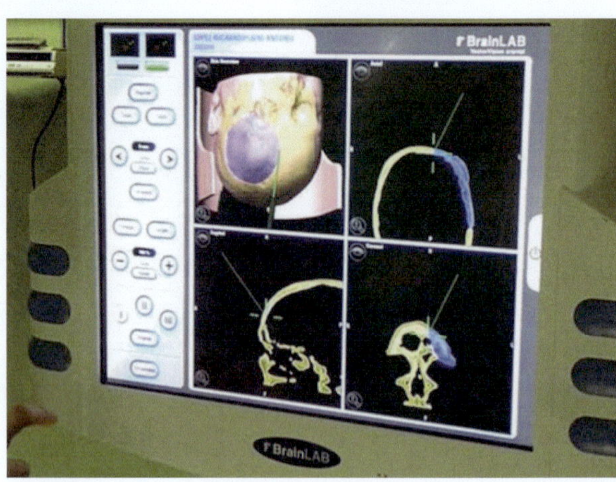

Fig. 3.28 Intraoperative navigation

Fig. 3.29 Surgical defect

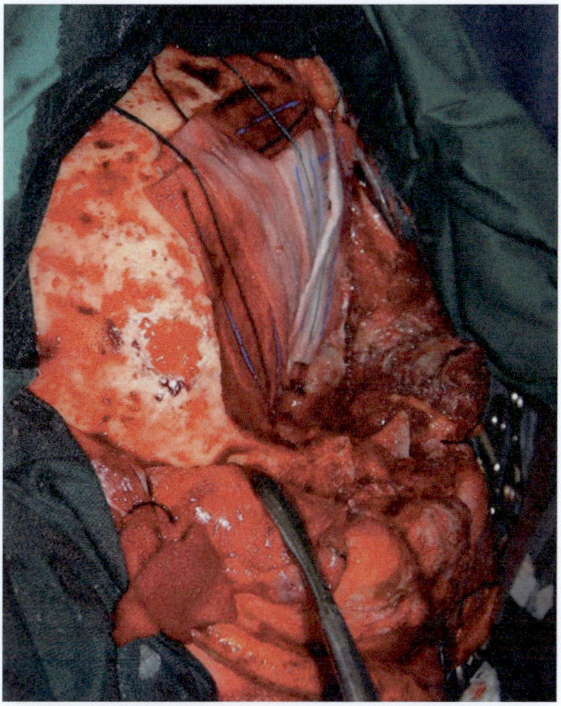

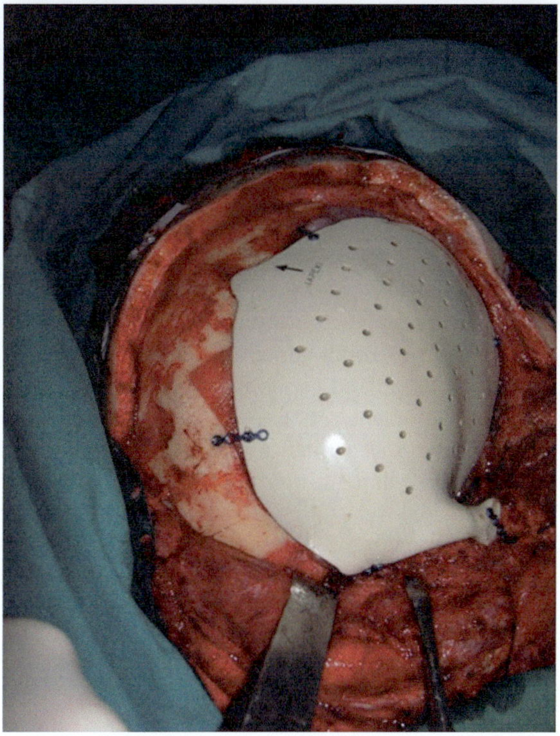

Fig. 3.30 PEEK prosthesis

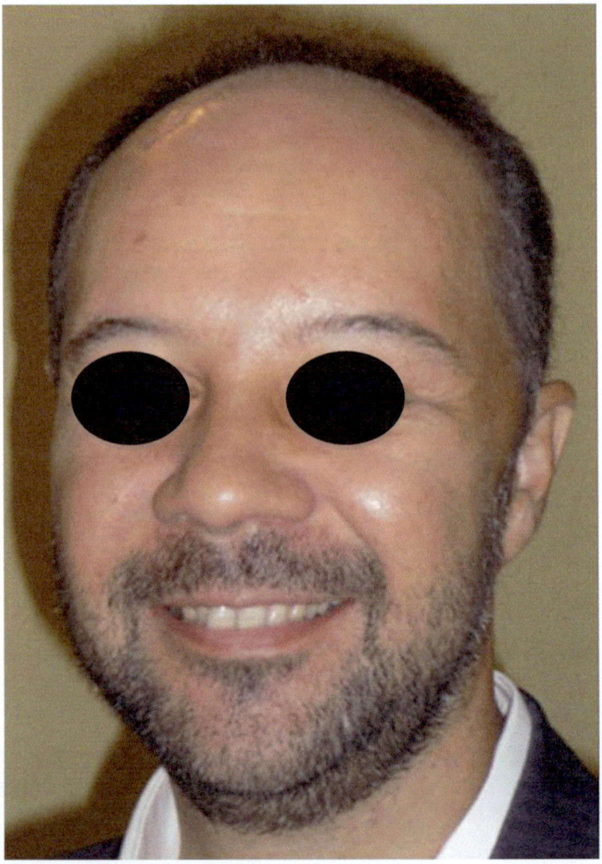

Fig. 3.31 Anteroposterior postoperative view

3.10 Repair of the Orbit

The orbital walls can be repaired using titanium mesh combined with good soft tissue coverage. Resection of intraorbital tissue can be limited to enucleation or removal of the orbital contents (exenteration) [20]. In enucleation, preservation of periorbital tissue and the conjunctival vascular bed enables placement of an ocular prosthesis; in exenteration, placement of a prosthesis requires the cavity to be filled using the flaps described above (temporalis muscle flap, galeal–pericranial flap, microvascular flap) in order to support the conjunctival sac (preserved or reconstructed using mucosal grafts), provided that the eyelids are preserved. In the case of exenteration combined with eyelid resection, the orbital cavity is filled with a musculocutaneous flap so that the skin component can be used to repair the eyelid defect or with a muscle flap covered with a free skin graft or a sliding cervicofacial skin flap [18]. In these cases, the flap can be covered using an ocular prosthesis with eyelid attachment, which can be fixed using implants placed on the underlying bone of the orbit.

3.11 Complications

In surgery of the cranio-orbital region involving the anterior cranial base, the main complications are associated with inappropriate reconstruction or failure of the reconstruction. The most severe complications arise from inadequate isolation of intracranial structures, opening of the dura mater, or production of dead space, all of which may be associated with life-threatening conditions such as cerebrospinal fluid leak, meningitis, brain abscesses, osteomyelitis, and vascular lesions [19]. The lack of appropriate reconstruction of the orbit can lead to ocular dystopia, diplopia, brain herniation into the orbit with transmission of the cerebral pulse to the orbital content, and facial disfigurement [1, 12]. Other complications, such as lesions of the superior branch of the facial nerve, may be due to inappropriate surgical approach or preparation of locoregional flaps such as the galeal–pericranial flap or temporalis muscle flap. Finally, both pedicle flaps and free flaps [21] themselves are affected by complications such as infection, dehiscence, and necrosis.

References

1. Shah JP, Bilsky MH, Patel SG. Malignant tumors of the skull base. Neurosurg Focus. 2002;13: 1–12.
2. Netter FH. Atlas de Anatomía Humana. 5th ed. Barcelona: Editorial Masson Elsevier; 2011.
3. Smith RR, Klopp CT, Williams JM. Surgical treatment of cancer of the frontal sinus and adjacent areas. Cancer. 1954;7(5):991–4.
4. Ketcham AS, Wilkins RH, Van Buren JM, Smith RR. A combined intracranial facial approach to the paranasal sinuses. Am J Surg. 1963;10:698–703.
5. Acero J, Navarro C. Midfacial translocation approaches, chap 21. In: Cappabianca P, Califano L, Iaconetta G, editors. Cranial, craniofacial and skull base surgery. Milan: Springer; 2010. p. 309–18.
6. Carrau RL, Kassam AB, Snyderman CH, Duvvuri U, Mintz A, Gardner P. Endoscopic transnasal anterior skull base resection for the treatment of sinonasal malignancies. Operative techniques. Otolaryngology. 2006;17(2):102–10.
7. Janecka IP, Tiedemann K. Skull base surgery: anatomy, biology and technology. Philadelphia: Lippincott-Raven Publishers; 1997.
8. Clauser L, Vinci R, Curioni C. Dismantling and reassembling of the facial skeleton in tumor surgery of the craniomaxillofacial area. History, surgical anatomy, and notes of surgical technique: part 1. J Craniofac Surg. 2000;11(4):318–25.
9. Hernandez-Altemir F. Transfacial access to the retromaxillary area. J Maxillofac Surg. 1986;14:165–70.
10. De Divitis O, Iacopino DG, Solari D, Stagno V, Grasso G. Chapter 2: Subfrontal approaches. In: Cappabianca P, Califano L, Iaconetta G, editors. Cranial, craniofacial and skull base surgery. Milan: Springer; 2010. p. 17–25.
11. Chang DW, Langstein HN, Gupta A, De Monte F, Do KA, Wang X, Robb G. Reconstructive management of cranial base defects after tumor ablation. Plast Reconstr Surg. 2001;107(6):1346–55.

12. Brusati R, Biglioli F, Mortini P. Chapter 23: Anterior cranial base reconstruction. In: Cappabianca P, Califano L, Iaconetta G, editors. Cranial, craniofacial and skull base surgery. Milan: Springer; 2010. p. 331–42.
13. Golovine SS. Procedure de cloture plastique de l'orbite apres l'exenteration. J Fr Ophtalmol. 1898;18:261–7.
14. Teknos JC, Smith TN, Day TA, Netterville JL, Burkey BB. Microvascular tissue transfer in reconstructing skull base defects: lessons learned. Laryngoscope. 2002;112:1871–6.
15. Rodriguez ED, Bluebond-Langner R, Park JE, Manson PN. Preservation of contour in periorbital and midfacial craniofacial microsurgery: reconstruction of the soft-tissue elements and skeletal buttresses. Plast Reconstr Surg. 2008;121(5):1738–47; discussion 1748.
16. Urken ML, Cheney ML. Free omentum and gastro-omentum. In: Urken ML, Cheney ML, Sullivan MJ, Biller HF, editors. Atlas of regional and free flaps for head and neck reconstruction. New York: Raven; 1995. p. 321–9.
17. Jalbert F, Boetto S, Nadon F, Lawers F, Schmidt E, Lopez R. One-step primary reconstruction for complex craniofacial resection with PEEK custom-made implants. J Craniomaxillofac Surg. 2014;42(2):141–8. doi:10.1016/j.jcms.2013.04.001. Epub 2013 May 18.
18. Cuesta-Gil M, Concejo C, Acero J, Navarro-Vila C, Ochandiano S. Repair of large orbito-cutaneous defects by combining two classical flaps. J CranioMaxillofac Surg. 2004;32(1):21–7.
19. Heth JA, Funk GF, Karnell LH, McCulloch TM, Traynelis VC, Nerad JA, Smith RB, et al. Free tissue transfer and local flap complications in anterior and anterolateral skull base surgery. Head Neck. 2002;24:901–11.
20. Acero J. Anterior cranio-facial tumors. Approaches and reconstruction guidelines. In: Mommaerts M, editors. Selected papers of the XX congress of the EACMFS. Bologna; 2008. p. 293–300.
21. Navarro-Cuellar C, Riba F, Guerra B, Pujol R, Herencia H, Navarro-Vila C. Reconstruction of the scalp with a free flap of omentum. Rev Esp Cirug Oral y Maxilofac. 2004;26:249–56. doi:10.4321/S1130-05582004000400006.

Reconstruction of Soft Tissue Defects Using Microsurgical Flaps

4

Ignacio Navarro Cuellar, Teresa González Otero,
José Alfonso Ruiz Cruz, and Carlos Navarro Vila

Abstract

Reconstructive surgery of the soft tissue of the head and neck is a challenge for the surgeon owing to the three-dimensional nature of the face and its tissues.

When deciding on a reconstructive technique, the traditional idea that the simplest reconstruction is usually the best should always be taken into account, as long as the basic tenets of functionality and cosmetic requirements are met. Therefore, defects that can be satisfactorily resolved using local or regional flaps should not be reconstructed using microsurgery. However, some patients need

I. Navarro Cuellar, MD, DDS, FEBOMS (✉)
Consultant at Oral and Maxillofacial Surgery Department,
Virgen de la Salud Hospital, Toledo, Spain
e-mail: nnavcu@hotmail.com

T. González Otero, MD, PhD, FEBOMS
Consultant at Oral and Maxillofacial Surgery Department,
La Paz University Hospital, Madrid, Spain
e-mail: gusarapillo2003@yahoo.es

J.A. Ruiz Cruz, MD, DDS, FEBOMS
Consultant at Oral and Maxillofacial Surgery Department,
University Hospital del Sur, Madrid, Spain
e-mail: jaruizcruz@gmail.com

C. Navarro Vila, MD, DMD, PhD, FEBOMS
Full professor, Medical Faculty Complutense University of Madrid, Madrid, Spain

Head of Oral and Maxillofacial Department Surgery, Gregorio Marañón General University Hospital, Madrid, Spain

Académico Correspondiente of the Royal National Academy of Medicine of Spain, Madrid, Spain
e-mail: cnavarro.vila@clinicanavarrovila.com

C. Navarro Vila (ed.), *Reconstructive Oral and Maxillofacial Surgery*,
DOI 10.1007/978-3-319-20487-1_4

greater tissue bulk, which can only be harvested from distant regions, and would therefore benefit from free flap-based reconstruction techniques.

This chapter addresses the microsurgical free flaps most commonly used for reconstruction of the soft tissue of the head and neck. Advantages and disadvantages are presented.

4.1 Introduction

The head and neck have a very particular three-dimensional structure that is formed by different types of tissue (skin, bone, and mucosa), thus making reconstruction especially difficult. In functional terms, several anatomical structures (e.g., the eyelids, lips, nose, and outer and inner ear) are difficult to reconstruct, yet their importance for the patient is undeniable. Reconstructive surgery attempts to minimize functional sequelae while maintaining the best appearance possible, since the face is what identifies patients to the rest of the world. Although different, these objectives are inseparable, and reconstructive surgery could not be considered successful if a patient who has made a functional recovery continues to have cosmetic sequelae that prevent him or her from leading a normal life. Similarly, a procedure cannot be considered successful if an acceptable cosmetic outcome is accompanied by markedly altered basic functions.

Free flaps and microsurgery have made it possible to reconstruct very extensive defects while minimizing functional, cosmetic, and psychological sequelae. Better recovery of functions such as swallowing, chewing, and lip competence, as well as satisfactory facial contour and general appearance, provides patients with a quicker and less traumatic return to a normal social life.

Based on the principle that "the best reconstruction is the simplest," free flaps are used to cover defects that are difficult to treat using free grafts and local or regional flaps. The main problem is the size of defect that warrants recourse to a free flap, and no consensus has been reached on the appropriate limit at which defects can be reconstructed using these techniques, since each anatomical region has its peculiarities and functions. Thus, an intraoral defect could require microsurgical reconstruction, whereas a defect of similar size affecting the skin could be treated with regional flaps.

Primary microsurgical reconstruction of soft tissue in the head and neck is generally used to repair the damage caused by ablative cancer surgery, whereas secondary reconstruction based on free flaps is usually associated with congenital defects or defects resulting from injury. Therefore, oncologic criteria aside, secondary reconstruction makes it possible to use techniques that do not involve the use or potential complications of free flaps. A clear example can be seen in post-traumatic defects of the scalp, where tissue expansion can lead to a successful outcome.

Finally, the patient must be made aware of the difference between the terms reconstruction and restoration. The defect can never be restored, since it is impossible to obtain tissue with exactly the same three-dimensional structure, functionality, and external appearance as the original tissue.

4.2 Determinants of Microsurgical Reconstruction

Appropriate selection of the patient is essential in microsurgical reconstruction. The flap is chosen based on a complete clinical history and knowledge of the defect to be reconstructed. Since life expectancy in developed countries has increased, patients with conditions requiring microsurgical reconstruction have greater associated morbidity.

According to Navarro and Arias [1], the factors to be considered when choosing free flaps are the following:

4.2.1 General Factors

4.2.1.1 Baseline Status

Patients with conditions that considerably affect the functioning of the heart, lungs, kidneys, vasculature, and liver are not good candidates for microsurgery.

4.2.1.2 Age

Age per se is not an exclusion criterion in elderly or pediatric patients, although associated conditions and active growth must be taken into account. Given the increase in life expectancy, microsurgical reconstruction is increasingly used in older patients.

4.2.1.3 History of Surgery or Injury

Previous surgery or injury at possible donor sites can determine the viability of the tissue to be transferred.

4.2.2 Vascular Factors

Cardiovascular risk factors such as diabetes, hypertension, dyslipidemia, and smoking can cause subclinical alterations that determine whether or not microvascular free flaps can be used. Arteriosclerosis should be taken into account when assessing and planning microvascular reconstruction. Images of the supra-aortic territory and extremities should be acquired for preoperative studies. Magnetic resonance angiography, computed tomography angiography, and echo Doppler can show the status of the vessels of the neck to be used for microsurgical anastomosis and the status of the vessels comprising the pedicle to be transferred. If anastomosis cannot be performed because of the absence of or disease affecting the vessels of the neck, venous grafts and loop grafts can be considered.

4.2.3 Factors Affecting the Recipient Defect/Site

4.2.3.1 Location of the Defect

If the defect is a skin defect, cosmetic subunits should be taken into account when resecting and transferring skin whose color is closest to that of the skin of the face. Reconstruction of mucosal defects is more complicated, since the type of tissue transferred is different. Both skin and muscle cover intraoral defects well and can even undergo metaplasia and mucosalization; however, they generally do not provide functionality or texture. Similarly, the presence of skin within the oral cavity can lead to hair growth or impede drainage of the salivary gland ducts.

4.2.3.2 Size of the Defect

The size of the defect is a key point when choosing the type of microvascular flap. In defects that do not require bulk, flaps can be planned with little fat and muscle, whereas larger defects generally require more tissue.

4.2.3.3 Three-Dimensional Nature of the Defect

In a single defect, it may be necessary to reconstruct both the skin and the mucosa or simply the mucosa on both sides of the oral cavity. Consequently, it may be necessary to use folded flaps, flaps with different skin paddles, chimeric flaps, sequential flaps, or even independent flaps.

4.2.3.4 Proximity of Vascular Structures

Reconstruction of a skin defect in the temporal region without using superficial temporal vessels is not the same as reconstructing a defect near the neck region, which could necessitate venous grafts.

4.2.3.5 Previous Surgery

Performing a secondary reconstruction on previously operated tissue is not easy. Postsurgical fibrosis and migration of structures are common complications of this type of intervention.

4.2.3.6 Previous Radiation Therapy/Chemotherapy

Dissection of structures is much more complicated and vascular fragility greater.

4.2.4 Factors Affecting the Donor Site

4.2.4.1 Type of Tissue to Be Transferred

Potential flaps include fasciocutaneous flaps, fascial flaps, myocutaneous flaps, and muscular flaps. Perforator flaps can be obtained above or below the fascia.

4.2.4.2 Length and Caliber of the Vascular Flap

These parameters can determine the choice between one flap and another.

4.2.4.3 Vascular Systems

Specific flaps such as the radial forearm fasciocutaneous flap have a superficial vascular system and a deeper vascular system.

4.2.4.4 Donor-Site Defect

The use of myocutaneous flaps can lead to muscle weakness and specific sequelae. It may be necessary to use skin grafts to close defects of the donor site, and the resulting scar may be visible.

4.2.4.5 Reconstruction by Phases

The use of prefabricated or prelaminated flaps may be indicated in secondary reconstructions.

4.3 Microvascular Flaps Used in the Reconstruction of Soft Tissue of the Head and Neck

Below, we present the free flaps that we consider most useful for microsurgical reconstruction of soft tissue defects of the head and neck. We discuss the vascular flaps, indications, advantages and disadvantages, and associated morbidity.

4.3.1 Radial Forearm Fasciocutaneous Flap

As reported by Yang et al. [2], the radial forearm flap is a classic, widely used flap for the reconstruction of soft tissue of the head and neck. It is versatile and pliable, has a long pedicle, and is easy to obtain.

4.3.1.1 Indications

The radial forearm flap is commonly used to reconstruct intraoral defects because it is thin, very pliable, and light in weight. It also maintains a steady volume over time. As for extraoral defects, it is indicated in the reconstruction of full-thickness defects of the cheek and cheek mucosa. It is used for the interior lining (because of its pliability) and frontal region (because of its thinness) following the principles of reconstruction based on cosmetic subunits. It is also used in the reconstruction of nasal defects (both externally and internally), as reported by Menick and Salibian [3].

4.3.1.2 Arterial Pedicle

The radial artery, which is responsible for the irrigation of the deep palmar arch, is 2.5 mm in diameter. It runs through the septum between the brachioradialis and flexor carpi radialis. The flap is supplied by the septocutaneous perforators.

4.3.1.3 Venous Pedicle

The venous pedicle is a double pedicle thanks to the venae comitantes of the radial artery (1–1.5 mm in diameter) that accompany it along the intermuscular septum to form the deep venous system and the cephalic vein (2–3.5 mm in diameter). It is independent of the arterial system and located in a suprafascial position, thus forming the superficial system.

4.3.1.4 Presurgical Planning

The nondominant arm is preferred. The Allen test must be performed to ensure that the ulnar artery can supply blood to the radial artery, thus demonstrating the presence of vascular anastomoses between the two systems. Echo Doppler provides more information on the caliber, location, and possible disorders of the arteries and veins. If the result of the Allen test is positive or the echo Doppler findings show an abnormality, this flap must not be used, since the supply to the first and second fingers of the hand could be compromised.

4.3.1.5 Tissue to Be Transferred

The tissue was traditionally harvested as a fasciocutaneous flap, and this continues to be the case. However, according to Biglioli et al. [4], other tissues can be included, for example, the superficial sensory nerves (lateral antebrachial cutaneous nerve) to provide sensory flaps, as well as muscles and tendons that provide volume and serve as bands in lip reconstruction, as described by Sasidaran et al. [5].

4.3.1.6 Morbidity

Grafts are usually necessary to cover the donor site (graft loss hinders healing), the resulting scar tends to be unsightly, and patients can be affected by sensory or motor disorders (owing to damage to or cutting of the sensory nerves or the radial nerve). The patient may no longer be able to tolerate cold owing to reduced blood supply.

4.3.1.7 Postsurgical Care

The hand should be immobilized for 10 days to enable the free skin graft to bond. Potential compartmental syndrome must be detected early, and the arm must remain raised for the first 3 days (Figs. 4.1, 4.2, 4.3, and 4.4).

An alternative to this flap is the ulnar forearm flap, which is based on the ulnar artery and its venae comitantes. It can be used in cases where the radial artery is

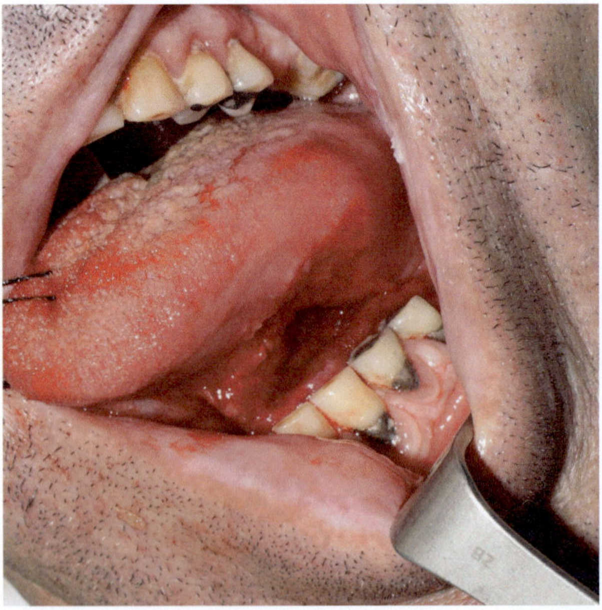

Fig. 4.1 Floor of the mouth and ventral tongue squamous cell carcinoma

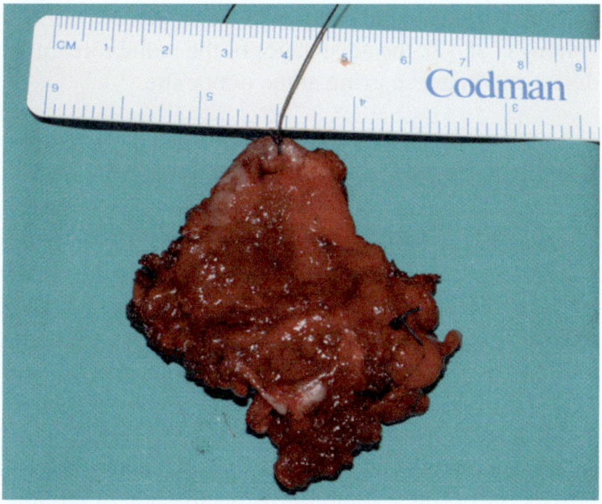

Fig. 4.2 Surgical specimen

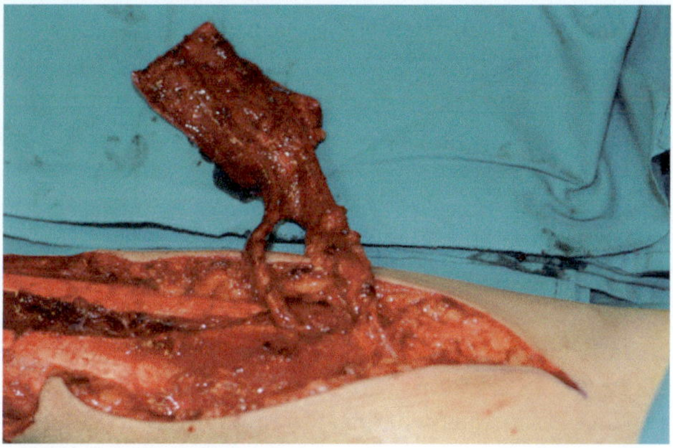

Fig. 4.3 Left antebrachial radial fasciocutaneous flap dissection

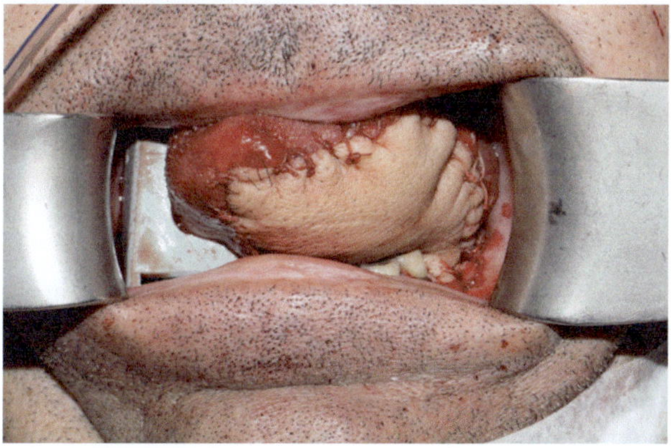

Fig. 4.4 Intraoperative clinical result

dominant in the supply to the forearm. According to Van Cann and Koole [6] and Antony et al. [7], the advantages of the radial forearm flap are a less severe cosmetic defect and better scarring at the donor site.

4.3.2 Anterolateral Thigh Flap (ALT)

First described by Song et al. [8], the ALT flap is a very useful perforator flap that is widely used in reconstruction procedures of the head and neck. The popularity of ALT flap led several authors, including Huang et al. [9], to reconsider continuing with the radial forearm flap. However, other authors use it to cover some of the indications of the myocutaneous abdominal rectus flap.

4.3.2.1 Indications

In our opinion, this flap should be used in cases where the radial forearm flap cannot provide sufficient volume for reconstruction of intraoral defects. It is a good option for reconstructing defects of the tongue stretching back to the oropharynx and cheek mucosa, extended hemiglossectomy, and full-thickness cheek defects where, in addition to reconstructing the skin and mucosa, the object of the procedure is to provide volume. As for extraoral defects, the ALT flap could be indicated in skin defects requiring large, bulkier flaps, such as those affecting the side of the face, the temporal region, and large defects of the scalp. According to Jiang et al. [10], the ALT can be harvested as a chimeric flap with multiple skin paddles.

4.3.2.2 Vascular Pedicle

The vascular pedicle of the ALT flap comprises the descending branch of the lateral femoral circumflex artery and its venae comitantes (approximately 2 mm in diameter), which are found in the septum between the vastus lateralis and femoris muscles. The perforators (approximately 0.5 mm in diameter) are mostly (85 %) musculocutaneous, whereas the remainder (15 %) are septocutaneous. The pedicle is dissected until the point where it leaves the lateral femoral circumflex artery. Lengths of up to 10 cm can be obtained.

4.3.2.3 Presurgical Planning

Doppler or echo Doppler is useful for locating the perforators. Lakhiani et al. [11] showed that most of the perforators are found in the middle third of the thigh, from the midpoint of a line that connects the anterior superior iliac spine and the supero-external part of the patella.

4.3.2.4 Tissue to Be Transferred

The ALT flap is harvested with the skin and subcutaneous cell tissue. The fascia is optional, although it is generally included. Suprafascial dissection is more cumbersome and complicated, although it spares the local anatomy and preserves muscle coverage. A sensory flap can be harvested by including branches of the lateral cutaneous nerve.

4.3.2.5 Morbidity

Harvesting the ALT flap has few complications, thus giving it an advantage over other flaps such as the rectus abdominis myocutaneous flap or the radial forearm flap, since it does not damage the abdominal wall or require major vascular axes to be sacrificed. It generally does not require free grafts, since it enables direct closure of defects measuring 8–9 cm. Leg extension and mobility are barely affected because they are compensated by the remaining extensor muscles. However, there is a possibility of loss of sensation in the thigh because of the damage to the lateral cutaneous femoral nerve. The unsightly scar left on the thigh is also a potential drawback.

4.3.2.6 Postsurgical Care

It is important to monitor for development of compartment syndrome (Figs. 4.5, 4.6, 4.7, 4.8, and 4.9).

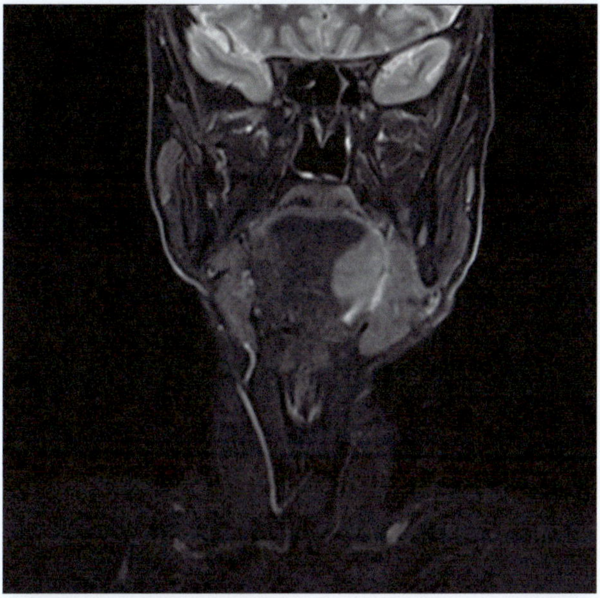

Fig. 4.5 MRI. Base of the tongue squamous cell carcinoma

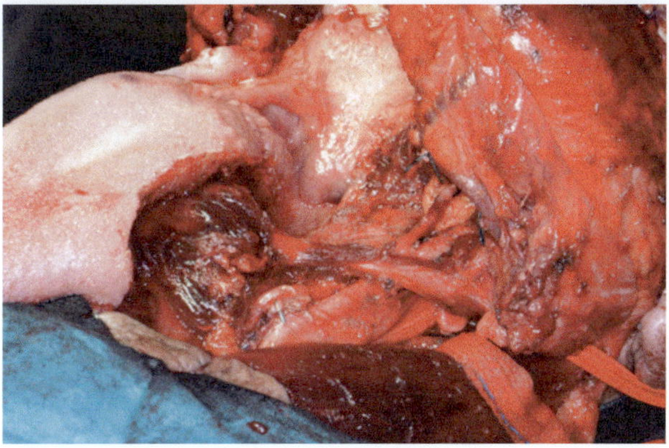

Fig. 4.6 Surgical defect after resection. Pull through cervical approach

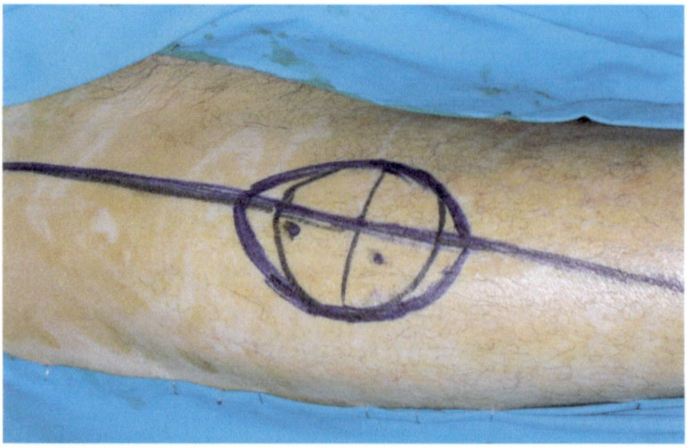

Fig. 4.7 ALT perforator flap design

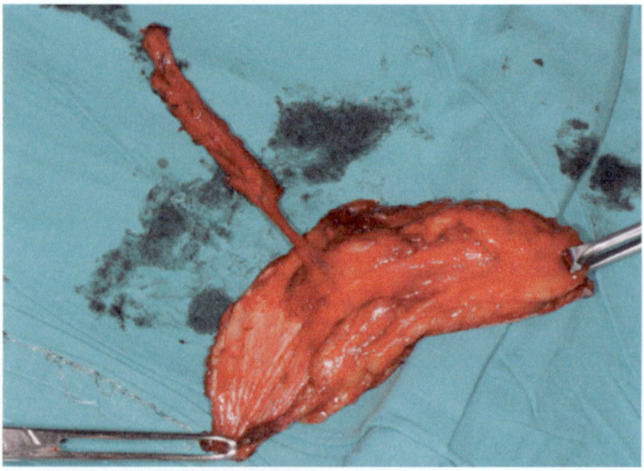

Fig. 4.8 Septocutaneous perforator flap

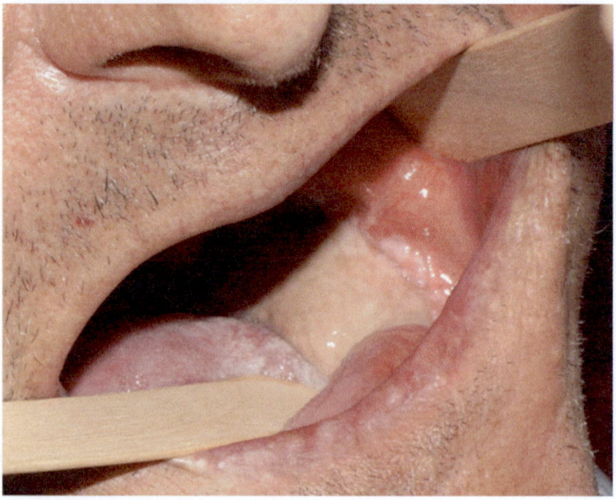

Fig. 4.9 One year postsurgery

The vastus lateralis flap is a variant of the ALT perforator flap. Dissection differs from that of the ALT, since it is necessary to locate the vascular pedicle without locating and isolating the perforators. It is necessary to follow the principles for dissection of the myocutaneous flaps, in which the skin and subcutaneous tissue are not separated from the underlying muscle. This flap is easier to harvest than the ALT flap, although it does require part of the vastus lateralis muscle to be sacrificed. Therefore, it is used for the reconstruction of three-dimensional defects requiring greater bulk, as reported by Engel et al. [12] after total glossectomy or to isolate the base of the skull or central nervous system. The vastus lateralis myocutaneous flap is a good alternative to the rectus abdominis myocutaneous flap (Figs. 4.10, 4.11, 4.12, 4.13, and 4.14).

Another variant of this flap is the adipofascial ALT, which is indicated for the reconstruction of defects of the intraoral and nasal mucosa [13].

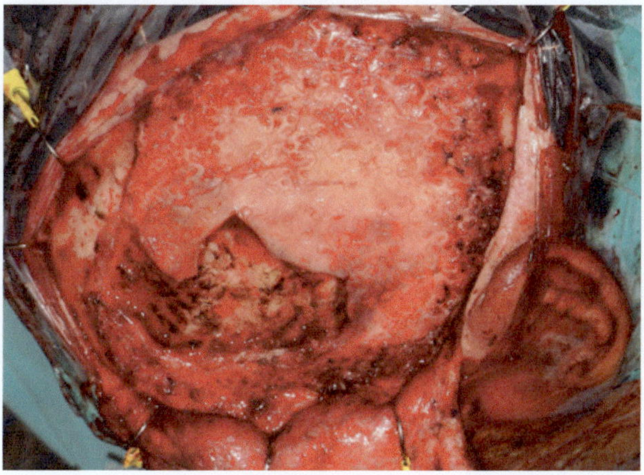

Fig. 4.10 Temporal defect associated to cerebrospinal fluid leak

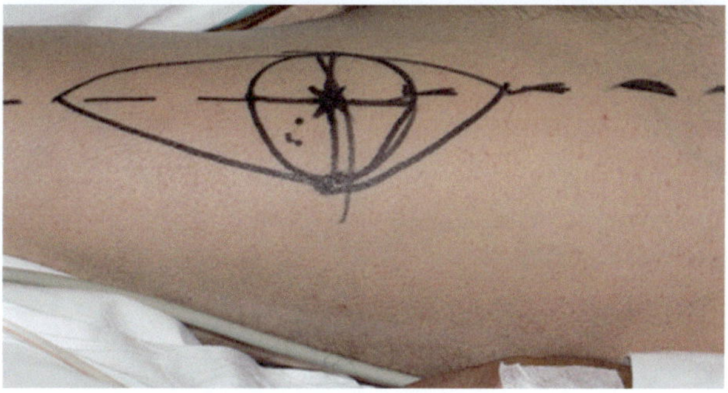

Fig. 4.11 Design of the myocutaneous vastus lateralis flap similar to the ALT perforator flap

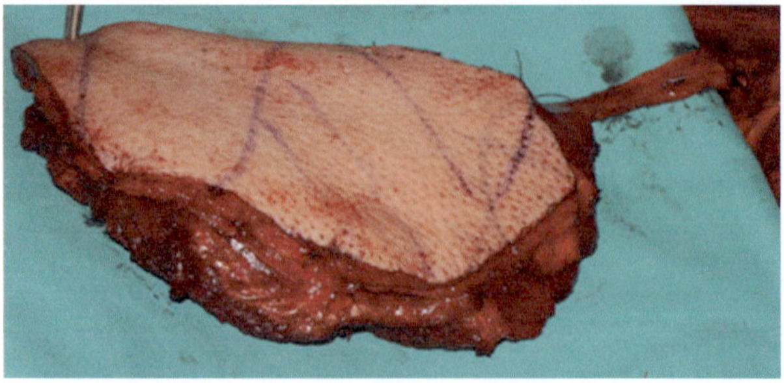

Fig. 4.12 Flap with muscular component

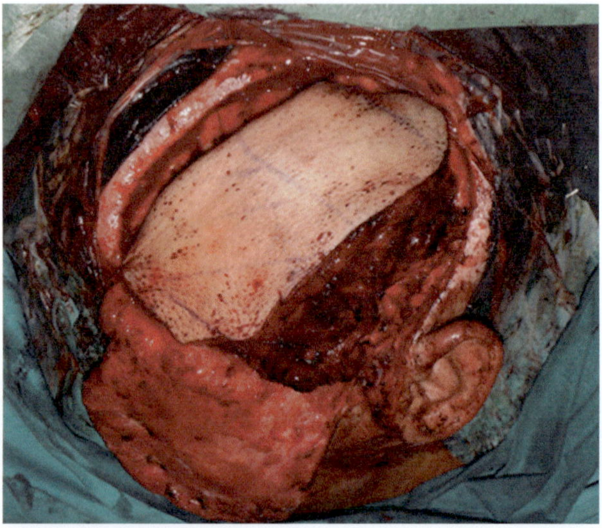

Fig. 4.13 Flap inset using the muscle to seal the leak

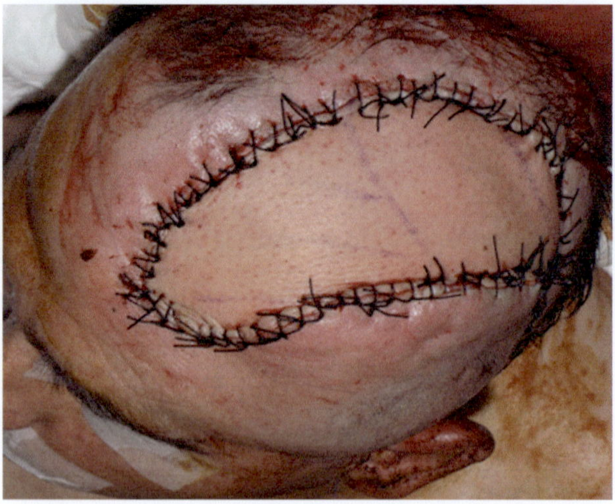

Fig. 4.14 Final intraoperative result

4.3.3 Rectus Abdominis Myocutaneous Flap

Pennington and Pelly [14] were the first to describe this flap, which is based on the deep inferior epigastric artery and vein. Together with the radial forearm flap, the rectus abdominis myocutaneous flap has been used for many years in the reconstruction of head and neck defects requiring considerable bulk. The use of perforator flaps and the possibility of including muscle in this type of flap mean that it has been less widely used.

4.3.3.1 Indications

The reconstruction of large intraoral defects, such as total glossectomy or type IV maxillectomy [15], that include orbital exenteration. It can be used in combination with the temporal myofascial flap. The rectus abdominis flap provides bulk to fill the middle third of the face, and the temporal myofascial flap is used to reconstruct the palate. As for extraoral reconstruction, the rectus abdominis myocutaneous flap is used mainly to seal bone defects at the base of the skull, which is isolated from the upper aerodigestive tract [16].

4.3.3.2 Vascular Pedicle

Deep inferior epigastric vessels. The caliber is usually around 3 mm. The greatest density of musculocutaneous perforators is found in the periumbilical region.

4.3.3.3 Presurgical Planning

This flap does not require specific assessment of the vasculature. However, it is important to determine whether the patient has previously undergone surgery of the abdominal region, especially in the iliac fossa, hypogastrium, and mesogastrium, since the pedicle could be damaged.

4.3.3.4 Tissue to Be Transferred

The rectus abdominis flap is generally a musculocutaneous flap. The skin paddle can be placed in several ways, although it is normally placed vertically over the longitudinal axis of the muscle. The whole muscle component can be transferred. It is important to respect the anterior fascia below the arcuate line.

4.3.3.5 Morbidity

The rectus abdominis flap should only be harvested after careful deliberation, since it is necessary to remove a basic muscle of the abdominal wall, whose flexor activity would therefore be compromised. When harvesting the flap, extra care must be taken not to accidentally open the peritoneal cavity. Abdominal hernia is another complication at the donor site. The use of synthetic mesh reduces the likelihood of hernia.

4.3.3.6 Postsurgical Care

The patient should wear a corset for a few weeks in order to a prevent hernia. Similarly, sporting activity should be suspended for about 2 months (Figs. 4.15, 4.16, 4.17, 4.18, 4.19, 4.20, and 4.21).

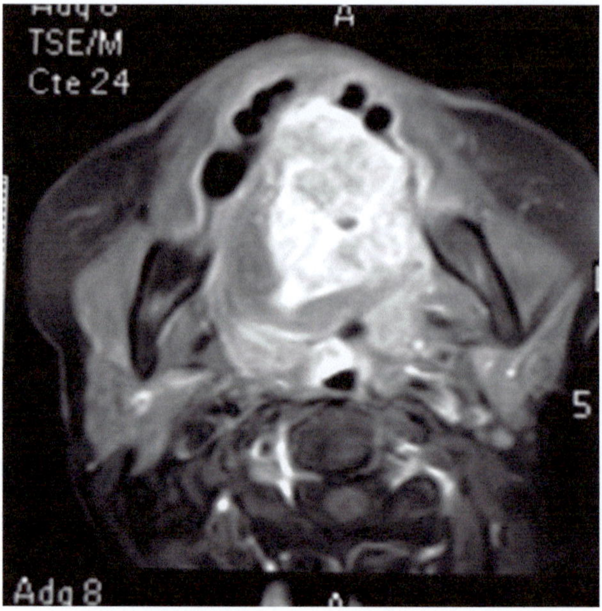

Fig. 4.15 Preoperative MRI

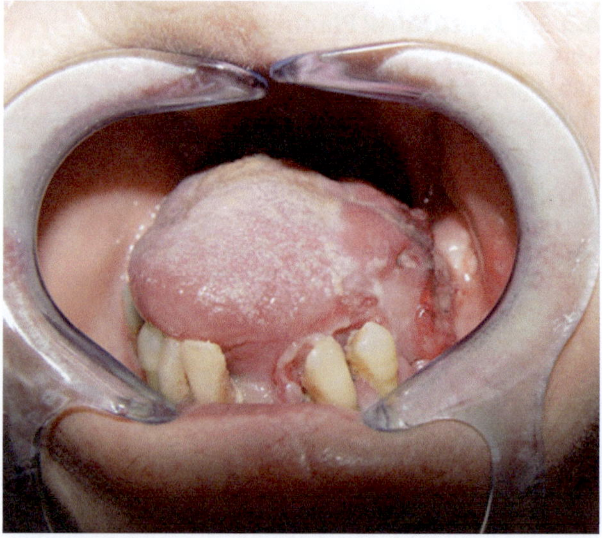

Fig. 4.16 Squamous cell carcinoma of the tongue

According to López-Arcas et al. [17], the deep inferior epigastric artery perforator flap is a perforator flap whose vascular axis is the same as that of the rectus abdominis myocutaneous flap, although it does not include muscle. It is widely used in breast reconstruction and constitutes yet another option for treating soft tissue defects in the head and neck. However, this flap has the drawback that it increases in volume when the patient gains weight.

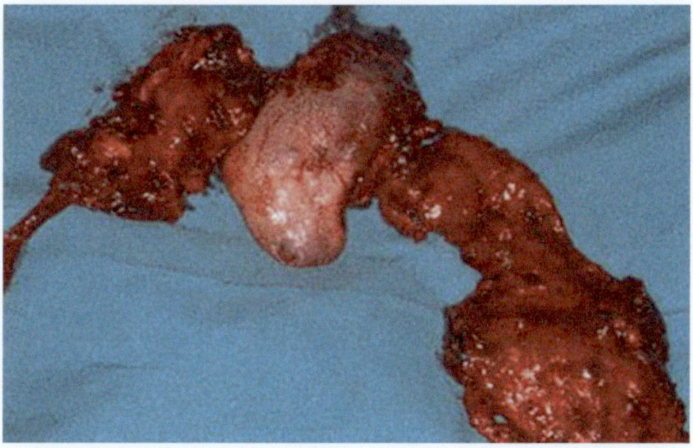

Fig. 4.17 Surgical specimen. Total glossectomy and bilateral neck dissection

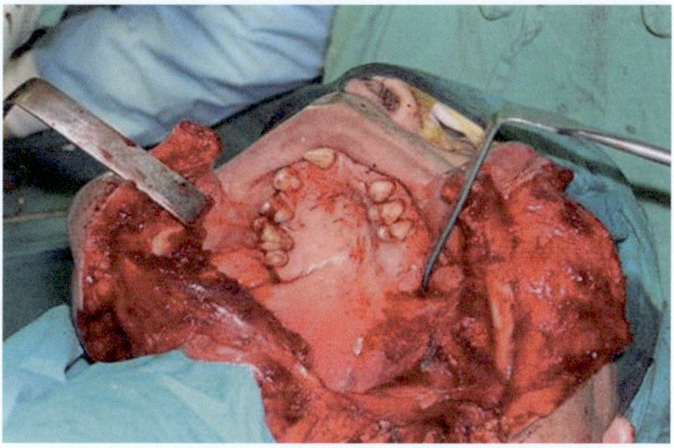

Fig. 4.18 Surgical defect

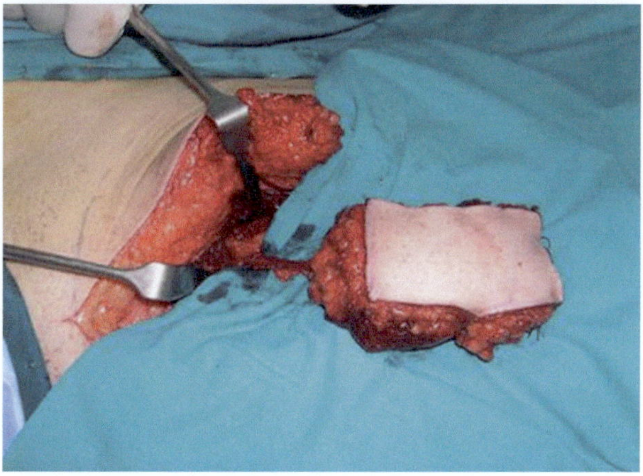

Fig. 4.19 Rectus abdominis flap

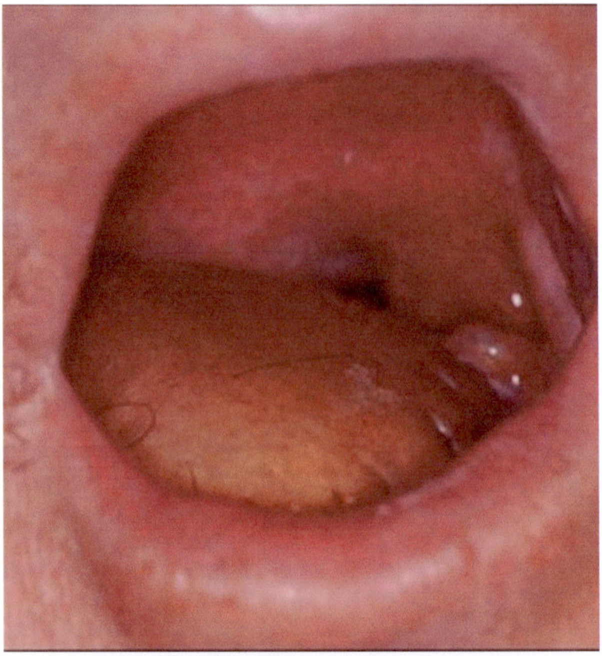

Fig. 4.20 Intraoral postoperative view

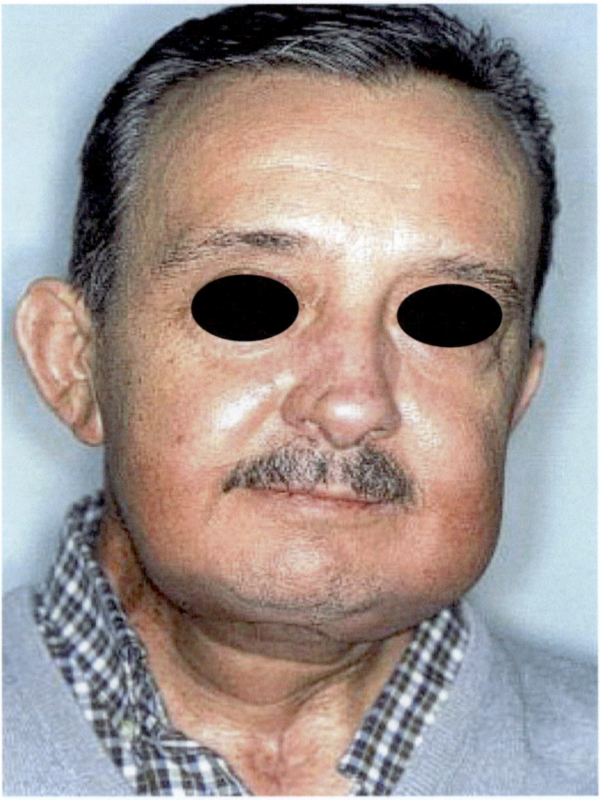

Fig. 4.21 1-year postoperative anteroposterior view

4.3.4 Latissimus Dorsi Flap

Although Tansini used the latissimus dorsi flap for the reconstruction of a chest wall defect, Watson et al. [18] were the first to use it as a free flap. The latissimus dorsi flap is one of the most widely used flaps for the reconstruction of large defects, since it provides a considerable amount of tissue and can be harvested as a free flap or pedicle flap. It can be used as a muscle or myocutaneous flap. Its main drawback is that it prevents work in 2 teams.

4.3.4.1 Indications

The latissimus dorsi flap was used by Kim et al. [19] to reconstruct scalp defects, both as a free flap and as a pedicle flap. It can be used for the reconstruction of large defects of the head and neck and full-thickness cheek defects, as well as for sealing the base of the skull. As a muscle flap, it is favored by Takushima et al. [20], who used it for dynamic reanimation of facial paralysis without having to turn to a 2-stage cross-face technique.

4.3.4.2 Vascular Pedicle

The pedicle is based on the thoracodorsal artery and venae comitantes, which are branches of the subscapular axis. Its diameter is 2–4 mm and it can be as long as 12 cm.

4.3.4.3 Presurgical Planning

It is necessary to rule out previous surgery at the donor site (the thoracodorsal vessels could have been ligated during axillary lymph node dissection). In the absence of previous surgery, no special preparation is necessary owing to the consistent vascular anatomy, although it is possible to use tests such as echo Doppler, which makes it possible to check that blood is flowing steadily through the vessels. If the flap is to be used for dynamic reanimation of facial paralysis, then its placement must be carefully planned.

4.3.4.4 Tissue to Be Transferred

The tissue to be transferred is usually a musculocutaneous flap for reconstructing defects caused by cancer or a muscle flap for sealing the base of the skull and for dynamic reanimation of facial paralysis (muscle, vessels, and thoracodorsal nerve).

4.3.4.5 Morbidity

The arm must be placed in lateral decubitus during surgery in order to prevent lesions of the brachial plexus. Internal rotation and adduction may be slightly altered. Transfer of this flap in children can lead to scoliosis and problems with the development of paravertebral muscle.

4.3.4.6 Postsurgical Care

The patient must undergo rehabilitation to correct muscle compensation (Figs. 4.22, 4.23, 4.24, 4.25, and 4.26).

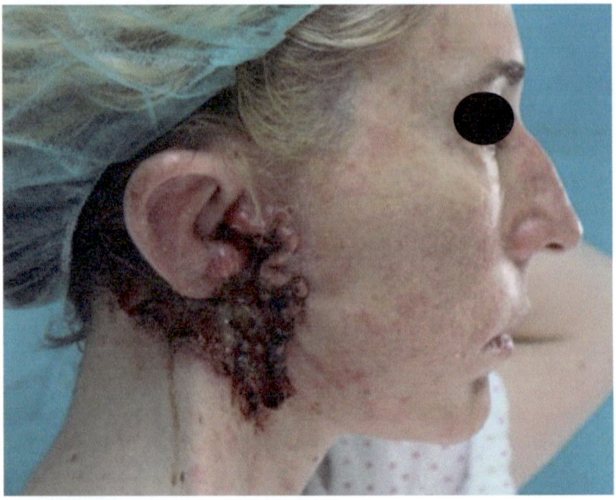

Fig. 4.22 Right auricular basal cell carcinoma

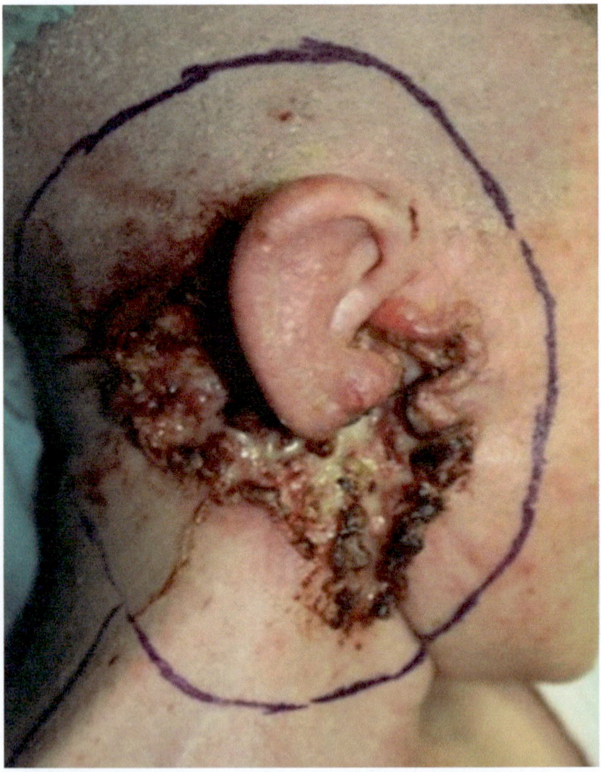

Fig. 4.23 Surgical resection design

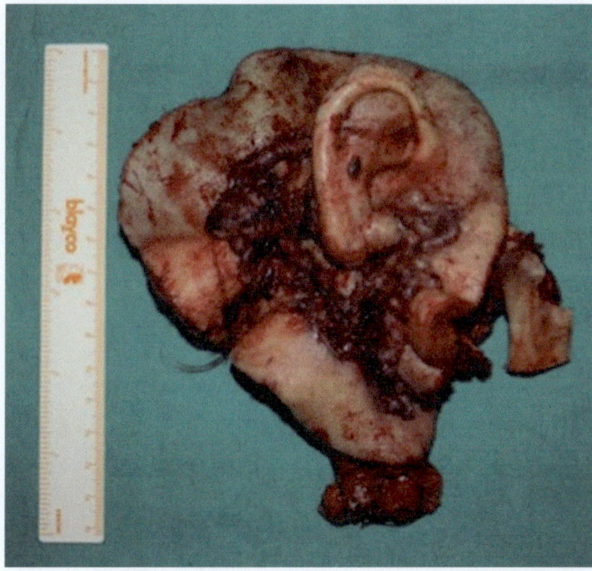

Fig. 4.24 Surgical specimen

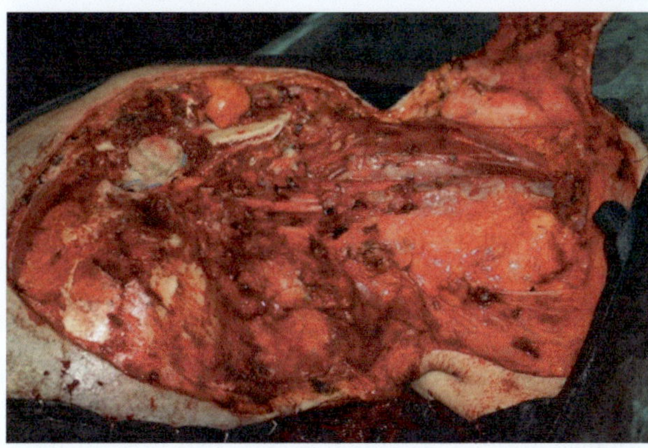

Fig. 4.25 Surgical defect

The thoracodorsal artery perforator flap is a variant of the myocutaneous latissimus dorsi flap that involves less muscle damage. Bach et al. [21] used this flap for the reconstruction of intraoral and oropharyngeal defects.

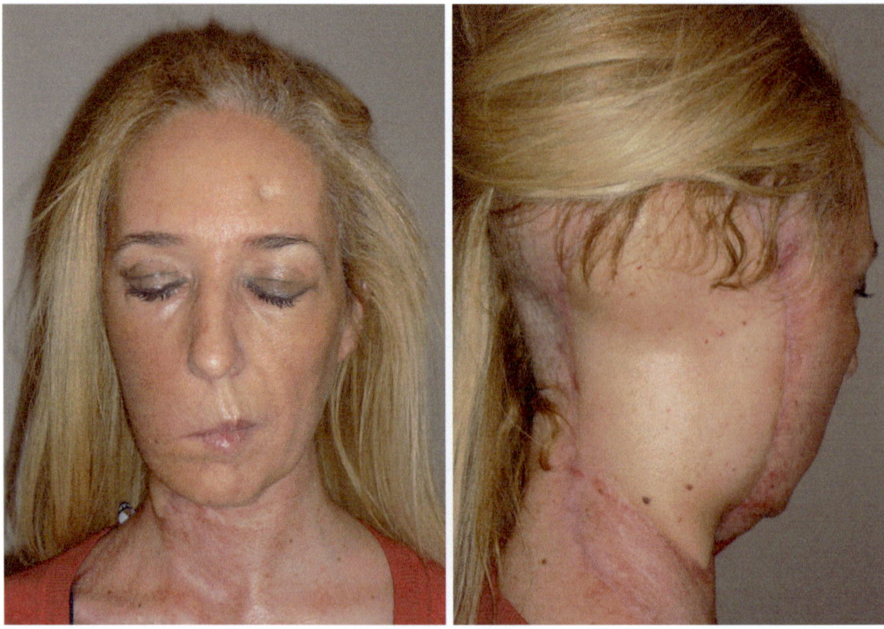

Fig. 4.26 Clinical appearance of the latissimus dorsi flap, 1 year postsurgery

4.3.5 Omentum Flap

The omentum flap was first used by McLean and Buncke [22] for the reconstruction of a scalp defect. It is both versatile and pliable and can therefore be easily adapted to the defect. However, given the associated abdominal morbidity, it is rarely used.

4.3.5.1 Indications

According to Ramzisham et al. [23], the main indication of the omentum flap in the head and neck was for reconstruction of scalp defects and for pharyngo-esophageal defects. This flap was also used to repair soft tissue in hemifacial microsomia and hemifacial atrophy (Parry-Romberg syndrome), although it has been abandoned because of the high frequency of reabsorption. It is possible to work in two teams: harvesting requires cooperation between general surgeons and digestive surgeons. In scalp reconstruction, the omentum flap should be combined with free skin grafts taken from the thigh or suprapubic region.

4.3.5.2 Vascular Pedicle

Gastroepiploic artery and venae comitantes. The pedicle can be harvested with the right or left gastroepiploic artery, although the right one is preferred for its length and diameter (1.5–3 mm).

4.3.5.3 Presurgical Planning

This flap should not be used if the patient has had previous abdominal surgery or infections such as appendicitis or cholecystitis that may have caused retraction of the omentum.

4.3.5.4 Tissue to Be Transferred

Greater omentum.

4.3.5.5 Morbidity

Conditions arising from a midline laparotomy such as adhesions, volvulus, peritonitis, and intra-abdominal abscesses.

4.3.5.6 Postsurgical Care

Compression of the skin graft for 7–10 days. An oral diet should be introduced gradually, and specific post-midline laparotomy care must be followed (Figs. 4.27, 4.28, 4.29, 4.30, 4.31, 4.32, and 4.33).

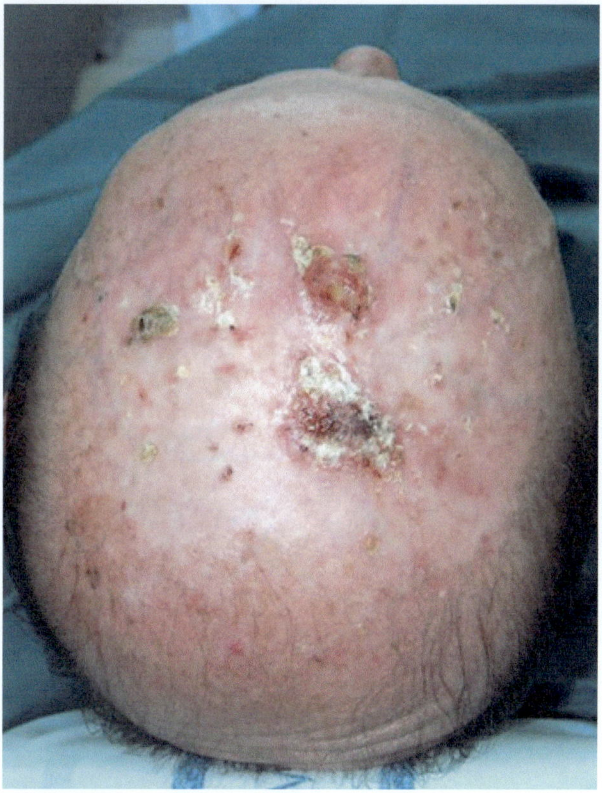

Fig. 4.27 Multiple basal cell carcinoma

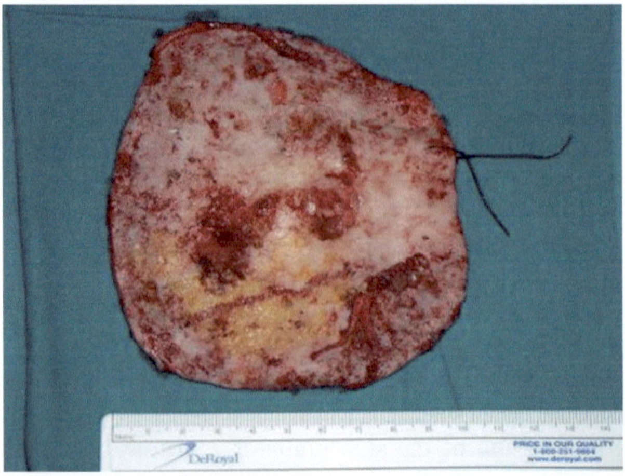

Fig. 4.28 Surgical specimen

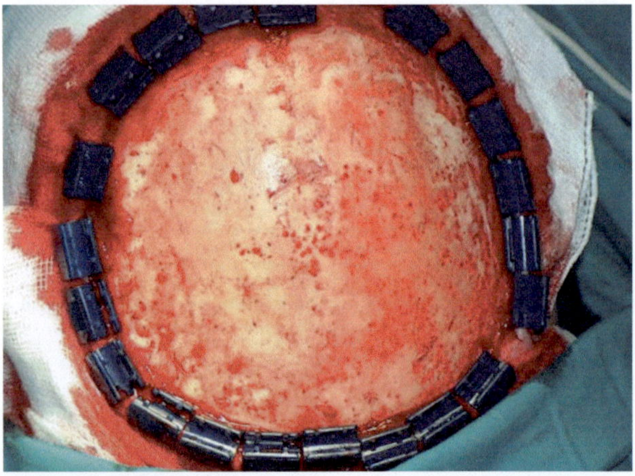

Fig. 4.29 Surgical defect

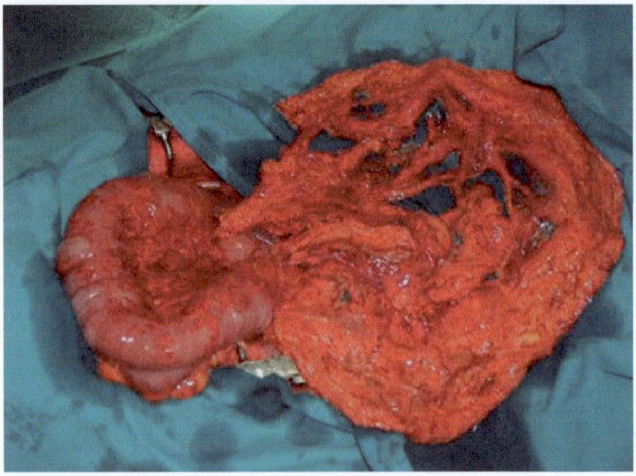

Fig. 4.30 Harvesting omentum flap

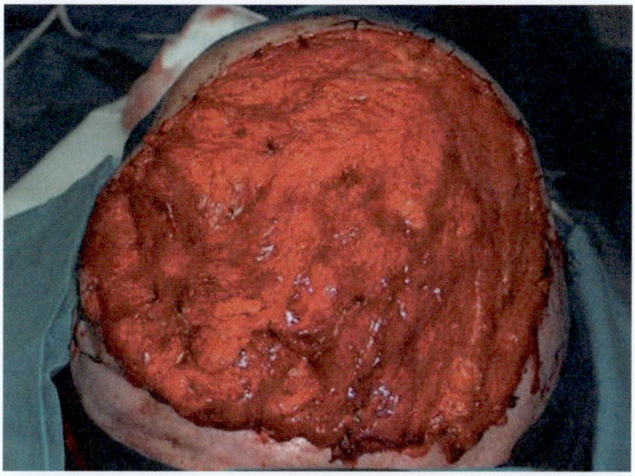

Fig. 4.31 Omentum flap adapted at the defect

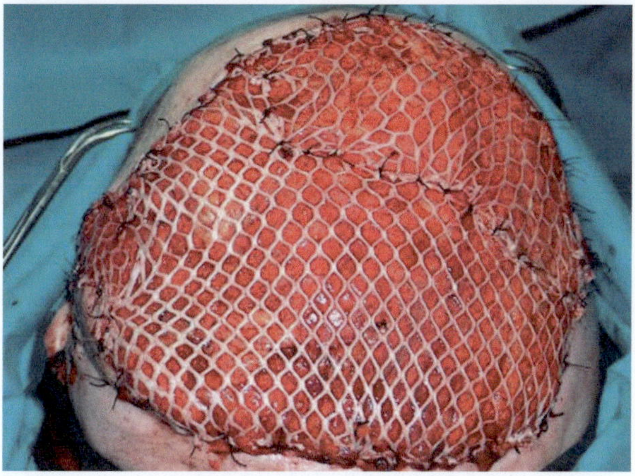

Fig. 4.32 Dermal graft over the omentum flap

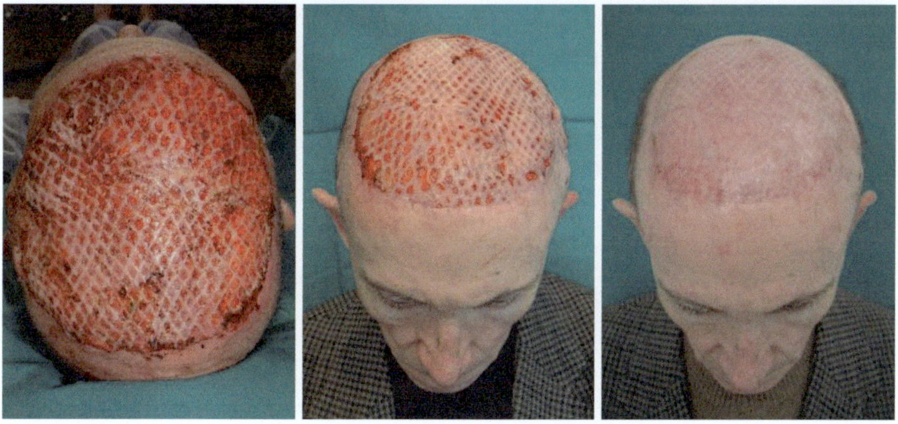

Fig. 4.33 Postoperative aspect 2 weeks, 3 weeks, and 7 weeks later

4.3.6 Other Free Flaps

- Lateral arm flap: This flap was described by Song et al. [24]. For some authors, such as Thankappan et al. [25], it is an alternative to the radial forearm fasciocutaneous flap or the ALT flap. Its pedicle, the posterior radial collateral artery, enables direct closure of the donor site. The length of the pedicle is acceptable, although its diameter is lower than that of the radial artery. In addition, dissection of this flap is cumbersome.
- Medial sural flap: This flap was first reported by Cabadas et al. in 2001 [26]. It is based on the medial sural artery and is now widely used in head and neck reconstruction (especially in reconstruction of the tongue) because it is both versatile and pliable. Dissection is more complicated than that of the flaps mentioned above, and some authors, such as He et al. [27], recommend previous vascular testing to better locate the pedicle and its perforators.

References

1. Navarro I, Arias J. Reconstrucciones craneomaxilofaciales complejas (cap 56). In: López Davis A, Martín Granizo R, editors. Cirugía oral y maxilofacial. Madrid: Panamericana; 2012. p. 630–49
2. Yang G, Chen B, Gao Y, et al. Forearm skin flap transplantation. Natl Med J China. 1981;61:139.
3. Menick FJ, Salibian A. Microvascular repair of heminasal, subtotal, and total nasal defects with a folded radial forearm flap and a full-thickness forehead flap. Plast Reconstr Surg. 2011;127(2):637–51.
4. Biglioli F, Liviero F, Frigerio A, Rezzonico A, Brusati R. Function of the sensate free forearm flap after partial glossectomy. J Craniomaxillofac Surg. 2006;34(6):332–9.
5. Sasidaran R, Zain MA, Basiron NH. Lip and oral commissure reconstruction with the radial forearm flap. Natl J Maxillofac Surg. 2012;3(1):21–4.
6. Van Cann EM, Koole R. The ulnar forearm free flap for the reconstruction of soft tissue defects in the head and neck area: free flap outcome and donor site outcome. Oral Surg Oral Med Oral Pathol Oral Radiol Endod. 2009;108:851–4.
7. Antony AK, Hootnick JL, Antony AK. Ulnar forearm free flaps in head and neck reconstruction: systematic review of the literature and a case report. Microsurgery. 2014;34(1): 68–75.
8. Song YG, Chen GZ, Song YL. The free thigh flap: a new free flap concept based on the septocutaneous artery. Br J Plast Surg. 1984;37:149–59.
9. Huang CH, Chen HC, Huang YL, Mardini S, Feng GM. Comparison of the radial forearm flap and the thinned anterolateral thigh cutaneous flap for reconstruction of tongue defects: an evaluation of donor-site morbidity. Plast Reconstr Surg. 2004;114:1704–10.
10. Jiang C, Guo F, Li N, Liu W, Su T, Chen X, Zheng L, Jian X. Multipaddled anterolateral thigh chimeric flap for reconstruction of complex defects in head and neck. PLoS One. 2014; 9(9): e106326. doi:10.1371/journal.pone.0106326.
11. Lakhiani C, Lee MR, Saint-Cyr M. Vascular anatomy of the anterolateral thigh flap: a systematic review. Plast Reconstr Surg. 2012;130(6):1254–68.
12. Engel H, Huang JJ, Lin CY, Lam W, Kao HK, Gazyakan E, Cheng MH. A strategic approach for tongue reconstruction to achieve predictable and improved functional and aesthetic outcomes. Plast Reconstr Surg. 2010;126(6):1967–77.
13. Revenaugh PC, Haffey TM, Seth R, Fritz MA. Anterolateral thigh adipofascial flap in mucosal reconstruction. JAMA Facial Plast Surg. 2014;16(6):395–9.

14. Pennington DG, Pelly AD. The rectus abdominis myocutaneous free flap. Br J Plast Surg. 1980;33(2):277–82.
15. Brown JS, Shaw RJ. Reconstruction of the maxilla and midface: introducing a new classification. Lancet Oncol. 2010;11:1001–8.
16. Herr MW, Lin DT. Microvascular free flaps in skull base reconstruction. Adv Otorhinolaryngol. 2013;74:81–91.
17. López-Arcas JM, Arias J, Morán MJ, Navarro I, Pingarrón L, Chamorro M, Burgueño M. The deep inferior epigastric artery perforator (DIEAP) flap for total glossectomy reconstruction. J Oral Maxillofac Surg. 2012;70(3):740–7.
18. Watson JS, Craig RD, Orton CI. The free latissimus dorsi myocutaneous flap. Plast Reconstr Surg. 1979;64(3):299–305.
19. Kim SW, Hwang KT, Kim JD, Kim YH. Reconstruction of postinfected scalp defects using latissimus dorsi perforator and myocutaneous free flaps. J Craniofac Surg. 2012;23(6):1615–9.
20. Takushima A, Harii K, Asato H, Kurita M, Shiraishi T. Fifteen-year survey of one-stage latissimus dorsi muscle transfer for treatment of longstanding facial paralysis. J Plast Reconstr Aesthet Surg. 2013;66(1):29–36.
21. Bach CA, Wagner I, Lachiver X, Guth A, Baglin AC, Chabolle F. The free thoracodorsal artery perforator flap in head and neck reconstruction. Eur Ann Otorhinolaryngol Head Neck Dis. 2012;129(3):167–71.
22. McLean DH, Buncke Jr HJ. Autotransplant of omentum to a large scalp defect, with microsurgical revascularization. Plast Reconstr Surg. 1972;49(3):268–74.
23. Ramzisham AR, Somasundaram S, Nasir ZM, Ali F, Das S. Successful free omental flap and skin graft reconstruction of scalp avulsion injury. Clin Ter. 2010;161(5):453–5.
24. Song R, Song Y, Yu Y, et al. The upper arm free flap. Clin Plast Surg. 1982;9:27–35.
25. Thankappan K, Kuriakose MA, Chatni SS, Sharan R, Trivedi NP, Vijayaraghavan S, Sharma M, Iyer S. Lateral arm free flap for oral tongue reconstruction: an analysis of surgical details, morbidity, and functional and aesthetic outcome. Ann Plast Surg. 2011;66:261–6.
26. Cavadas PC, Sanz-Giménez-Rico JR, Gutierrez-de la Cámara A. The medial sural artery perforator free flap. Plast Reconstr Surg. 2001;108:1609–15.
27. He Y, Jin SF, Zhang ZY, Feng SQ, Zhang CP, Zhang YX. A prospective study of medial sural artery perforator flap with computed tomographic angiography-aided design in tongue reconstruction. J Oral Maxillofac Surg. 2014;72(11):2351–65.

Reconstruction of Soft Tissue Defects with Regional Flaps

5

José Ignacio Salmerón Escobar, José Alfonso Ruiz Cruz, Ana María López López, and Carlos Navarro Vila

Abstract

Regional flaps are pedicle flaps obtained from anatomical regions close to the defect to be constructed. Their advantages over pedicle flaps are similarity with the skin adjacent to the defect (color, texture, and hair), the speed with which they can be harvested, and the lower cost, lower comorbidity, and lower personnel and infrastructure requirements. Their disadvantages are their limited size, limited distance between the donor site and the receptor site, and lower predictability when preparing compound flaps with bone. Regional flaps can sometimes be combined with microvascular free flaps for the reconstruction of complex defects.

J.I. Salmerón Escobar, MD, PhD, FEBOMS (✉)
Associate professor, Medical Faculty Complutense University of Madrid, Madrid, Spain

Consultant at Oral and Maxillofacial Surgery Department, Gregorio Marañón General University Hospital, Madrid, Spain
e-mail: jisalmeron@telefonica.net

J.A. Ruiz Cruz, MD, DDS, FEBOMS
Consultant at Oral and Maxillofacial Surgery Department, University Hospital del Sur, Madrid, Spain
e-mail: jaruizcruz@gmail.com

A.M. López López, MD, DDS, FEBOMS
Consultant at Oral and Maxillofacial Surgery Department, Miguel Servet University Hospital, Zaragoza, Spain
e-mail: anitalopez@gmail.com

C. Navarro Vila, MD, DMD, PhD, FEBOMS
Full professor, Medical Faculty Complutense University of Madrid, Madrid, Spain

Head of Oral and Maxillofacial Department Surgery, Gregorio Marañón General University Hospital, Madrid, Spain

Académico Correspondiente of the Royal National Academy of Medicine of Spain, Madrid, Spain
e-mail: cnavarro.vila@clinicanavarrovila.com

C. Navarro Vila (ed.), *Reconstructive Oral and Maxillofacial Surgery*,
DOI 10.1007/978-3-319-20487-1_5

5.1 Temporalis Muscle Flap

5.1.1 Introduction

The temporalis muscle was first used as a flap in 1898 by Golovine [1] to fill the space left after orbital exenteration. Since then, it has been used in the head and neck, mainly for reconstruction of the oral cavity [2], face, preauricular region [3], and scalp, as well as for surgery to treat facial paralysis, especially that affecting traction of the upper eyelid and oral commissure.

5.1.2 Vascularization

The temporalis flap receives 3–4 branches of the internal maxillary artery and the temporal artery. The branches of the maxillary artery can separate into the anterior deep temporal artery, posterior deep temporal artery, and the accessory deep temporal artery. Alternatively, they can supply the muscle from a common trunk of the maxillary artery. The maxillary artery supplies the anterior and medial portions of the temporalis muscle, as well as the deepest part of the muscle [4].

The blood supply from the temporal artery is more constant than that of the maxillary artery. It reaches the temporalis muscle where it becomes the middle temporal artery [5] and supplies blood to the middle and posterior third of the temporalis muscle surface.

The superficial temporal vein, which drains the temporal vein, and the deep temporal vein are responsible for venous drainage of the temporalis muscle along the course of the temporal and maxillary arteries, respectively (Fig. 5.1).

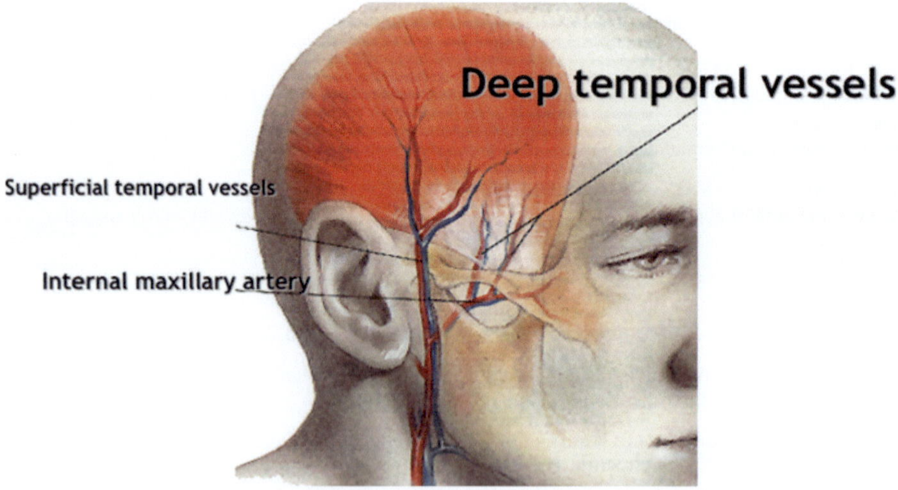

Fig. 5.1 Vascular pedicle

5.1.3 Indications

The temporalis myofascial flap can be used in whole or in part depending on the area and volume of the defect and on the functional requirements of the reconstruction to be used for facial paralysis.

Given its anatomical proximity and considerable versatility, the temporalis myofascial flap is very useful for treating defects of the oral cavity [6]. Disinsertion of the muscle and rotation medially toward the zygomatic arch enable reconstruction to be performed from the maxillary midline in patients whose health status or older age contraindicates microsurgery with bone tissue. The temporalis myofascial flap is very useful for reducing the dead space remaining after orbital exenteration. It provides volume and reduces the risk of cerebrospinal fluid leak [7]. These are our preferred indications for this flap.

The temporalis myofascial flap can also be useful for the reconstruction of other defects of the middle third such as the malar region, orbital border, and oroantral fistulas.

The temporalis myofascial flap plays an important role in patients with facial paralysis for whom a microvascular muscle flap cannot be used. It enables traction of the oral commissure in order to create a smile despite the lesion of the buccal branch of the facial nerve. It is also possible to pull the frontal region upward, thus enabling the patient to raise the eyebrows and correcting the defect resulting from lesion of the frontal branch of the facial nerve [8]. Innervation of the temporalis muscle by the trigeminal nerve has the drawback that for the dynamic outcome to be aesthetically pleasing and symmetrical, the patient must undergo rehabilitation and a learning process, since the facial nerve is responsible for mobilizing the muscles of facial expression on the healthy side. The trigeminal nerve is sensory and supplies the muscles of mastication but not those of facial expression (Fig. 5.2).

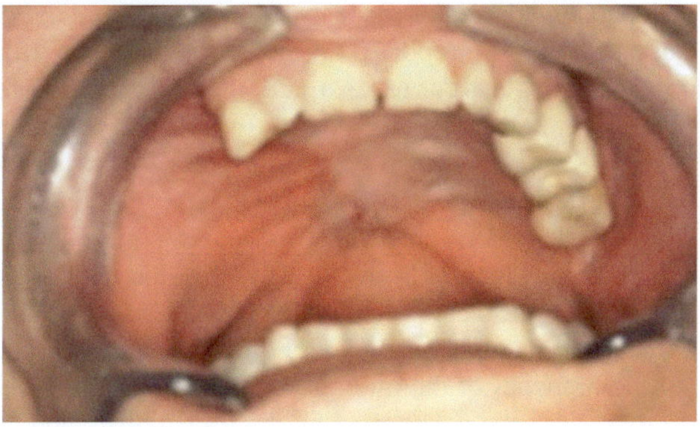

Fig. 5.2 Reconstruction of the right palate with temporalis muscle flap

5.1.4 Complications

The temporalis muscle flap is very predictable, with the result that associated complications are very uncommon. Potential complications include hemorrhage, hematoma, and seroma. In dentulous patients, every effort must be made to ensure that the flap does not interfere with occlusion in order to prevent vascular complications arising from involuntary mechanical pressure on the part of the patient.

Clinical follow-up requires physical examination of the flap, since it may be affected by partial or complete necrosis, although this is uncommon. The veins are more commonly compromised than the arteries. Care must be taken when turning the flap to prevent the pedicle from twisting and when sliding it medially toward the zygomatic arch for reconstruction of intraoral defects. If the flap is compromised, the arch should be cut and repositioned with plates and screws once the maneuver has been completed.

Knowledge of the anatomy of the facial nerve is essential during shaping of these flaps, since there is a risk of damaging the facial nerve, especially the frontal branch.

A drawback of the temporalis myofascial flap is the cosmetic defect in the temporal fossa. Throughout history, various materials have been used to avoid the unsightly defect resulting from the loss of tissue in the temporal region. The materials used include autologous bone grafts, bone cement (methyl methacrylate, hydroxyapatite), porous high-density polyethylene prostheses [9, 10], preformed acrylic prostheses, and titanium mesh [11]. All of these materials are susceptible to infection and exposure.

5.2 Pectoralis Myocutaneous Flap

5.2.1 Introduction

The pectoralis myocutaneous flap was first used in 1979 by Ariyan to transplant pedunculated tissue for reconstruction of head and neck defects [12]. Later, in 1980, Cuono and Ariyan reported on the inclusion of the fifth rib in the pectoralis osteomyocutaneous flap for reconstruction of composite defects [13].

5.2.2 Vascularization

The pectoralis major has two distinct vascular territories. The more cranial region is supplied by the pectoral branch of the thoracoacromial artery and the muscular branches of the first, second, and third perforating branches of the intercostal arteries and branches of the internal thoracic artery [14]. The more caudal region of the pectoralis muscle is supplied by the fourth, fifth, and sixth perforating branches of the internal thoracic artery [15].

Venous drainage of the pectoralis major is by venae comitantes that follow the course of the arteries of the same name (see above) before emptying into the axillary vein [16].

5.2.3 Indications

Since the end of the twentieth century, the pectoralis flap has been used to resolve major tissue defects of the head and neck. With the advent of new microsurgical reconstruction techniques, we can now provide the quantity and type of tissue necessary with better functional and cosmetic outcome [17]. Therefore, this flap has been relegated to the role of "rescue" flap, for use in patients with defects of the middle third or intraoral and cervical defects in which microvascular free flaps and pharyngeal-laryngeal reconstructive surgery are not used [18]. It can prove useful for the reconstruction of total glossectomy in patients who are not candidates for microsurgical free flaps such as the rectus abdominis flap or anterolateral thigh flap.

Within the oral cavity, it is possible to reconstruct both cranial and ipsilateral soft palate defects. Outside the oral cavity, it is possible to cover skin and soft tissue defects in the orbitozygomatic region [19]. The flap can be used with the muscle pedicle external to the skin of the neck in patients with associated comorbidities. If no complications have arisen 3 weeks after surgery, the flap pedicle can be cut in order to improve the appearance of the face and facilitate the patient's return to a normal social life (Figs. 5.3, 5.4, 5.5, 5.6, and 5.7).

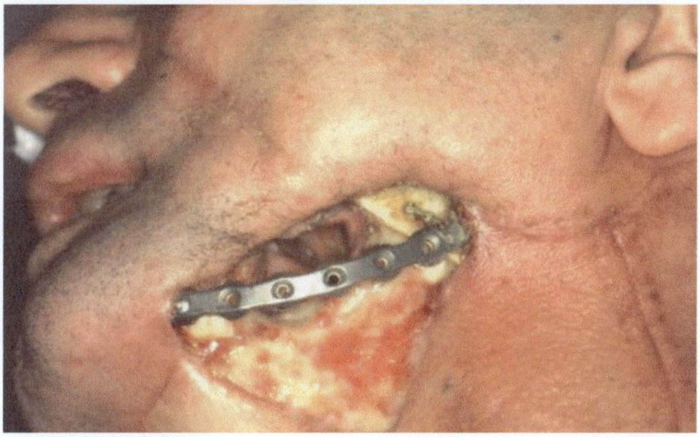

Fig. 5.3 Preoperative defect

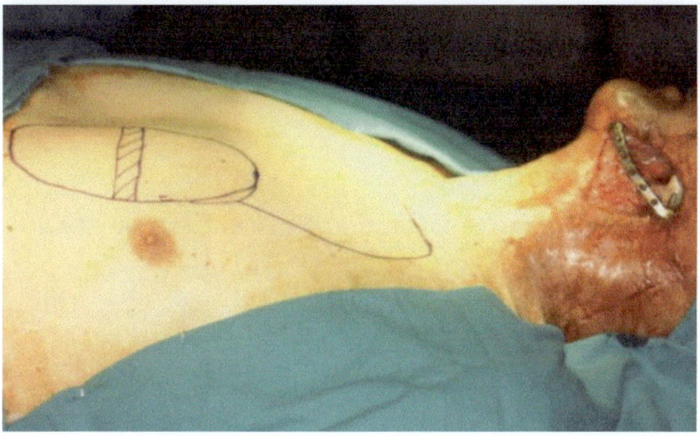

Fig. 5.4 Pectoralis muscle flap design

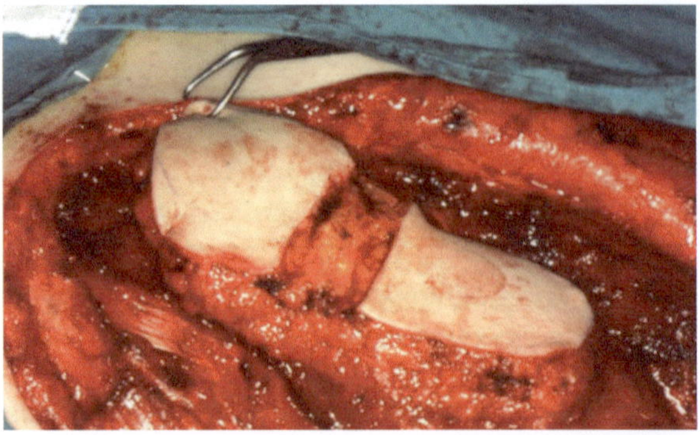

Fig. 5.5 Pectoralis muscle flap with de-epithelialized area

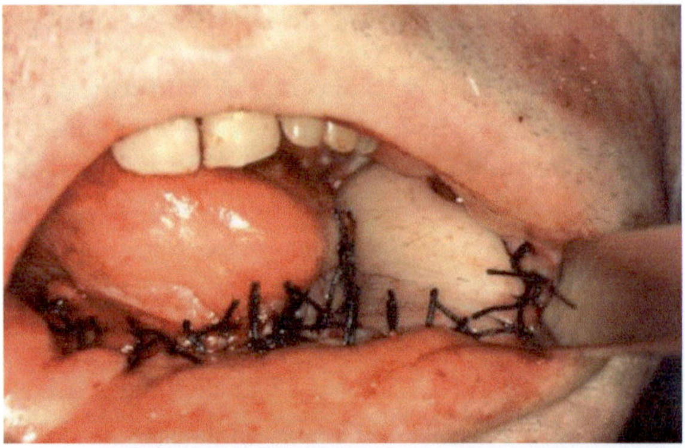

Fig. 5.6 Intraoral reconstruction

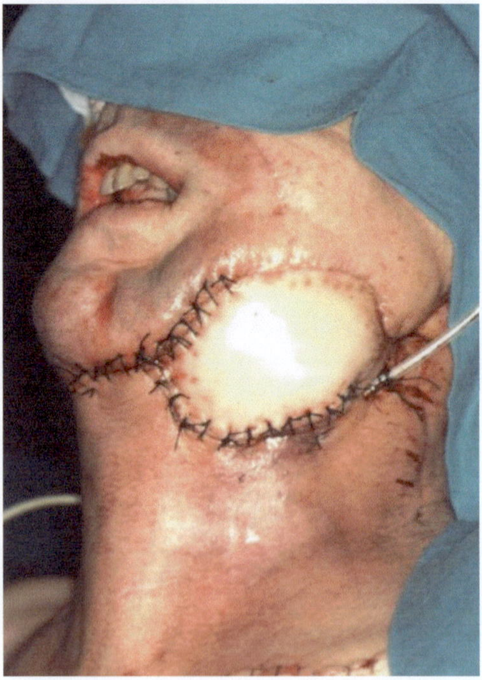

Fig. 5.7 External reconstruction

5.2.4 Complications

The pectoralis flap carries a high risk of partial necrosis of the skin paddle and of the underlying muscle, as well as of orocutaneous and pharyngocutaneous fistula. Total necrosis of the flap is unusual, although areas of peripheral epidermolysis are common.

The flap carries a high risk of wound dehiscence, especially in women and in patients aged over 60 years because of the force of gravity and the increase in fatty tissue. If there is a communication with the oral cavity, the risk of infection along the subcutaneous course of the flap increases considerably [17].

5.3 Latissimus Dorsi Myocutaneous Flap

5.3.1 Introduction

The latissimus dorsi myocutaneous flap was used for the first time in head and neck reconstruction by Quillen in 1978 [20], although it has been used in breast reconstruction since the beginning of the twentieth century.

The flap can be free or pedicled. Its almost constant anatomy and the wide caliber of the vessels of the pedicle make it a predictable option for reconstruction. It can be harvested as a muscle flap, musculocutaneous flap, or osteomyocutaneous flap. It contributes a large area of vascularized tissue and volume. The muscle commonly atrophies, although occasionally it will be necessary to use secondary thinning procedures and contour correction [21].

The skin island can be designed in different directions depending on which best suits the reconstruction. Moreover, the scarce variability of the regional and vascular anatomy means that the subscapular system can be used to obtain many free or pedicle flaps for the reconstruction of complex soft tissue and bone defects (Fig. 5.8).

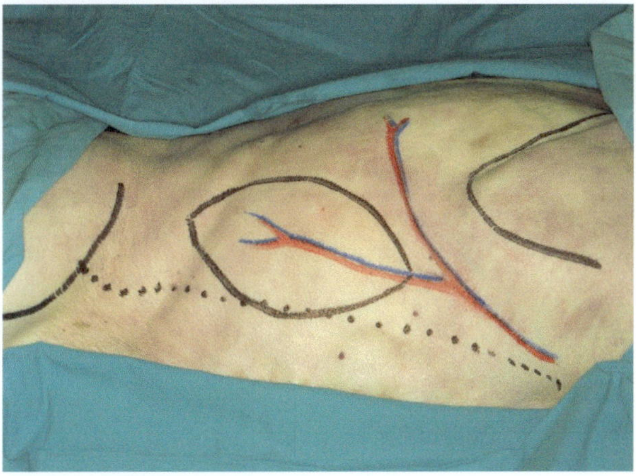

Fig. 5.8 Surgical design

5.3.2 Vascularization

The main flap is formed cranially by the thoracodorsal vein and artery and medially by the circumflex scapular artery in the mid part. Both are branches of the subscapular artery. Additionally, the latissimus dorsi is supplied by the posterior intercostal perforators and perforating branches of the subscapular artery [22]. The most caudal part of the muscle is supplied by branches of the lumbar arteries.

The veins of the scapular system accompany each artery in groups of 2, except in the section of the thoracodorsal artery, where venous return is through a single thoracodorsal vein.

5.3.3 Indications

Given that the latissimus dorsi flap is a pedicle flap, it can be used to cover soft tissue defects in the cervical region. It can also be used to cover defects of the temporal and occipital scalp. This flap can also prove suitable for the reconstruction of tissue defects in the oral cavity, including glossectomy [23, 24], although this is not its

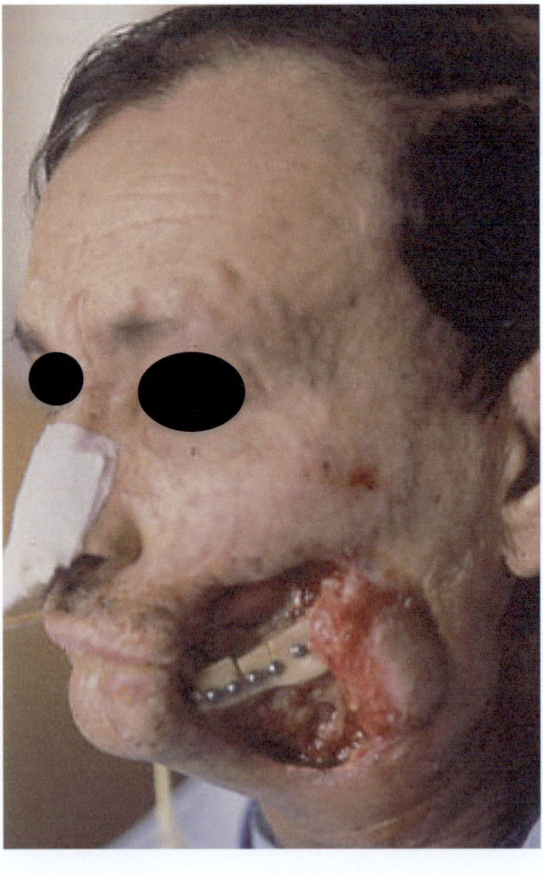

Fig. 5.9 Preoperative defect

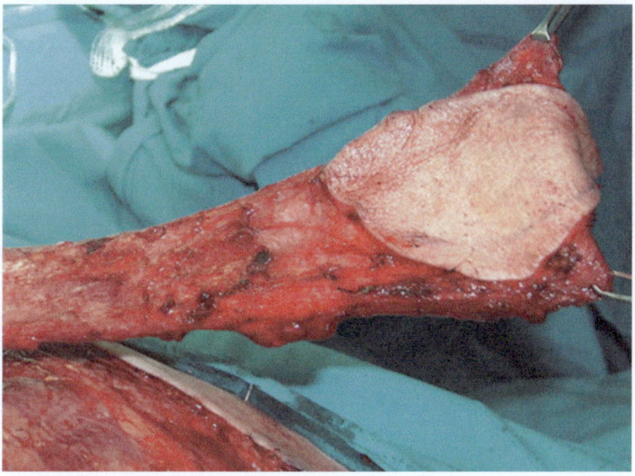

Fig. 5.10 Isolated flap

Fig. 5.11 Postoperative view

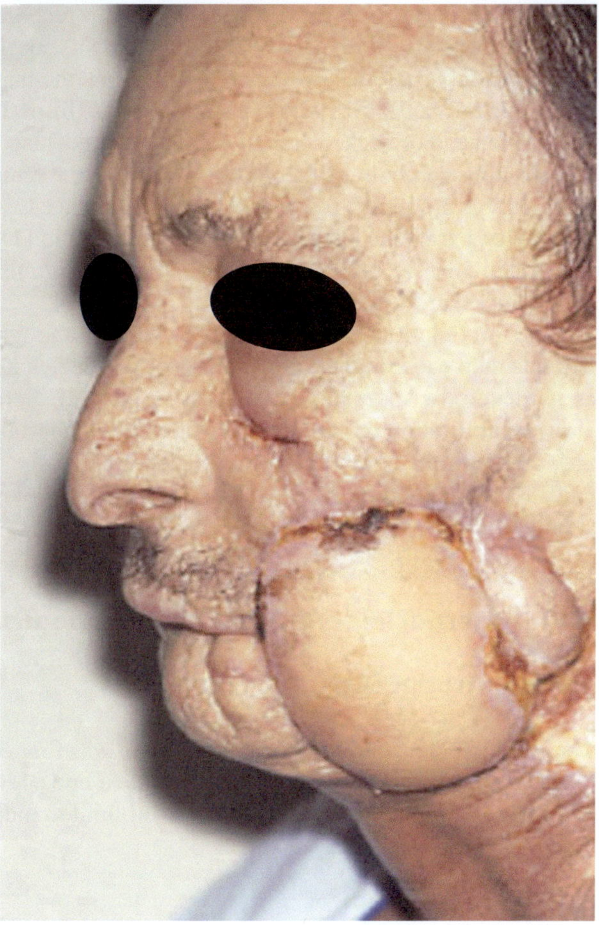

most frequent use. Given advances in microsurgical techniques, the latissimus dorsi flap is now reserved for medically compromised patients who are to undergo reconstruction with a free flap, patients who require large reconstructions, and patients without cervical vessels for microsuture [24].

Today, the latissimus dorsi myocutaneous flap is the first choice for many surgeons in scalp reconstruction because it is reliable and easy to harvest and has a large surface area [25]. Very often, because of problems with the length between the pedicle and the area to be reconstructed, a free latissimus dorsi flap with microsurgery techniques is preferred [26]. Thus, distance is no longer a disadvantage, and the risk of wound dehiscence from accidental traction of the pedicle with neck movements is reduced (Figs. 5.9, 5.10, and 5.11).

5.3.4 Complications

As with any flap, the latissimus dorsi myocutaneous flap carries a risk of vascular compromise, either by arterial ischemia or, more frequently, venous damage. Given the wide caliber of the vessels of this flap, these complications are not frequent. The most caudal part of the muscle, which in scalp reconstruction is the most cranial, carries a greater risk of necrosis because the vascularization of the lower third is from the lumbar arteries, which are cut to rotate the flap.

As this is a bulky flap whose pedicle ascends from the donor site to the recipient site on the head or neck, a certain risk of wound dehiscence is expected. Other risks include infection both of the donor site and of the recipient site—especially if the oral cavity is the area to be repaired—and fistula in cases of communication with the oral cavity, parafacial sinuses, or cerebrospinal fluid [27]. In such cases, the borders of the flap and the neighboring tissue should be completely sealed. Seromas and hematomas can form [28].

Loss of function is not normally severe, although this may be the case for patients who use crutches to walk or need a wheelchair and for professionals such as gardeners or sportspeople such as golfers. If there are no contraindications, early rehabilitation of the shoulder should be undertaken within the first week of the intervention. If the shoulder is immobilized for longer periods, the patient tends to adopt antalgic postures that considerably delay normal functioning of the shoulder [29].

5.4 Sternocleidomastoid Myocutaneous Flap

5.4.1 Introduction

The sternocleidomastoid myocutaneous flap was first described by Owens in 1955 [30]. Since then, the use of this flap has been considered controversial, and it has been relegated to adjuvant procedures with limited indications. It can be used as a myocutaneous flap and as an osteomyocutaneous flap if clavicle bone tissue is included.

5.4.2 Vascularization

The main blood supply is from a branch of the superior thyroid artery. However, the occipital artery is largely responsible for the supply of the cranial third of the muscle. In addition, the middle third sometimes receives direct branches from the external carotid artery. The caudal third can receive its supply from the suprascapular artery, cervical transverse artery, the thyrocervical trunk, and the superficial cervical artery [31]. The skin paddle is vascularized by myocutaneous perforators (veins and arteries) [32]. Given that venous return runs parallel to arterial return, the flap can be used cranially or caudally as a pedicle flap.

5.4.3 Indications

Since it was first described, the sternocleidomastoid flap has been heavily criticized because of the safety risk in tumors of the head and neck: the course of the muscle is close to the cervical lymph node chains II, III, IV, and V. Furthermore, partial necrosis of the raised skin paddle is common, affecting 20–52 % of all flaps harvested [33].

This flap is has been used mainly as a partial muscle flap after parotidectomy. It is placed between the skin and the branches of the facial nerve, thus reducing the risk of Frey syndrome [34–36] and the resulting cosmetic defect [35], although the superficial muscular aponeurotic system flap is now more generally used. The sternocleidomastoid flap can also provide bulk and improve contour after a resection. Its volume can be increased by rotation.

The flap can be used for the reconstruction of the floor of the mouth and the tongue, as well as for intraoral, cervical, and facial structures caudal to the zygomatic arch [37]. Greater knowledge of the vascular anatomy of this muscle has made it possible to improve the harvesting technique, thus enabling the flap to be converted to a pedicle perforator flap and improving the arc of rotation of the pedicle. Consequently, as we can be more selective with the quantity of tissue to be transferred, the survival rate of the skin paddle is increased [38].

We use the sternocleidomastoid flap very occasionally to increase facial volume in 3-dimensional reconstructions. Although this is not the flap of choice for mandibular reconstruction, an osteomyocutaneous flap can be harvested based on the insertion in the clavicle. Thus, a longitudinal section of the clavicle can be made, and dental implants can be placed either immediately or at a later date [39]. Given the morbidity associated with resection of the clavicle, we have never used the sternocleidomastoid flap in this way (Figs. 5.12, 5.13, 5.14, and 5.15).

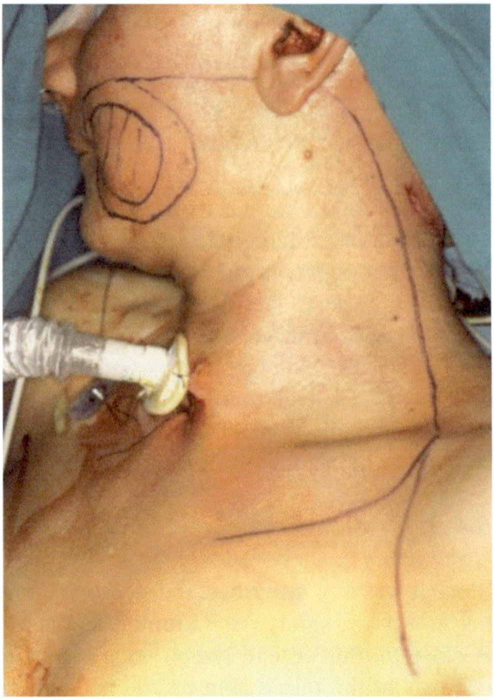

Fig. 5.12 Surgical design

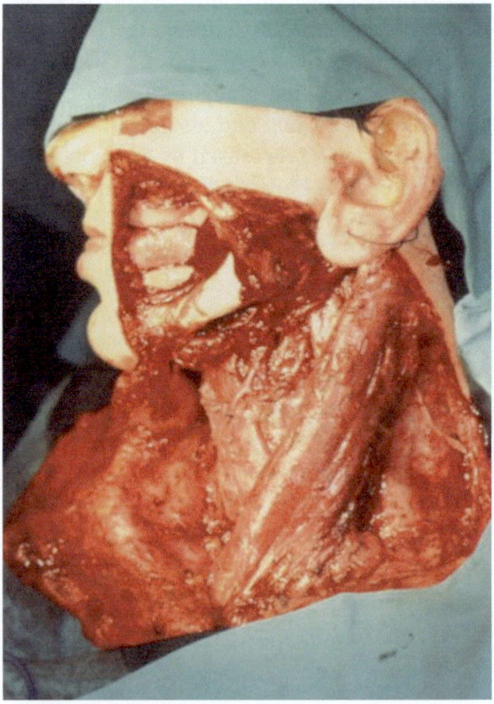

Fig. 5.13 Surgical defect

5.4.4 Complications

Before harvesting this flap, it is necessary to locate the spinal accessory nerve, which must be spared. Injury of the spinal accessory nerve can affect trapezius muscle function, and problems with rotation, elevation, and adduction of the arm have been reported, as have atrophy and pain in the arm [40].

As with any other flap, the sternocleidomastoid flap can be affected by total or partial necrosis. Total necrosis is uncommon, except in patients who receive radiation therapy as a complementary treatment. Partial necrosis of the skin paddle is quite common. As mentioned above, this complication can be reduced if the flap is harvested as a perforator flap [41].

In the case of intraoral reconstruction, there is a risk of orocutaneous fistula and wound dehiscence, although this risk can be reduced by suturing the flap on several planes. In addition, it is recommended to attach the flap to the bone using a suspension suture and insist on postural measures during the first week after surgery.

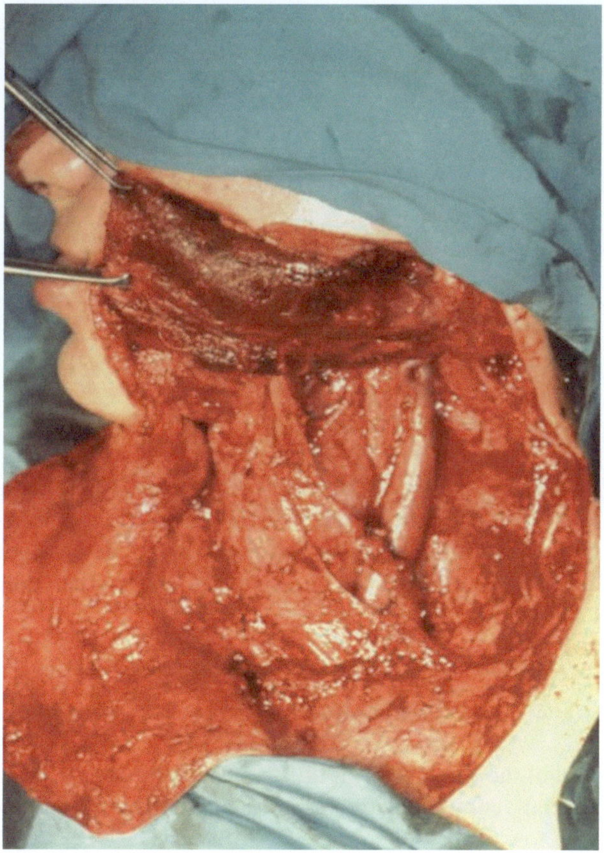

Fig. 5.14 Sternocleidomastoid muscle providing bulk to the face

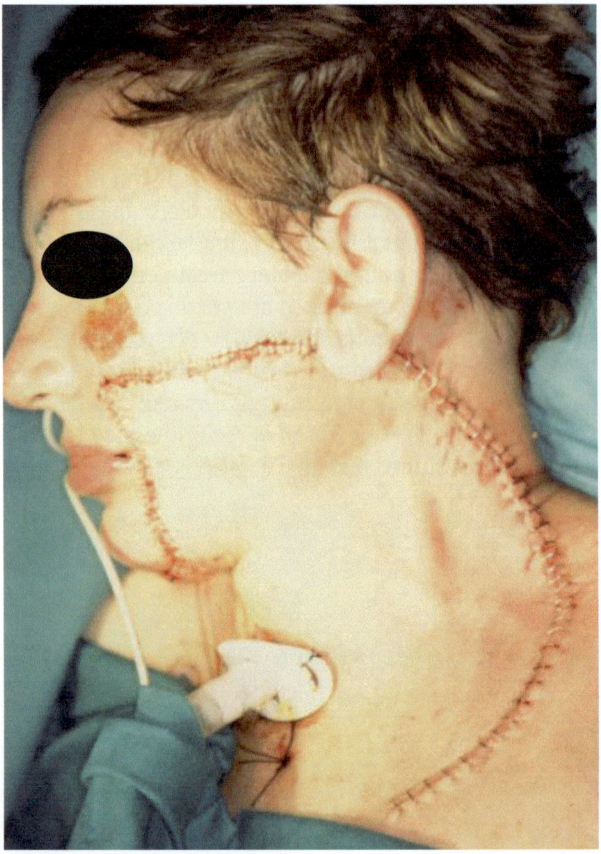

Fig. 5.15 Immediate postoperative aspect

5.5 Cervicopectoral Skin Flap

5.5.1 Introduction

The cervicopectoral flap was first described by Becker in 1978 for the reconstruction of head and neck defects [42]. It is well vascularized and has a large skin surface. In addition, its color, texture, and thickness and the disposition of the adnexa are very similar to those of the surrounding tissue. The cosmetic outcome is excellent [43].

5.5.2 Vascularization

One of the advantages of this flap is that it uses the local blood supply from various arterial-venous perforators; consequently, the risk of complete necrosis of the flap is very low [44].

The upper third, from the ala to the chin, is supplied by perforating branches of the facial artery. The perforators of the superior thyroid artery supply the middle part of the flap (cervical region). The vascular network formed by the cervical transverse artery supplies the caudal part of the flap, which includes the neck and chest [45]. The flap is also supplied by blood from the anterior thoracic vessels of the internal mammary artery [46].

5.5.3 Indications

The cervicopectoral flap is the first choice for skin defects that do not require tissue bulk. Although a cervicofacial flap may be sufficient for malar lesions, the cervicopectoral flap is better for more extensive or cranial lesions, since it can completely cover the wound remaining after extirpation of the lesions in the orbit, malar region, parotid region, masseteric region, and chin, as well as in simple reconstruction of the lip [47]. The incision used for this flap can also be used to perform an ipsilateral cervical dissection, thus saving time, reducing morbidity, and providing a more extensive surgical field. In addition, the surgical plane of this flap coincides with that of the flap taken for parotidectomy and cervical dissection [46]. The flap is simple and easy to harvest.

If additional volume is necessary, the cervicopectoral flap can be combined with free muscle flaps, such as the rectus abdominis, or pedicle flaps, such as the pectoral flap, which can then be covered with the cervicopectoral flap. This approach provides volume and is cosmetically acceptable after large resections. The combination is very commonly used in orbital exenteration, where a temporal myofascial flap can be combined with the cervicofacial flap [48]. Its greatest advantage is that it provides an extensive area of skin whose color and texture are similar to those of the face, thus leading to a very acceptable cosmetic outcome (Figs. 5.16, 5.17, 5.18, 5.19, 5.20, and 5.21).

5.5.4 Complications

The cervicopectoral flap is frequently affected by superficial epidermolysis [47], although complete necrosis is extremely rare. Scars at the donor site, very old age,

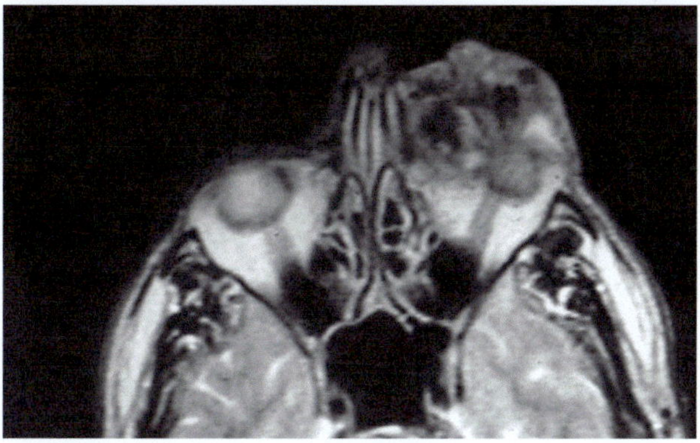

Fig. 5.16 MRI of the tumor

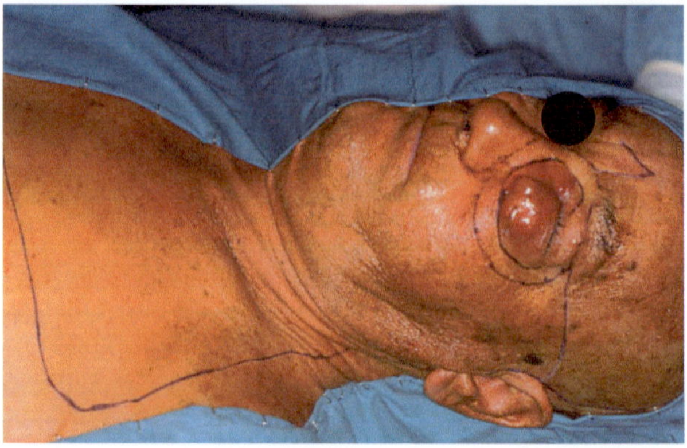

Fig. 5.17 Cervicopectoral design

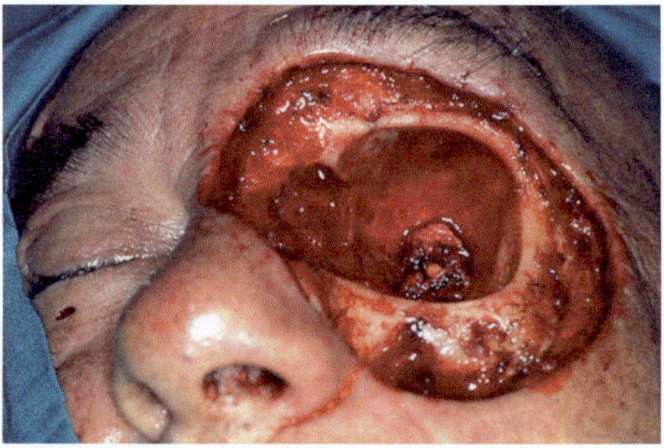

Fig. 5.18 Surgical defect

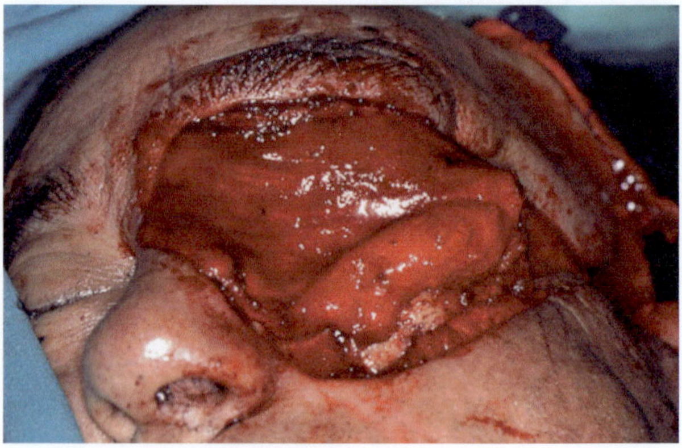

Fig. 5.19 Temporalis muscle flap filling the orbit

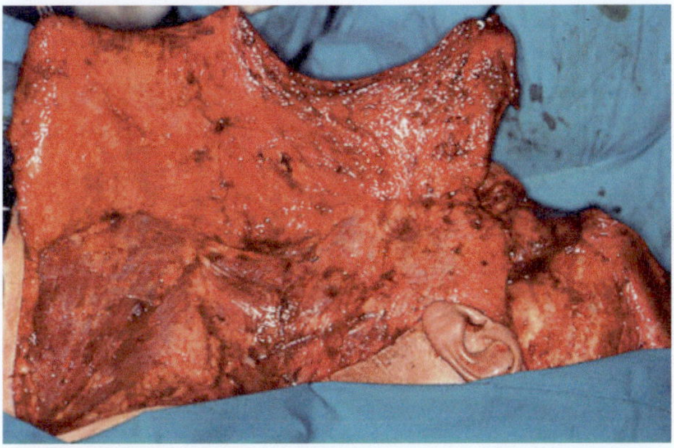

Fig. 5.20 Elevation of the flap

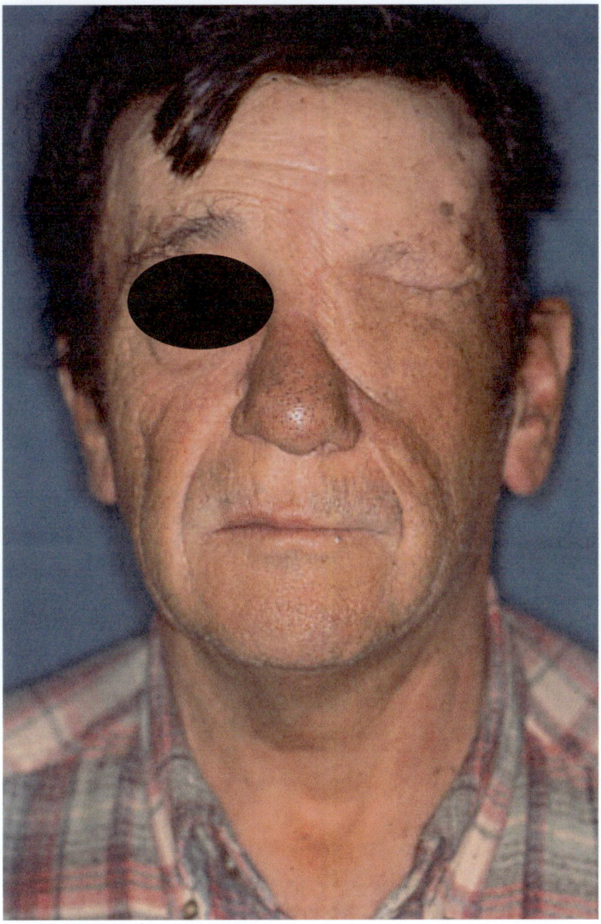

Fig. 5.21 Final result

and heavy smoking constitute relative contraindications for this flap, since all these factors increase the risk of vascular complications. In the case of epidermolysis, the most likely outcome is that the tissue will scar after second intention healing. Given that the donor site is extensive, there is a risk of hemorrhage, hematoma, and infection.

5.6 Nasolabial Flap

5.6.1 Introduction

The nasolabial flap is a small and predictable flap that is easy to harvest [49]. It can be used for the reconstruction of small defects of the oral cavity, tongue, malar region, commissures, tip of the nose, ala, and lower eyelid [50]. It can be pedicled caudally or cranially and can be used bilaterally depending on the area of tissue to be repaired [51].

5.6.2 Vascularization

The flap is supplied by the angular artery, the infraorbital artery, and the transverse facial artery. This complete supply means that the flap can be obtained as a random or axial flap.

Depending on where the tissue from the nasolabial region is to be placed, the flap can be pedicled to the different vessels that supply it. Thus, the flap can be pedicled superiorly, with the blood supply based on the infraorbital artery, and inferiorly from the angular artery. Lastly, it can be pedicled both medially and laterally after the transverse facial artery [52].

5.6.3 Indications

The nasolabial flap is indicated for small soft tissue defects. If the flap is near the midline, two flaps can be obtained, thus enabling closure of larger midline defects [51]. Its main indication is for defects of the floor of the mouth.

The flap is easy to harvest and leaves a very discreet cosmetic defect, since the scar is camouflaged by the nasolabial groove. It is very useful for the reconstruction of intraoral soft tissue and even the tongue. In men, intraoral reconstruction has the drawback that the flap transports hair. Once the flap has settled, laser technology can be used to prevent hair growth.

In combined defects (bone and soft tissue), the nasolabial flap can be used to cover the bone flap. For example, in defects of the symphysis, bone tissue can be reconstructed using a microvascular iliac crest flap, teeth can be reconstructed with immediate placement of implants on an implant-supported prosthesis, and soft tissue can be reconstructed with a bilateral nasolabial flap [53], thus obviating dissection of the inferior oblique muscle with the iliac crest and reducing the comorbidity of the procedure.

Given its anatomical proximity and versatility, which provide multiple options for blood supply, and color similar to that of the nose [54], the nasolabial flap enables different combinations for repair of soft tissue [55, 56]. In combination with other flaps, it serves as a therapeutic tool for the reconstruction of the lips and perioral tissue [57] (Figs. 5.22, 5.23, 5.24, and 5.25).

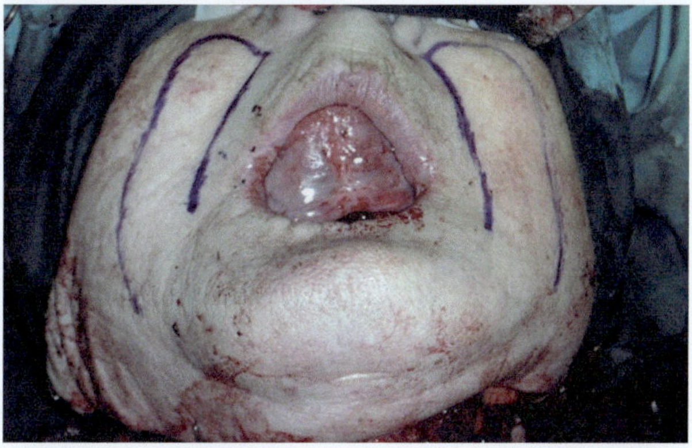

Fig. 5.22 Nasolabial flap design

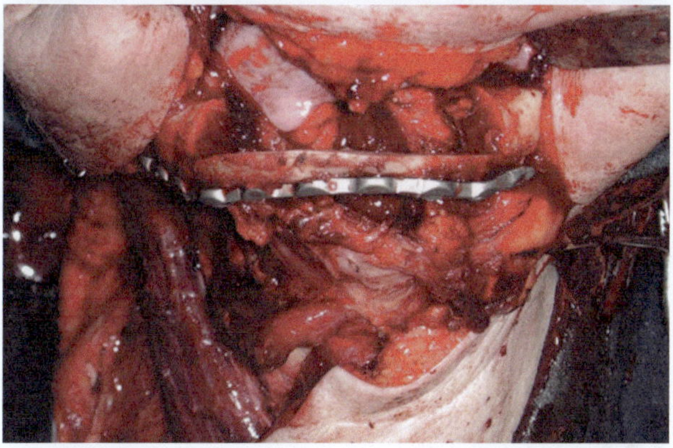

Fig. 5.23 Surgical defect

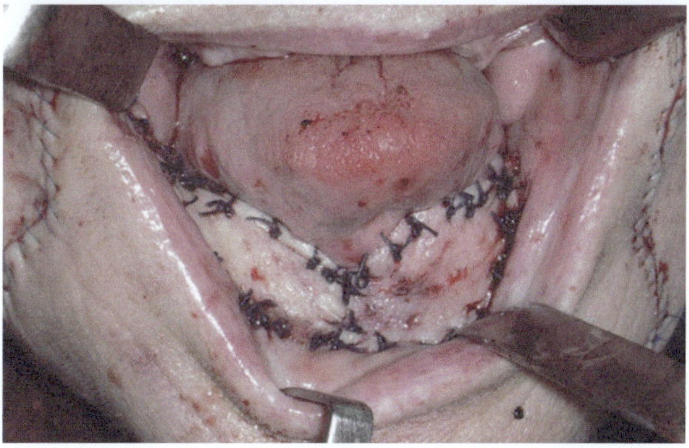

Fig. 5.24 Intraoperative view

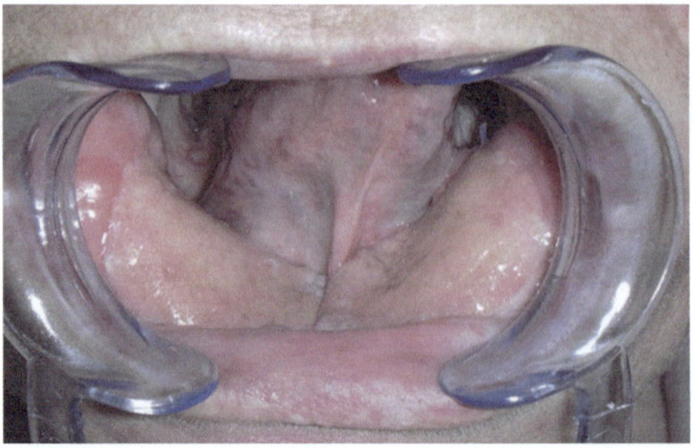

Fig. 5.25 6 months postoperative

5.6.4 Complications

Detractors of this flap highlight the disadvantage that it leaves a scar on the face. In fact, in patients with no history of hypertrophic or keloid scarring, the scar is barely visible, since it is camouflaged by the nasolabial groove. The cosmetic outcome is satisfactory or very satisfactory for most patients [58].

The risk of wound dehiscence is greater if the flap is used for reconstruction of mobile and intraoral soft tissue, as in the case of tongue reconstruction. Infection of the donor site is rare, since the area exposed during harvesting is small and highly vascularized [49]. Superficial epidermolysis is possible, as are partial necrosis and total necrosis, although the latter is uncommon.

If the flap is used for reconstruction of the infraorbital area, a safety margin of 7 mm from the medial canthus should be left in order to reduce the risk of ectropion [59].

5.7 Buccinator Flap

5.7.1 Introduction

The buccinator flap was first described by Reychler [60] as a myomucosal island flap. It has excellent texture, color, and pliability for reconstruction of intraoral soft tissue defects that are small in area and thickness. Closure of the donor site may be direct and not require an extraoral incision. The flap can be harvested as a mucosal, muscular, or myomucosal flap.

5.7.2 Vascularization

The buccinator muscle is supplied by branches of the facial, internal maxillary, and infraorbital arteries.

The facial artery is the main vessel supplying the buccinator muscle. The buccal artery, a posterior branch of the facial artery, supplies the posterior half, and the inferior buccal and anterior buccal arteries, both of which are branches of the facial artery, supply the inferior and anterior regions [61].

The branches of the internal maxillary artery that supply blood to the buccinator are the buccal artery and the posterior superior alveolar artery. The buccal artery supplies blood to the posterior part of the muscle, whereas the posterosuperior alveolar artery participates in the supply of the posterior superior region [62].

Lastly, the anterior superior region of the buccinator is also supplied by small branches of the infraorbital artery.

All of these vessels converge to form an anastomosis that enables several pedicle flaps to be harvested. On the lateral surface of the muscle, a venous anastomotic system forms the buccal plexus that drains into the facial vein, namely, the pterygoid plexus.

5.7.3 Indications

The buccinator flap can be attached anteriorly, posteriorly, or superiorly. A myomucosal island flap is also possible. The flap obtained is delimited cranially by the parotid duct, anteriorly by the oral commissure, and posteriorly by the pterygomandibular ligament [61].

It can be used for reconstruction of the nasal cavity [63], hard palate [64], soft palate [65], dental alveolus, upper lip, maxillary antrum, and floor of the orbit if it is attached superiorly. When it is attached inferiorly, it can be used to reconstruct the floor of the mouth, lateral border of the tongue [66], mandibular vestibule [67], tonsillar fossa, and lower lip [68]. The island flap described by Zhao et al. [39] makes it possible to reconstruct defects of the lateral wall of the pharynx and of the base of the tongue [41].

The buccinator flap can also be used in combination with other flaps, since it is thin and pliable, and its appearance is similar to that of the tissue to be reconstructed. It can be used to cover the bone tissue of a microvascular osteomyocutaneous fibula flap [69]. The resulting appearance for subsequent placement of implants is very similar to that of the original mandible.

5.7.4 Complications

Although the blood supply to the buccinator flap is good, there is a risk of partial or total necrosis. It is important to ensure that the pedicle is not accidentally compressed by occlusion [70]. The risk of vascular compromise is greater in patients with a compromised facial artery (e.g., those who have undergone cervical dissection).

In cases of insufficient hemostasis, there is a risk of hemorrhage and hematoma, which is relatively frequent in such a well-vascularized area [71].

The anatomical relationship with the facial nerve requires the dissection to be made in the appropriate plane in order to prevent temporary or permanent lesion of the nerve, especially of the marginal and buccal branches.

If the upper limit of the dissection is not respected, there is a risk of stenosis of the parotid duct. The donor site should not be closed with tension sutures, since this can lead to retraction of the scar and undesirable cosmetic alterations.

If the flap is attached, the pedicle can be cut after 3 weeks to ensure greater cosmetic and functional quality of life.

5.8 Platysma Flap

5.8.1 Introduction

The platysma myocutaneous flap was first described in the English-language literature in 1978 by Futrell et al. [72]. It is simple to harvest and is useful for covering tissue defects of the neck, oral cavity, and lower third.

5.8.2 Vascularization

The main blood supply is via the submental artery. Branches of the posterior auricular, occipital, facial, superior thyroid, and subclavian arteries also supply the platysma and the superficial skin of the flap [73].

5.8.3 Indications

The platysma flap is easy to harvest, although it does not provide large areas of skin. It can be attached caudally or cranially [74] and is useful for defects of the neck and lower third.

This flap can be used to repair defects of the anterior floor of the mouth [75, 73], tongue, and pharynx [76]. It can be used as an alternative to the superficial muscular-aponeurotic system flap after parotidectomy [77]. It could also prove useful for reconstruction of the wall of the airways and digestive tract [78].

The platysma flap is not suitable for patients who have undergone radiation therapy (head and neck), ligation of the facial artery, or radical dissection, since there is a high risk of necrosis.

5.8.4 Postsurgical Recommendations

In general, the drainage placed for neck surgery can also serve to prevent the formation of hematomas and seromas. As with all treatments of the neck, it is essential to be alert to hemorrhaging that may lead to compression of the airway and respiratory insufficiency.

The supine position should be avoided. It is generally preferable that the patient be seated or with the bed raised to reduce pressure and thus reduce inflammation and edema in the neck.

In defects of the cheek, malar region, tongue, and floor of the mouth that are distant from the pedicle, every attempt should be made to ensure that the pedicle is not tense. Therefore, posture should be managed, and the patient and his/her family should receive information on how to avoid movements that place the pedicle in tension.

5.8.5 Complications

One of the reasons the platysma flap is disliked by many surgeons is the relatively low rate of venous return (7–30 %) [79]. Arterial complications are more unusual. Hemorrhaging and hematomas can occur.

Since there is a risk of cutaneous fistula in defects of the oral cavity or airway, complete closure should be ensured by suturing on several planes.

5.9 Palatal Flap

5.9.1 Introduction

The palatal flap was first used by Millard in 1962 [80] to treat a cleft palate. It is a predictable and simple flap that can be harvested quickly. The main drawback of the palatal flap is that direct closure of the donor site is not possible, although given that the underlying tissue is bone, there is no tissue contraction, and second intention scarring is favorable. In addition, the pedicle is short, although it can be lengthened if it is freed from the bony canal.

5.9.2 Vascularization

The blood supply is from the major palatine artery, which anastomoses medially and anteriorly with the nasopalatine artery. An extensive arterial-venous plexus is also formed with the branches of the contralateral palatine artery [81], thus making it possible to obtain a mucoperiosteal flap of almost the whole mucosa pedicled to the greater palatine artery. The flap can also be pedicled to the nasopalatine artery [82] and even with random vascularization [83] if a suitable length/width ratio is maintained.

5.9.3 Indications

The palatal flap is mostly used to close oroantral communication [84] of any cause. Fistulas of up to 5 mm can resolve spontaneously; however, larger fistulas must be completely sealed, preferably on two planes. A major advantage of this flap is that it provides keratinized mucosa for the recipient site [85].

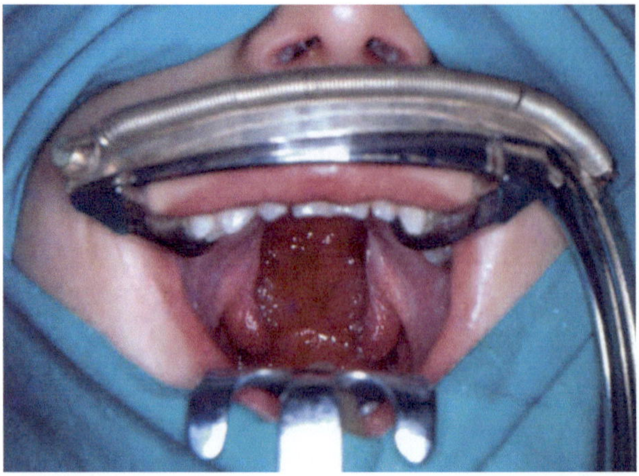

Fig. 5.26 Palatal defect

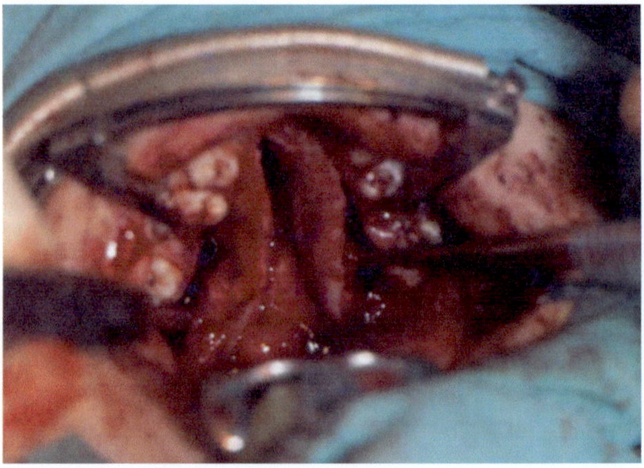

Fig. 5.27 Palatal flap

As mentioned above, this flap is useful for repairing a cleft palate [86] and, less commonly, it can be used to resolve defects of the base of the skull [87]. Lee proposed a technique for reconstructing oroantral communication defect and using a delayed autologous bone graft for subsequent placement of implants [88] (Figs. 5.26, 5.27, and 5.28).

5.9.4 Complications

The most frequent complications are hemorrhage, which is due to the abundant blood supply in the palate and the impossibility of primary closure at the donor site. This hemorrhage is easily controlled with local compression [89].

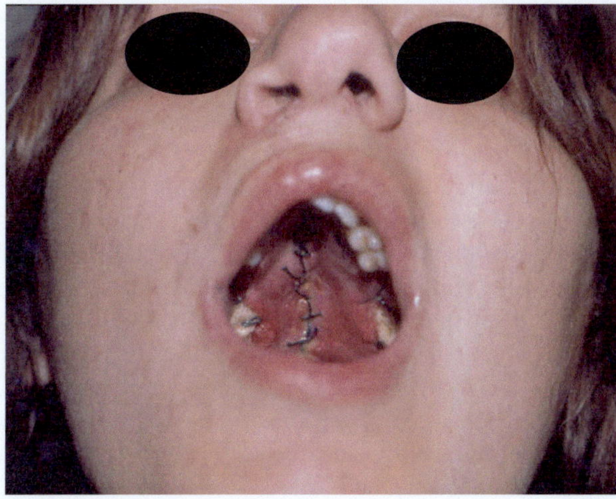

Fig. 5.28 Postoperative view

Pain and discomfort at the donor site—which heals by second intention—can be resolved by applying triamcinolone and topical lidocaine gel.

Although complete necrosis of the flap is very rare, partial necrosis is observed in 5–10 % of patients. Given that the defect sometimes closes despite the necrosis, it may not be necessary to perform additional procedures after withdrawing the necrotized tissue. The risk of necrosis is greater in patients who have received radiation therapy to the head and neck, patients who have previously received palatal flaps (which can compromise the blood supply to the flap), or when the internal maxillary artery or external carotid artery has been ligated.

5.10 Submental Flap

5.10.1 Introduction

The submental flap is a relatively new flap that was first described by Martin et al. [90] at the end of the twentieth century. Since then, it has been increasingly used because it is widely accepted by patients, it is anatomically close to the oral cavity and face, and it is quick and easy to harvest.

5.10.2 Vascularization

The flap is supplied by the submental artery, which is a branch of the facial artery [91]. An arterial anastomotic network can be found between the submental arteries. Venous drainage is to the facial vein.

5.10.3 Indications

The submental flap has a long pedicle [92] that arises very close to the floor of the mouth; therefore, it can be used to reconstruct intraoral and facial defects without tension. Furthermore, the resulting scar is discreet and generally very well accepted [93]. Another advantage of using this flap for intraoral and facial reconstruction is that the skin is thin and adapts easily to the defect. It has also been used as a microvascular free flap [94], although this is not its most habitual application.

The main drawback of the submental flap is that the submental region is at the level of the neck most commonly affected by dissemination of lymph node tumors [95] in patients with cancer of the oral cavity. There is a risk of recurrence of the tumor in the flap if the neck has not been appropriately dissected during the first procedure. The other disadvantage of this flap affects men undergoing reconstruction of the oral cavity, since beard hair grows in the reconstructed area. However, this disadvantage can be resolved if the flap is de-epithelialized [96].

Despite these drawbacks, the submental flap is a very versatile option. It is used mainly for reconstruction of the floor of the mouth and the oral cavity. It is particularly useful for reconstruction of the tongue and alveolar ridge and can be combined with mandibular bone tissue, thus making it an osteomyocutaneous flap for the reconstruction of inferior lateral maxillary defects [97]. However, the submental flap is not our preferred technique for this type of defect.

In addition to its application in the oral cavity, the submental flap can be used to reconstruct defects of the face, lips [98], parapharyngeal space, and parotid region.

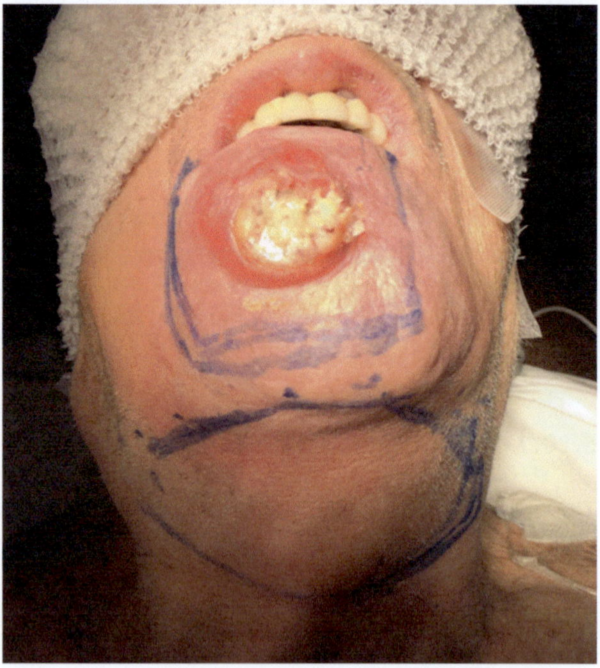

Fig. 5.29 Anteroposterior view of the tumor

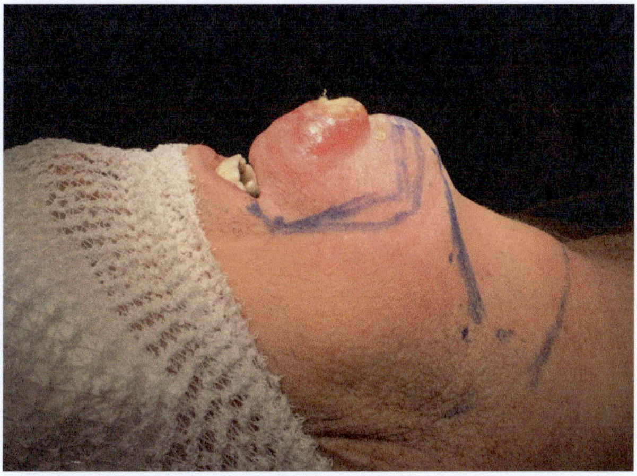

Fig. 5.30 Lateral view of the tumor

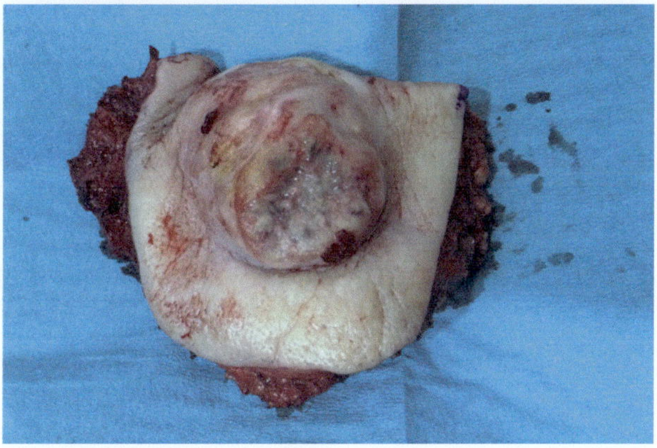

Fig. 5.31 surgical specimen

It can be combined with microvascular bone flaps [99] and even with free bone grafts [100] for defects involving bone and soft tissue. Two skin paddles can also be obtained for reconstruction of thickness defects at the masseter [101].

When used with retrograde flow, this flap can play a role in the reconstruction of defects of the temporal region, orbit, and even frontal region [91, 102] (Figs. 5.29, 5.30, 5.31, 5.32, 5.33, and 5.34).

5.10.4 Complications

The submental flap is not subject to high rates of necrosis, although the risk of necrosis does increase considerably in patients who have received radiation therapy (neck or floor of the mouth) or undergone previous cervical surgery and when the facial artery has been ligated. In order to protect the pedicle and reduce the risk of torsion, mylohyoid muscle tissue and tissue from the digastric muscle belly can be incorporated to surround the pedicle [96].

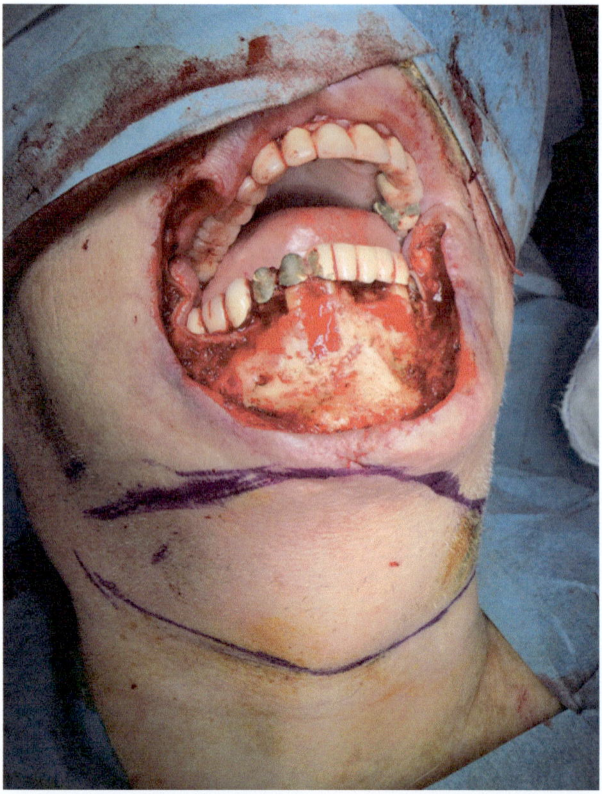

Fig. 5.32 Surgical defect and flap design

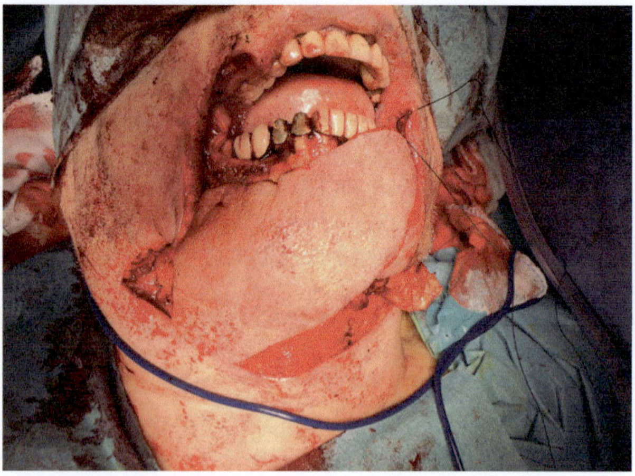

Fig. 5.33 Intraoperative position of the flap

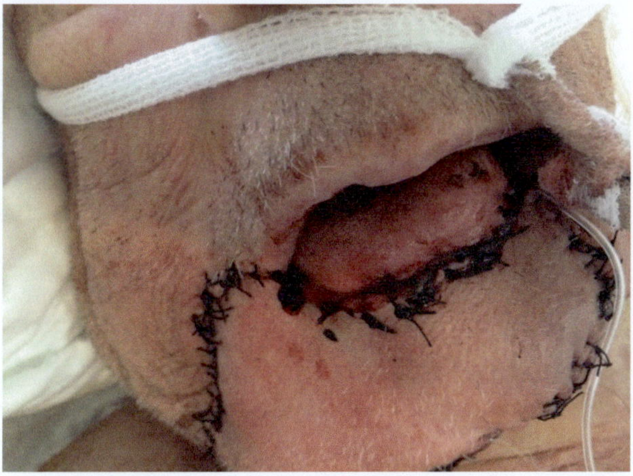

Fig. 5.34 Postoperative view

The flap is subject to hematoma, wound dehiscence, and infection. The risk of infection and wound dehiscence is considerably greater in reconstruction of defects of the oral cavity.

Given the closeness of the pedicle to the marginal branch of the facial nerve, there is a 1.1 % risk of lesion in this branch [103].

References

1. Golovine S. Procédé de cloture plastique de l'orbite après l'exentération. Arch Ophthalmol. 1898;18:679–80.
2. Bradley P, Brockbank J. The temporalis muscle flap in oral reconstruction. A cadaveric, animal and clinical study. J Maxillofac Surg. 1981;9(3):139–45.
3. Demirdover C, Sahin B, Vayvada H, Oztan HY. The versatile use of temporoparietal fascial flap. Int J Med Sci. 2011;8(5):362–8.
4. Elazab EEB, Abdel-Hameed FAM. The arterial supply of the temporalis muscle. Surg Radiol Anat. 2006;28(3):241–7.
5. Corrêa MB, Wafae GC, Pereira LA, Wafae N, Ruiz CR. Arterial branches to the temporal 530 muscle. Ital J Anat Embryol. 2008;113(2):109–15.
6. Upton J, Ferraro N, Healy G, Khouri R, Merrell C. The use of prefabricated fascial flaps for lining of the oral and nasal cavities. Plast Reconstr Surg. 1994;94(5):573–9.
7. Torroni A, Cervelli D, Gasparini G, Grussu F, Moro A, Marianetti TM, et al. Anterior retrograde approach to the myofascial temporalis muscle for the orbital reconstruction: series of 9 consecutive cases. Ann Plast Surg. 2015;74:37–42.
8. Viterbo F, Romão A, Brock RS, Joethy J. Facial reanimation utilizing combined orthodromic temporalis muscle flap and end-to-side cross-face nerve grafts. Aesthetic Plast Surg. 2014; 38(4):788–95.
9. Eldaly A, Magdy EA, Nour YA, Gaafar AH. Temporalis myofascial flap for primary cranial base reconstruction after tumor resection. Skull Base. 2008;18(4):253–63.

10. Rapidis AD, Day TA. The use of temporal polyethylene implant after temporalis myofascial flap transposition: clinical and radiographic results from its use in 21 patients. J Oral Maxillofac Surg. 2006;64(1):12–22.
11. Lipira A, Limbrick D, Haughey B, Custer P, Chicoine MR. Titanium mesh reconstruction to maintain scalp contour after temporalis musculofascial flap reconstruction of the floor of the middle cranial fossa: a technical note and report of two cases. Skull Base. 2009;19(4):303–9.
12. Ariyan S. The pectoralis major myocutaneous flap. A versatile flap for reconstruction in the head and neck. Plast Reconstr Surg. 1979;63(1):73–81.
13. Cuono CB, Ariyan S. Immediate reconstruction of a composite mandibular defect with a regional osteomusculocutaneous flap. Plast Reconstr Surg. 1980;65(4):477–84.
14. Prakash K, Saniya K. Anatomical study of pectoral nerves and its implications in surgery. J Clin Diagn Res. 2014;8(7):AC01–5.
15. Rikimaru H, Kiyokawa K, Inoue Y, Tai Y. Three-dimensional anatomical vascular distribution in the pectoralis major myocutaneous flap. Plast Reconstr Surg. 2005;115(5):1342–52; discussion 1353–4.
16. Rikimaru H, Kiyokawa K, Watanabe K, Koga N, Nishi Y, Sakamoto A. New method of preparing a pectoralis major myocutaneous flap with a skin paddle that includes the third intercostal perforating branch of the internal thoracic artery. Plast Reconstr Surg. 2009;123(4):1220–8.
17. Liu R, Gullane P, Brown D, Irish J. Pectoralis major myocutaneous pedicled flap in head and neck reconstruction: retrospective review of indications and results in 244 consecutive cases at the Toronto General Hospital. J Otolaryngol. 2001;30(1):34–40.
18. Elfeky AE, Nasr WF, Khazbak A, Abdelrahman MS, Allam ZA, Gareer WY, et al. Hypopharyngeal reconstruction: a comparison of three alternatives. Eur Arch Otorhinolaryngol. 2014 Sep 27. [Epub ahead of print].
19. Pingarron L, Ruiz J, Rey J, Maniegas L, Roson S, Martinez D. Subclavicular pectoralis major myocutaneous flap for optimal reconstruction of large orbitozygomatic defects: a case report. Craniomaxillofac Trauma Reconstr. 2014;7(3):245–8.
20. Quillen CG, Shearin JC, Georgiade NG. Use of the latissimus dorsi myocutaneous island flap for reconstruction in the head and neck area: case report. Plast Reconstr Surg. 1978;62(1):113–7.
21. Lessard L, Tahiri Y. Complex scalp, skull, and dural defect reconstruction using a turnover "tournedos" myocutaneous free flap. J Craniofac Surg. 2013;24(1):62–5.
22. Antohi N, Stan V, Huian C, Nae S. Poststernotomy wound management by debridement and pedicle flaps reconstruction. Chirurgia (Bucur). 2014;109(5):670–7.
23. Ong HS, Ji T, Zhang CP. The pedicled latissimus dorsi myocutaneous flap in head and neck reconstruction. Oral Maxillofac Surg Clin North Am. 2014;26(3):427–34.
24. Rigby MH, Hayden RE. Regional flaps: a move to simpler reconstructive options in the head and neck. Curr Opin Otolaryngol Head Neck Surg. 2014;22(5):401–6.
25. Neligan PC. Head and neck reconstruction. Plast Reconstr Surg. 2013;131(2):260e–9.
26. Fowler NM, Futran ND. Achievements in scalp reconstruction. Curr Opin Otolaryngol Head Neck Surg. 2014;22(2):127–30.
27. Frederick JW, Sweeny L, Carroll WR, Peters GE, Rosenthal EL. Outcomes in head and neck reconstruction by surgical site and donor site. Laryngoscope. 2013;123(7):1612–7.
28. Ou K-L, Dai Y-H, Wang H-J, Chen T-M, Dai N-T, Chang S-C, et al. The lower trapezius musculocutaneous flap for head and neck reconstruction: two decades of clinical experience. Ann Plast Surg. 2013;71 Suppl 1:S48–54.
29. Vucak MC, Masic T, Hassouba M, Hatibovic H, Babajic E. Reconstructive option of extensive head and neck defects in cancer surgery. Med Arch (Sarajevo, Bosnia Herzegovina). 2013;67(4):275–7.
30. Owens N. A compound neck pedicle designed for the repair of massive facial defects: formation, development and application. Plast Reconstr Surg (1946). 1955;15(5):369–89.

31. Leclère FM, Vacher C, Benchaa T. Blood supply to the human sternocleidomastoid muscle and its clinical implications for mandible reconstruction. Laryngoscope. 2012;122(11):2402–6.
32. Jabaley ME, Heckler FR, Wallace WH, Knott LH. Sternocleidomastoid regional flaps: a new look at an old concept. Br J Plast Surg. 1979;32(2):106–13.
33. Ariyan S. Further experiences with the sternocleidomastoid myocutaneous flap: a clinical appraisal of 31 cases. Plast Reconstr Surg. 1997;99(1):61–9.
34. Liu DY, Tian XJ, Li C, Sun SS, Xiong YH, Zeng X-T. The sternocleidomastoid muscle flap for the prevention of Frey syndrome and cosmetic deformity following parotidectomy: a systematic review and meta-analysis. Oncol Lett. 2013;5(4):1335–42.
35. Sanabria A, Kowalski LP, Bradley PJ, Hartl DM, Bradford CR, de Bree R, et al. Sternocleidomastoid muscle flap in preventing Frey's syndrome after parotidectomy: a systematic review. Head Neck. 2012;34(4):589–98.
36. Wei D, Liu J, Zhao W, Zhu H, Li Z, Wang H. Use of the versatile sternocleidomastoid flap in oral and maxillofacial surgery: our experience. Br J Oral Maxillofac Surg. 2013;51(8):742–6.
37. O'Brien B. A muscle-skin pedicle for total reconstruction of the lower lip; case report. Plast Reconstr Surg. 1970;45(4):395–9.
38. Khazaeni K, Rajati M, Shahabi A, Mashhadi L. Use of a sternocleidomastoid myocutaneous flap based on the sternocleidomastoid branch of the superior thyroid artery to reconstruct extensive cheek defects. Aesthetic Plast Surg. 2013;37(6):1167–70.
39. Zhao W, Zhu H, Xu J, Wang H. Using sternocleidomastoid-clavicle myocutaneous flap to reconstruct compound operative defect of oral carcinoma. Hua Xi Kou Qiang Yi Xue Za Zhi. 2011;29(5):537–41.
40. Windfuhr JP. Malpractice claims and unintentional outcome of tonsil surgery and other standard procedures in otorhinolaryngology. GMS Curr Top Otorhinolaryngol Head Neck Surg. 2013;12:Doc08.
41. Khan K, Hinckley V, Cassell O, Silva P, Winter S, Potter M. A novel use of the facial artery based buccinator musculo-mucosal island flap for reconstruction of the oropharynx. J Plast Reconstr Aesthet Surg. 2013;66(10):1365–8.
42. Becker DW. A cervicopectoral rotation flap for cheek coverage. Plast Reconstr Surg. 1978;61(6):868–70.
43. Blackwell KE, Buchbinder D, Biller HF, Urken ML. Reconstruction of massive defects in the head and neck: the role of simultaneous distant and regional flaps. Head Neck. 1997;19(7):620–8.
44. Lazaridis N, Tilaveridis I, Dalambiras S, Iordanidis S. The fasciocutaneous cervicopectoral rotation flap for lower cheek reconstruction: report of three cases. J Oral Maxillofac Surg. 1997;55(10):1166–71.
45. Vinh VQ, Ogawa R, Iwakiri I, Hyakusoku H, Tanuma K. Clinical and anatomical study of cervicopectoral superthin flaps. Plast Reconstr Surg. 2007;119(5):1464–71.
46. Anand AG, Amedee RG, Butcher RB. Reconstruction of large lateral facial defects utilizing variations of the cervicopectoral rotation flap. Ochsner J. 2008;8(4):186–90.
47. Bianchi B, Ferri A, Ferrari S, Copelli C, Poli T, Sesenna E. Free and locoregional flap associations in the reconstruction of extensive head and neck defects. Int J Oral Maxillofac Surg. 2008;37(8):723–9.
48. Soler-Presas F, Cuesta-Gil M, Borja-Morant A, Concejo-Cútoli C, Acero-Sanz J, Navarro-Vila C. Midface soft tissue reconstruction with the facio-cervico-pectoral flap. J Craniomaxillofac Surg. 1997;25(1):39–45.
49. Braasch DC, Lam D, Oh ES. Maxillofacial reconstruction with nasolabial and facial artery musculomucosal flaps. Oral Maxillofac Surg Clin North Am. 2014;26(3):327–33.
50. Chitlangia P, Kumuran E, Sabitha KS. Use of nasolabial flap in intra and extraoral reconstruction: our experience with 40 cases. J Maxillofac Oral Surg. 2012;11(4):451–4.
51. Deora SS, Nanjappa M, Kumaraswamy SV. Bilateral pedicled nasolabial flaps for the anterior alveolus mandibular defect: a review. J Maxillofac Oral Surg. 2010;9(4):385–8.

52. Singh S, Singh RK, Pandey M. Nasolabial flap reconstruction in oral cancer. World J Surg Oncol. 2012;10(1):227.
53. Navarro Cuellar C, Caicoya SJO, Acero Sanz JJ, Navarro Cuellar I, Muela CM, Navarro Vila C. Mandibular reconstruction with iliac crest free flap, nasolabial flap, and osseointegrated implants. J Oral Maxillofac Surg. 2014;72(6):1226.e1–15.
54. Weathers WM, Wolfswinkel EM, Nguyen H, Thornton JF. Expanded uses for the nasolabial flap. Semin Plast Surg. 2013;27(2):104–9.
55. Bi H, Xing X, Li J. Nasolabial-alar crease: a natural line to facilitate transposition of the nasolabial flap for lower nasal reconstruction. Ann Plast Surg. 2014;73(5):520–4.
56. Shim H-C, Kim G, Choi J-H, Kim J-H, Kim E-J, Park H-J, et al. The reverse nasolabial flap with a cartilage graft for the repair of a full-thickness alar defect: a single-stage procedure. Ann Dermatol. 2014;26(3):377–80.
57. Minagawa T, Maeda T, Shioya R. Esthetic and safe lower lip reconstruction of an asymmetric defect due to cancer resection: a modified Webster method combined with a nasolabial flap. J Oral Maxillofac Surg. 2011;69(6):e256–9.
58. El-Marakby HH, Fouad FA, Ali AH. One stage reconstruction of the floor of the mouth with a subcutaneous pedicled nasolabial flap. J Egypt Natl Canc Inst. 2012;24(2):71–6.
59. Alonso-Rodriguez E, Cebrian-Carretero J, Moran-Soto M, Burgueno-Garcia M. Versatility of nasolabial flaps in oral cavity reconstructions. Med Oral Patol Oral Cir Bucal. 2014;19(5):e525–30.
60. Reychler H. The island flap of the buccinator muscle. Acta Stomatol Belg. 1988;85(1):63–8.
61. Szeto C, Yoo J, Busato G-M, Franklin J, Fung K, Nichols A. The buccinator flap: a review of current clinical applications. Curr Opin Otolaryngol Head Neck Surg. 2011;19(4):257–62.
62. Rahpeyma A, Khajehahmadi S, Rezvani HN. Pedicle length in the inferiorly based buccinator myomucosal island flap: a cadaveric study. Int J Oral Maxillofac Surg. 2014;43(2): 173–6.
63. Kim GG, Hang AX, Mitchell CA, Zanation AM. Pedicled extranasal flaps in skull base reconstruction. Adv Otorhinolaryngol. 2013;74:71–80.
64. Franco D, Rocha D, Arnaut M, Freitas R, Alonso N. Versatility of the buccinator myomucosal flap in atypical palate reconstructions. J Craniomaxillofac Surg. 2014;42:1310–4. doi:10.1016/j.jcms.2014.03.016. Epub 2014 Apr 2.
65. Hens G, Sell D, Pinkstone M, Birch MJ, Hay N, Sommerlad BC, et al. Palate lengthening by buccinator myomucosal flaps for velopharyngeal insufficiency. Cleft Palate Craniofac J. 2013;50(5):e84–91.
66. Woo SH, Jeong H-S, Kim JP, Park JJ, Ryu J, Baek C-H. Buccinator myomucosal flap for reconstruction of glossectomy defects. Otolaryngol Head Neck Surg. 2013;149(2): 226–31.
67. Licameli GR, Dolan R. Buccinator musculomucosal flap: applications in intraoral reconstruction. Arch Otolaryngol Head Neck Surg. 1998;124(1):69–72.
68. González García R, Naval Gías L, Rodríguez Campo FJ, Escorial Hernández V, Martos PL, Sastre Pérez J, et al. Colgajo miomucoso de buccinador en la reconstrucción de defectos del área maxilofacial. Rev Española Cirugía Oral y Maxilofac. 2005;4:197–205.
69. González-García R, Ruiz-Laza L, Manzano D, Román-Romero L, Moreno C, Monje F. Buccinator myomucosal flap as soft tissue covering for vascularized free fibular flap in anterior maxillary bony defects. J Oral Maxillofac Surg. 2010;68(4):927–30.
70. Massarelli O, Baj A, Gobbi R, Soma D, Marelli S, De Riu G, et al. Cheek mucosa: a versatile donor site of myomucosal flaps. Technical and functional considerations. Head Neck. 2013;35(1):109–17.
71. Van Lierop AC, Fagan JJ. Buccinator myomucosal flap: clinical results and review of anatomy, surgical technique and applications. J Laryngol Otol. 2008;122(2):181–7.
72. Futrell JW, Johns ME, Edgerton MT, Cantrell RW, Fitz-Hugh GS. Platysma myocutaneous flap for intraoral reconstruction. Am J Surg. 1978;136(4):504–7.
73. Hurwitz DJ, Rabson JA, Futrell JW. The anatomic basis for the platysma skin flap. Plast Reconstr Surg. 1983;72(3):302–14.

74. Savoldelli C, Castillo L, Guevara N, Santini J, Odin G. The superior pedicled platysma-myocutaneous flap. Rev Stomatol Chir Maxillofac. 2008;109(2):98–102.
75. Emsen IM. Using platysma myocutaneous flap with Z-plasty for head and neck reconstruction. J Craniofac Surg. 2014;25:e559–60.
76. Eckardt AM. Platysma myocutaneous flap – its current role in reconstructive surgery of oral soft tissue defects. J Korean Assoc Oral Maxillofac Surg. 2013;39(1):3–8.
77. Wang WH, Zhu J, Li M, Xia B, Xu B. Usefulness of platysma muscle flap following superficial parotidectomy. J Craniomaxillofac Surg. 2013;41(1):10–4.
78. Akaraviputh T, Angkurawaranon C, Phanchaipetch T, Lohsiriwat V, Nimmanwudipong T, Chinswangwatanakul V, et al. Platysma myocutaneous flap interposition in surgical management of large acquired post-traumatic tracheoesophageal fistula: a case report. Int J Surg Case Rep. 2014;5(5):282–6. Surgical Associates Ltd.
79. Baur DA, Williams J, Alakaily X. The platysma myocutaneous flap. Oral Maxillofac Surg Clin North Am. 2014;26(3):381–7.
80. Millard DR. Wide and/or short cleft palate. Plast Reconstr Surg Transplant Bull. 1962;29: 40–57.
81. Garner JM, Wein RO. Use of the palatal flap for closure of an oronasal fistula. Am J Otolaryngol. 2006;27(4):268–70.
82. Hernando J, Gallego L, Junquera L, Villarreal P. Oroantral communications. A retrospective analysis. Med Oral Patol Oral Cir Bucal. 2010;15(3):e499–503.
83. Lee JJ, Kok SH, Chang HH, Yang PJ, Hahn LJ, Kuo YS. Repair of oroantral communications in the third molar region by random palatal flap. Int J Oral Maxillofac Surg. 2002;31(6): 677–80.
84. Martinez-Garcia A, Bueno JM. Incisive vessel-based palatal flap for the reconstruction of anterior maxillary soft tissues. Int J Periodontics Restorative Dent. 2011;31(1):83–9.
85. Jamali JA. Palatal flap. Oral Maxillofac Surg Clin North Am. 2014;26(3):305–11.
86. Millard DR, Seider HA. The versatile palatal island flap: its use in soft palate reconstruction and nasopharyngeal and choanal atresia. Br J Plast Surg. 1977;30(4):300–5.
87. Oliver CL, Hackman TG, Carrau RL, Snyderman CH, Kassam AB, Prevedello DM, et al. Palatal flap modifications allow pedicled reconstruction of the skull base. Laryngoscope. 2008;118(12):2102–6.
88. Lee B-K. One-stage operation of large oroantral fistula closure, sinus lifting, and autogenous bone grafting for dental implant installation. Oral Surg Oral Med Oral Pathol Oral Radiol Endod. 2008;105(6):707–13.
89. Ward BB. The palatal flap. Oral Maxillofac Surg Clin North Am. 2003;15(4):467–73, v.
90. Martin D, Pascal JF, Baudet J, Mondie JM, Farhat JB, Athoum A, et al. The submental island flap: a new donor site. Anatomy and clinical applications as a free or pedicled flap. Plast Reconstr Surg. 1993;92(5):867–73.
91. Cheng A, Bui T. Submental island flap. Oral Maxillofac Surg Clin North Am. 2014;26(3): 371–9.
92. Ferrari S, Copelli C, Bianchi B, Magri AS, Ferri A, Varazzani A, et al. The submental island flap: pedicle elongation and indications in head and neck reconstruction. J Craniomaxillofac Surg. 2014;42(6):1005–9.
93. Safdar J, Liu F-Y, Moosa Y, Xu Z-F, Li Z-N, Sun C-F, et al. Submental versus platysma flap for the reconstruction of complex facial defects following resection of head and neck tumors. Pak J Med Sci. 2014;30(4):739–44.
94. Burić N, Krasić D, Pesić Z, Jovanović G. Microvascular submental island flap prelaminated with oral mucosa in reconstruction of the lateral defect of nose. Med Pregl. 2010;63(9–10): 723–7.
95. Howard BE, Nagel TH, Donald CB, Hinni ML, Hayden RE. Oncologic safety of the submental flap for reconstruction in oral cavity malignancies. Otolaryngol Head Neck Surg. 2014;150(4):558–62.
96. Rahpeyma A, Khajehahmadi S. Oral reconstruction with submental flap. Ann Maxillofac Surg. 2013;3(2):144–7.

97. Chen W-L, Ye J-T, Yang Z-H, Huang Z-Q, Zhang D-M, Wang K. Reverse facial artery-submental artery mandibular osteomuscular flap for the reconstruction of maxillary defects following the removal of benign tumors. Head Neck. 2009;31(6):725–31.
98. Martin D, Coeugniet E, Ladu G, Mahoudeau C. Use of a submental flap for reconstruction of both lips in a complex case of mutilation. Ann Chir Plast Esthet. 2013;58(6):704–7.
99. Bianchi B, Ferri A, Ferrari S, Copelli C, Ferri T, Sesenna E. Iliac crest free flap and submental island flap for maxillary reconstruction. J Plast Surg Hand Surg. 2013;47(6):538–42.
100. Rahpeyma A, Khajehahmadi S. Onlay bone grafting simultaneous with facial soft tissue augmentation in a hemifacial microsomia patient using de-epithelialized orthograde submental flap: a technical note. Ann Stomatol (Roma). 2014;5(1):30–3.
101. Chow T-L, Choi C-Y, Ho L-I, Fung S-C. The use of bipaddled submental flap for reconstructing composite buccal defect. J Maxillofac Oral Surg. 2014;13(1):75–7.
102. Wang J-G, Chen W-L, Ye H-S, Yang Z-H, Chai Q. Reverse facial artery-submental artery deepithelialised submental island flap to reconstruct maxillary defects following cancer ablation. J Craniomaxillofac Surg. 2011;39(7):499–502.
103. Bertrand B, Foletti J-M, Noël W, Duron J-B, Bardot J. Submental island flap: a review of the literature. Ann Chir Plast Esthet. 2015;60:44–53.

Functional Implant-Supported Dental Rehabilitation in Oncologic Patients

6

Santiago Jose Ochandiano Caicoya, Carlos Navarro Cuellar, Julio Acero Sanz, and Carlos Navarro Vila

Abstract

Functional restoration of the oral cavity after ablative surgery to treat cancer is one of the main challenges facing the head and neck surgeon. Reconstruction of teeth and bone and rehabilitation of occlusion play a key role in restoring quality of life. Osseointegrated implants have revolutionized reconstructive treatment in patients with cancer of the oral cavity, since they enable stabilization of dental prostheses.

S.J. Ochandiano Caicoya, MD, DDS, FEBOMS (✉)
Consultant at Oral and Maxillofacial Surgery Department, Gregorio Marañón General University Hospital, Madrid, Spain
e-mail: sochandiano@hotmail.com

C. Navarro Cuellar, MD, DDS, FEBOMS

Associate Professor Medical Faculty, Complutense University of Madrid, Madrid, Spain

Consultant at Oral and Maxillofacial Surgery Department, Gregorio Marañón General University Hospital, Madrid, Spain
e-mail: cnavarrocuellar@gmail.com

J. Acero Sanz, MD, DDS, PhD, FEBOMS
Head of Oral and Maxillofacial Surgery Department, Ramón y Cajal University Hospital, Madrid, Spain

Associate Professor of Alcalá University of Madrid, Madrid, Spain
e-mail: j-acero@telefonica.net

C. Navarro Vila, MD, DMD, PhD, FEBOMS
Full Professor Medical Faculty, Complutense University of Madrid, Madrid, Spain

Head of Oral and Maxillofacial Department Surgery, Gregorio Marañón General University Hospital, Madrid, Spain

Académico Correspondiente of the Royal National Academy of Medicine of Spain, Madrid, Spain
e-mail: cnavarro.vila@clinicanavarrovila.com

C. Navarro Vila (ed.), *Reconstructive Oral and Maxillofacial Surgery*,
DOI 10.1007/978-3-319-20487-1_6

Our surgical team analyzes the situation of each patient and assesses the need for extraction in completely or partially edentulous patients, the indication for implants to support prostheses, and the placement of implants in a primary or secondary procedure.

Functional restoration of the oral cavity after ablative surgery to treat cancer is one of the main challenges facing the head and neck surgeon [1].

Tumor resection entails a loss of the normal anatomical structure (shape and volume), which can be corrected using microsurgical or pedicle free flaps to reconstruct lost tissue with similar tissue. Defects must be addressed on an individual basis depending on whether they comprise bone and soft tissue or simply soft tissue. Reconstruction can be based on bone, soft tissue, or both. Reconstruction techniques have made it possible to design several types of flap (skin, muscle, and bone) that enable 3-dimensional repair of oromandibular defects resulting from tumor resection. Although reconstruction of mandibular continuity defects improves facial harmony, restoration of function requires dental rehabilitation [2].

Restoring function is very difficult, even with appropriate anatomic reconstruction.

The oral cavity and the lower facial third are key areas when restoring cosmesis and function. When facial anatomy is altered, important social functions such as chewing, swallowing, and phonation are irreversibly affected. Combination with radiation therapy can worsen complications and functional alterations [3].

In 1991, Urken [4] stated that the objectives of functional reconstruction were the following:

- Primary restoration of bone continuity with rigid fixed vascularized bone
- Immediate placement of osseointegrated implants in order to ensure rapid rehabilitation of occlusion
- Placement of thin and pliable tissue for reconstruction of the floor of the mouth and tongue
- Restoration of sensation in soft tissue: labial sensation and competence, restoration of sensation in intraoral tissue

Therefore, reconstruction of teeth and bone and rehabilitation of occlusion play a key role in restoring quality of life. Unlike reconstruction of other parts of the oral cavity, repair of the osseodental unit also has the enormous advantage that the dental rehabilitation and occlusion achieved are similar to before resection; in other words, the patient's ability to chew is much the same as before surgery. In 2006, Roumanas et al. [5] showed that tumor resection was followed by a considerable reduction in the ability to chew. However, this function was restored after microsurgical reconstruction and conventional dental rehabilitation of both the affected and the nonaffected side. Furthermore, if dental rehabilitation is with prostheses placed on implants, recovery of function is much better on both sides. The improvement in function is statistically significant.

Osseointegrated implants have revolutionized reconstructive treatment in patients with cancer of the oral cavity, since they enable stabilization of dental prostheses. Thus, we can achieve real cosmetic and functional rehabilitation. Placement of osseointegrated dental implants in patients with defects of the maxillofacial region has been common practice for the last 5 years. Riediger [4] was the first author to fit delayed implants in microsurgical flaps and Urken [4] the first to fit implants immediately during the bone reconstruction procedure.

The patient must be made aware of the immediate and delayed effects of radiation therapy on the oral cavity. One of the earliest effects (during the first or second week) is intense mucositis, followed by xerostomia (loss of up to 99 % of normal salivary flow), loss of the sensation of taste, and aggressive caries. Later effects include trismus and fibrosis, which further complicate appropriate rehabilitation of oral function [6].

The support, retention, and stability of a dental prosthesis after surgery and radiation therapy can be severely altered, and bone regeneration is also diminished; therefore, conventional prostheses offer no real solutions to cancer patients.

Implant-supported and implant-retained rehabilitation is the only valid alternative when restoring cosmesis and function.

Few studies provide long-term results in large patient populations. One of the reasons for this lack of data is that long-term survival continues to be low, despite advances in surgery and adjuvant therapy. In this chapter, we will address several controversial issues concerning the effect on implants of factors such as radiation therapy, the reconstructive method used, the type of bone flap, optimal time for fitting implants, and the approach to dental rehabilitation.

We present our experience in dental rehabilitation of cancer patients at the Oral and Maxillofacial Surgery Department, Hospital General Universitario Gregorio Marañón, Madrid, Spain, over the last 24 years (1990–2014). The study population includes 216 patients (155 men, 61 women) who received a total of 1665 implants.

Eighty-five percent of the patients were treated for malignant neoplasm; the most common tumor was squamous cell cancer. The remaining 15 % were treated for odontogenic tumors, mainly ameloblastoma. As for location, 21 cases involved the maxilla, and the remainder the mandible, lower alveolar ridge, gums, buccal mucosa, tongue, floor of the mouth, and oropharynx.

Mean age was 52 years (range, 18–84 years). Follow-up of the implants and dental rehabilitation ranged between 9 months and 23 years.

Of the 216 patients, 199 were treated with dental prostheses. Rehabilitation was impossible in 17 patients (death immediately after surgery, locoregional recurrence, early distant metastasis, lack of patient cooperation, and severe functional and anatomic limitations).

We used free microsurgical grafts in 135 patients, fibula flaps in 68, iliac crest flaps in 41, radial forearm flaps in 17, scapula flaps in 3, rectus abdominis flaps in 3, and anterolateral thigh flaps in 3. We used pectoralis major pedicle flaps in 18 patients, trapezius osteomyocutaneous flaps in 16, and temporalis muscle flaps in 10. The reconstruction was performed with local nasolabial flaps, buccinator flaps, or direct closure in 19 cases. In 11 cases, the patients were not treated using surgery, but with radiation therapy with(out) adjuvant chemotherapy administered systemically or intra-arterially. Finally, we used vertical and horizontal distraction osteogenesis in five cases for both the maxilla and the mandible. In a group of five patients with maxillary tumors (Brown type I and II, unilateral and bilateral), soft tissue was reconstructed and closed without using bone, and the occlusion was restored by means of zygomatic implants to support and retain the dental prostheses.

Until 1999, we used cylindrical hydroxyapatite-coated impacted implants (408 implants). From 1999 onwards, we used titanium screw implants, and from 2006 until the present, we have used RBM-treated screw implants (MG Osseous, Mozo-Grau®). All the implants had the external hex connection.

Adjuvant radiation therapy was administered to 149 patients (69 %). A total of 1113 implants were fitted during the primary procedure (ablative and reconstructive surgery, before radiation therapy [507 implants]) or during the secondary procedure (at least 12 months after radiation therapy [606 implants]). We used hyperbaric oxygen before fitting the implants in only three patients. With respect to the results of osseointegration in patients who received radiation therapy, we can observe a difference between pre-2006 results and subsequent results. Until 2006, we used hydroxyapatite-coated implants or plasma-coated titanium implants in 57 patients (342 implants [160 primary, 182 secondary]). The success rate was 96.2 % (6 failures in 160) in the primary implants and 88.47 % (21 failures in 182) in the secondary implants. From 2006 onwards, we used 771 RBM-coated implants (Mozo-Grau®) in order to improve the position and orientation of the implant depending on the prosthesis chosen for each patient. Thus, slightly under half were fitted during the primary procedure (347/771), and the remainder during the secondary procedure (424/771). The success rate of osseointegration in this group from 2006 onwards was 94.25 %, with no significant differences between the primary and secondary groups.

The osseointegration period in patients not receiving radiation therapy was of the usual duration, i.e., 3 months for the mandible and four for the maxilla. However, this period was twice as long in patients undergoing radiation therapy. The second phase was with local anesthesia at the outpatient clinic. In patients who had received radiation therapy, we tried to ensure that this phase was minimally traumatic, with incisions as small as possible and minimal detachment of gum tissue.

In 45 % of cases, the implants were fitted in the bony component of the flap; in the remaining 55 %, they were fitted in the remnant bone.

The best results were observed for microsurgical bone flaps. Thus, the success rate was 92–94 % for the fibula flap and iliac crest flap and almost 90 % for the scapula flap. The poorest results (30 % failure rate) were recorded for the trapezius osteomyocutaneous flap, in which two-thirds of implants were fitted after radiation therapy. Implants fitted in remnant bone were successful in 80–90 % of cases. We found poorer results for osseointegration in the maxilla than in the mandible, although the differences were not significant. Zygomatic implants performed particularly well, even in patients who underwent radiation therapy, among whom the success rate was 100 %.

Of all the implants fitted, 15 % (250/1665) could not hold prostheses. We can distinguish between two subgroups. The first subgroup comprised 17 patients with 51 implants who could not undergo rehabilitation because of locoregional recurrence, second primary cancer, distance metastasis, flap loss, or death from causes not associated with the tumor. The second group comprised 199 implants that could not be used because of poor positioning and patients whose rehabilitation was possible but not functional because of limited tongue movement, severe trismus, labial incompetence, dysphagia, and lack of patient cooperation in long-term maintenance. Consequently, in some cases, the prosthesis had to be withdrawn.

Three weeks after the second phase, we took impressions using customized open impression trays.

The rehabilitation technique has varied in recent years. During the initial phase, our usual choice was overdentures; however, during the last 8 years, we have used fixed screws. We sometimes use metal–porcelain structures, the most common design being fixed hybrid metal–resin prostheses with no mucous support or acrylic flanges that hide soft tissue, thus making it easier to detect recurrence. Our experience from the last 24 years shows that 70 % of our prostheses were fixed and 30 % movable overdentures. However, from 2006 onwards, the number of fixed prostheses increased to the extent that this approach is now used in 90 % of cases.

The success rate of osseointegration is almost 90 % in the 216 cancer patients we treated with implants, including patients who received radiation therapy and those who did not. Most failures were not due to poor osseointegration but to loss of the patient because of recurrences, second primary cancer, metastasis, or lack of cooperation during follow-up. Of the 216 patients selected for implants, 199 reached the prosthesis phase. Prostheses were supported in the vast majority of patients, although during the initial phases of our experience, poorly positioned sleeping implants were more common than now. Despite successful osseointegration and suitable dental rehabilitation, the prostheses had to be removed in ten patients because of poor functional outcome in chewing and swallowing due to severe trismus, lingual incompetence, and loss of tongue mobility.

Data from our series are shown in Table 6.1.

6.1 Discussion

The discussion is based on our experience.

6.1.1 What Type of Implant Should Be Used: Smooth Machined Surface, Rough Surface, or Very Rough Surface?

Few studies have examined the effect of surface, size, or length to ensure better osseointegration in cancer patients.

In 2007, Nelson et al. [7] used four-implant systems in 93 cancer patients. Two had a smooth machined surface (Bränemark®, Steri-Oss®) and two had a rough surface (Camlog®, Straumann®). No significant differences were found in the success rate of osseointegration.

In 2010, Heberer et al. [8] studied 20 cancer patients who received radiation therapy with adjuvant chemotherapy. Six months after adjuvant therapy, a total of 120 modified and conventional sandblasted acid-etched implants were fitted in the

Table 6.1 Dental Implants placed at Gregorio Marañón General University Hospital

Bone resection	No of cases	Reconstructive technique	Radiotherapy	Implants	Implants in bone flaps	Implants in remnant bone	Primary implants	Osseointegrated implants	Failed implants
Segmental mandibular	68	Fibula flap	419	581	406	175	0 %	550 (94.8 %)	31
Segmental mandibular	41	Iliac crest flap (deep circumflex iliac artery)	278	399	283	116	399 (100 %)	369 (92.6 %)	30
Segmental mandibular	18	Pectoralis major flap	59	101	0	101	24 (23.7 %)	87 (86 %)	14
No resection or marginal mandibular	17	Radial forearm flap	89	134	0	134	33 (25 %)	118 (88 %)	16
Segmental mandibular	16	Osteomyocutaneous trapezius flap	81	88	52	36	27 (31 %)	61 (69 %)	26 (29.5 %)
Hemimaxillectomy or less	10	Temporalis flap	41	66	0	66	0 %	49 (75 %)	17
High maxillectomy	5	Zygomatic implants and soft tissue closure	3	13		13	3 (25 %)	100 % zygoma	0
Any resection or no bone resection	19	Local soft tissue flap (nasolabial, buccinator, direct closure)	43	141		141	17 (12 %)	131 (93 %)	10
Marginal or segmental mandibular	3	Scapular flap	9	17	5	12	0 %	15 (88 %)	2
Any soft tissue resection or no bone resection	6	Rectus abdominis flap, ALT flap	26	36	4	32	4 (11 %)	28 (77 %)	8
Marginal mandibular or maxillary	3	Vertical distraction osteogenesis	0	16	7	9	0 %	14 (88 %)	2

Bone resection	No of cases	Reconstructive technique	Radiotherapy	Implants	Implants in bone flaps	Implants in remnant bone	Primary implants	Osseointegrated implants	Failed implants
Segmental mandibular	2	Horizontal distraction osteogenesis	0	8	7	1	0 %	7	1
No surgery. RT+ – chemo, intra-arterial chemo + RT	11	Chemo + RT	65	65	0	65	0 %	53 (82 %)	12
	216		1113 (149 patients)	1665	764 (45 %)	901 (55 %)	507	1496 (89.84 %)	169

mandible of all 20 patients. The mean success rate at 1 year was 96 % for the conventional implants and 100 % for the modified implants. Both surfaces presented bone loss at the implant shoulder (0.3–0.4 mm). The authors concluded that both surfaces were highly successful in irradiated bone and that the results for the modified surface were better because they were more hydrophilic and had high surface energy.

In 2011, Buddula et al. [9] performed a 21-year retrospective study of 48 patients with 271 implants fitted in areas that had received a minimum of 50 Gy and concluded that the smooth machined surface implants failed 2.9 times more than those with a rough surface. In addition, the machined surface implants failed more frequently in the maxilla than in the mandible and more in posterior than in anterior sectors. Smooth implants with a diameter of ≤3.75 mm failed more frequently than those with a diameter of ≥4 mm. However, in the rough implants, no association was found between failure and location (maxilla-mandible, anterior-posterior), bone quality, or implant diameter and length.

In 2012, Fenlon et al. [10] analyzed 41 patients with 145 implants fitted on 47 flaps and concluded that the survival of implants with a microrough surface is better that that of implants with a macrorough or smooth surface.

In 2014, Gander et al. [11] reported results for 136 microrough Astra® implants placed in 33 patients, 21 of whom had received radiation therapy at least 1 year before the implants were fitted. In this subgroup, 12 of 84 implants failed. The differences between these patients and those who did not receive radiation therapy were not significant.

The initial results of our experience with hydroxyapatite-coated impacted implants (until 1999) were very good in terms of osseointegration, even in irradiated bone. However, we did observe a progressive loss of load-bearing implants, as described by Albrektssön [12], mainly owing to treatment-refractory peri-implantitis. We believe that once this implant becomes contaminated, the surface roughness hampers treatment considerably and cannot prevent peri-implant bone loss.

Therefore, in 2006 we decided to switch to screwed models with a rough titanium surface. The new RBM-treated surfaces, which have a mean roughness of 1.4 Ra, have led to osseointegration rates close to those of noncancer patients, even in patients who have received radiation therapy. No progressive loss of load-bearing implants was observed during follow-up. Furthermore, peri-implantitis is much less frequent.

6.1.2 Which Type of Prosthesis Is Preferred in Cancer Patients?

No consensus has been reached on which is the best prosthesis for rehabilitation of cancer patients. In fact, several authors report on surgical outcome and osseointegration of implants, although few report successful functional rehabilitation. In 2008, Smölka et al. [13] reported that successful osseointegration of implants is one thing, whereas the ability of implants to support a genuinely useful and functional prosthesis is another. The authors found that a 92 % success rate fell to 42.9 % owing to factors such as recurrence and lack of patient cooperation.

The ideal prosthesis in cancer patients is one that prevents lesions of the soft tissue while simultaneously providing appropriate support, retention, and stability. Therefore, in our opinion, prostheses should be implant retained and implant supported. In 1999, Weischer and Mohr [14] described how they modified their rehabilitation protocol in cancer patients during the 1990s. The authors switched from combined mucosa-implant-supported prostheses to exclusively implant-supported prostheses owing to mucosal lesions associated with the prosthesis in patients who had undergone radiation therapy, mainly osteoradionecrosis that began through infection of traumatic mucosal ulcers.

In 2006, Garrett et al. [15] defended their use of overdentures in preference to implants in cancer patients. They gave the following explanations for their preference:

1. By sacrificing the marginal nerve and inferior dental nerve during ablation, the lower lip retracts, thus compromising speech and closure to prevent the escape of saliva. The flange of the overdenture repositions the lower lip towards the front, thus improving congruence with the upper lip.
2. The flange of the prosthesis improves facial appearance by supporting and projecting the lip in the same way as the tooth or the original alveolar ridge.
3. The overdenture enables better daily hygiene and maintenance, thus minimizing problems affecting the soft tissue.
4. In cases where function and mobility of the tongue are compromised, a removable prosthesis allows the teeth to be placed more posteriorly, thus enabling better management of the food bolus by the remnant tongue.
5. Removable prostheses are much less expensive than fixed prostheses.

In 2007, Nelson et al. [7] reported results from the rehabilitation of 93 cancer patients (68 with rigid bar-retained overdentures and 25 with fixed implant-supported prostheses). Problems with the overdenture retention clip in 11 of the 68 patients required regular management. Moreover, in two patients, movement of the prosthesis led to mucosal ulcers. No maintenance complications were detected in the patients with fixed implant-supported prostheses; therefore, the authors recommended using fixed prostheses where possible.

By contrast, Kovacs [16] and Linsen et al. [17] (in 2000 and 2009, respectively) found no differences between overdentures and fixed prostheses in terms of which was the best prosthetic solution.

Mancha de la Plata et al. [18] found a better cosmetic and functional outcome with fixed screwed prosthesis in their series of 30 patients who had undergone radiation therapy. In 2014, Fang et al. [19], on the other hand, found a better functional and cosmetic outcome with removable prostheses, since these better compensated for soft tissue defects, although they also reported several advantages of fixed rehabilitation, stating that the ideal prosthetic solution should be carefully designed on an individual basis.

We currently favor implant-supported implant-retained fixed rehabilitation, with neither contact nor support from the mucosa. This is the approach of choice in 90 % of the patients we treat. We only use overdentures when we have fewer than four implants per dental arch, in cases of large soft tissue defect (poor tongue mobility, defective lip support), or when there is a considerable increase in the interarch space that forces us to use excessively bulky fixed structures.

The occlusion of choice in fixed prosthesis is that which is mutually protected with minimum contact in the cantilevered areas; in the case of removable prosthesis, we prefer balanced occlusion.

6.1.3 How Many Implants Should Be Fitted? Does Anatomic Location Affect the Success of the Implant?

The consensus in the literature is that to avoid gum lesions and ensure an adequate fit of implant-supported and implant-retained prostheses, it is necessary to fit 4–6 implants per arch [20, 21].

In fibula-based reconstructions, Smölka et al. [13] recommend at least five implants for fixed rehabilitation with "Bränemark-like" ceramic or resin structures. With fewer implants, it is possible to use overdentures with bar or ball attachments (O-ring) or telescopic overdentures. Magnetic abutments are not recommended.

The ideal number of implants for overdentures is the same as for noncancer patients and has been reported to be between two and four [47, 22].

The anatomic location of the implant seems to be important in patients undergoing radiation therapy. Thus, Visch et al. [23] conclude that location is the dominant variable when assessing the success of osseointegration. Better outcomes have been reported in the mandible than in the maxilla and in anterior rather than posterior sectors. Nooh et al [24] offer an overall success rate of 78.9 % in the maxilla and 93.3 % in the mandible. This better outcome in the mandible is generally attributed to the greater bone density and better blood supply in this area [25]. Several studies report 100 % success with implants fitted in the maxilla [8] or similar results for both the maxilla and the mandible [7].

In our department, therefore, the ideal minimum number of implants to ensure fixed rehabilitation is 4–6; when there are fewer, we recommend overdentures. As we generally try to use fixed prostheses, we fit between four and six implants in the edentulous mandible and six in the edentulous maxilla.

We generally fit the implants in the anterior sector; in the posterior sector, we usually fit the last implant in the area of the first and second premolars. Therefore, our rehabilitation procedures usually involve a single premolar and a molar. Although implants can be fitted more distally, such an approach is not useful in prosthetic terms, since these areas are difficult to access owing to limited mouth opening. In addition, hygiene and maintenance are somewhat complicated in the posterior areas for the same reason. Therefore, we generally try to avoid these areas.

6.1.4 Does Radiation Therapy Affect Osseointegration of Implants in Cancer Patients?

In the initial era of implant surgery, radiation therapy was considered an absolute contraindication when fitting implants [26].

Ionizing radiation produces energy that damages or destroys cells by impairing nuclear DNA or altering the molecular characteristics of isolated cells. Radiation therapy in the oral cavity leads to changes in the bone and soft tissue. It affects bone cells and vascularization and reduces remodeling ability through damage to osteoblasts, osteocytes, and osteoclasts. In the case of osteoblasts and osteocytes, the ability of new bone to divide and synthesize is diminished. However, the osteoclasts continue to reabsorb to the extent that bone loss is faster than new bone formation. Radiation damages vessels first through hyperemia, then by endarteritis, thrombosis, and progressive occlusion until the capillaries are obliterated. Consequently, the number of bone marrow cells and bone vascularization are diminished, leading to fibrosis and fatty degeneration of bone marrow.

In the case of soft tissue, oral mucosa, gums, and glands, radiation therapy leads to inflammation, altered salivary composition, reduced amount of saliva, gum detachment, and changes in oral flora. Consequently, function is worsened and the risk of osteonecrosis increases.

Recent systematic reviews show that the risk of osteoradionecrosis is low (2 %) and that this complication is more likely during the first 2 years after radiation therapy. The risk increases with the number of procedures affecting the bone, such as tooth extraction, and in patients with poor oral health and hygiene [27, 28].

In experimental animal studies, Arnold et al. [29] used rat femur and Brasseur et al. [30] used dog mandible to show that the capacity for remodeling and osseointegration was not affected in animals that first receive implants and then radiation therapy. The results were in fact poorer in animals that first received radiation therapy and then implants. Furthermore, mineral distribution and porosity were more heterogeneous in irradiated bone. Despite these effects in dogs, osteons form correctly and osseointegration is achieved, even in bone that is irradiated before implants are fitted, provided that the implants are fitted at a later period (6 months after radiation therapy is complete according to Brasseur et al.). Schweiger [31] found similar results with dog mandibles and concluded that osseointegration was possible. By contrast, Larsen et al. [32] recorded a poorer performance with rabbit tibia and a reduction in the osseointegration surface of the implant in irradiated bone not treated with hyperbaric oxygen.

In a human postmortem histopathology study, Bolind et al. [33] examined implants fitted in irradiated bone and showed that osseointegration had occurred. These authors calculated that the mean contact surface was only 40 %: the normal percentage in nonirradiated bone was 80 % for the mandible and 60 % for the maxilla. A positive correlation was found between the figure for bone–implant contact and time between radiation therapy and placement of the implants. The authors concluded that if sufficient time is left after radiation therapy, human bone can recover part of its capacity for remodeling and achieve osseointegration.

In 2009, Ihde et al. [34] carried out a literature review of all experimental animal studies and studies of patients who had received radiation therapy and implants. They concluded that patients who receive radiation therapy have a two- to threefold greater relative risk of losing implants than nonirradiated patients.

The osseointegration surface (peri-implant trabecular bone) was analyzed by Marxand Morales [35] after 4 months in transplanted bone, normal mandible, and irradiated bone. Seventy-two percent of the implant–bone interface in transplanted bone was occupied by new bone tissue. New bone tissue accounted for 50 % of normal bone and 40 % of irradiated bone; in both cases, the tissue was sufficient to support occlusal loading. Based on Marx [36], hyperbaric oxygen was used to induce neoangiogenesis and increase fibroblast activity, thus ensuring increased partial pressure of oxygen in previously hypoxemic and ischemic irradiated areas. The standard protocol comprises 30 sessions (20 before implantation and 10 after surgery) with hyperbaric oxygen (100 %, at 2.4 atm, 90 min per session).

The series presented by Taylor and Worthington [37] in 1993 comprised 21 implants in previously irradiated mandibular bone. No implants were lost at the end of follow-up (3–7 years).

The series reported in 1998 by Niimi et al. [38] comprised 228 implants placed in irradiated maxillas in the United States and Japan. The success rate was 98 % in the case of irradiated mandibles that underwent hyperbaric oxygen therapy. The corresponding success rate in the upper jaw was 72 %. Ali et al. [39] reported a 60 % success rate in the upper jaw and a 100 % success rate in the lower jaw. In the study by Eckert et al. [40], the survival rate was 64 % in the maxilla and 99 % in the mandible.

In 2007, Nelson et al. [7] studied 93 patients, 29 of whom had undergone radiation therapy. Implant survival in the radiation therapy group was 84 % at 46 months and 54 % at 13 years. No statistically significant differences in osseointegration were found between patients who had received radiation therapy and those who had not.

Linsen et al. [17] found a 94 % implant survival rate in irradiated bone after 10 years. The authors stated that failure occurred mainly during the osseointegration phase (some months immediately after the implants were fitted) and that osteoradionecrosis associated with implants was exceptional.

In their retrospective study of 48 patients who received implants in previously irradiated bone (≥50 Gy), Buddula et al. [41] recorded survival rates of 98.9, 89.9, and 72.3 % at 1, 5, and 10 years, suggesting that osseointegration was progressively lost over the years. Furthermore, failure was much more common in the maxilla than in the mandible (success rate of 80.5 % in the maxilla vs. 93.6 % in the mandible at 5 years). No differences were found between implants fitted on irradiated remnant bone or irradiated flap bone.

In their series of 335 implants and 30 patients, Mancha de la Plata et al. [18] recorded osseointegration in 92.6 % of cases at 5 years in patients who had previously received radiation therapy. In the subgroup of patients with osteoradionecrosis, the success rate fell to 48.3 %.

In 2013, Chambrone et al. [42] carried out a systematic review of implants fitted in irradiated native bone (not flaps) and concluded that radiation therapy has a clearly negative effect on implant survival. They found a 174 % greater possibility of failure when the implants were fitted in irradiated bone. Furthermore, implants fitted in the maxilla had a 496 % greater risk of failure than those fitted in the mandible. Treatment with hyperbaric oxygen provided no survival benefit for implants in cancer patients.

In 2013, Tanaka et al. [25] reviewed and updated findings for implants in cancer patients who had received radiation therapy and found a success rate that increased from 74.4 to 98.9 % and was greater than 84 % in most studies. Both implants and rehabilitation with prostheses were successful.

Zheng et al. [43] proposed three different approaches to improve the condition of irradiated bone: hyperbaric oxygen, bone morphogenetic protein (BMP-2), and osteogenic growth peptide. The authors warned that there was no evidence in favor of these approaches and that they should be used on an individual basis.

An interesting observation was made by Gander et al. [11] in their study of 21 patients who had received radiation therapy that the radiation technique can affect osseointegration, since six implants failed in the only two patients who received conventional radiotherapy. Only six failures of osseointegration were recorded in the remaining 19 patients, who received intensity-modulated radiation therapy.

In our series, the overall success of osseointegration for implants fitted in irradiated bone was very high, close to 95 %, consistent with results in the literature for patients who did not receive hyperbaric oxygen. Most failures in patients who have received radiation therapy are due to locoregional recurrence, distant metastasis, second primary cancer, or diseases other than cancer.

The risk of osteoradionecrosis in the mandible after placement of implants was minimal in our series. We detected mandibular necrosis associated with an implant in only two patients. In both cases, pain and an orocervical fistula were observed in the parasymphysis. In one of these cases, hyperbaric oxygen was used before surgery to treat the complication, which involved withdrawal of the implant and curettage of the area affected accompanied by appropriate long-term antibiotic therapy. The complication resolved with no further sequelae.

6.1.5 When Should Implants Be Fitted? When Is the Optimal Time for the Second Phase?

Prosthodontic rehabilitation of cancer patients should be planned as a normal part of treatment and therefore included in the treatment schedule before ablative surgery.

The cancer team choose the optimal therapeutic approach based on the following:

- The characteristics of the tumor (histology, TNM classification, and imaging studies [computed tomography])
- The defect of the bone and soft tissue after ablative surgery
- The appropriate method of reconstruction to repair the defect and restore function
- The potential need for complementary radiation therapy

The prosthodontics team can estimate the effects of these factors on oral function and the potential difficulties involved in fitting a prosthesis (loss of the neutral zone, i.e., the available dynamic space for fitting a prosthesis between the lip, cheek, and tongue, as well as alterations in tongue mobility, lip closure, and mandibular mobility) [3].

Once the anatomic alteration expected after ablative surgery is known and reconstruction of contour and function is planned, the dental prosthesis must be chosen. Ideally, this is implant supported, and the optimal position for the implants depends on the prosthesis to be fitted.

The experience of the cancer team makes it possible to move from the initial situation, in which implants are placed where feasible, to one where choice and optimal placement of the microsurgical flap depend on prosthodontic rehabilitation and the implants that will make it possible. In other words, the reconstruction of soft and hard tissue should be guided by function and occlusal rehabilitation.

There is no consensus in the literature on the ideal time for placement of an implant. Depending on the relationship between administration of radiation therapy and placement of implants, a primary implant is defined as that which is placed before radiation therapy (during ablative and reconstructive surgery) and a secondary implant as that which is placed in tissue that has already been irradiated, irrespective of whether administration was recent or not.

When the need for adjuvant radiation therapy is foreseeable, many authors recommend primary implants [44, 45]. The advantages they report are as follows:

- The time from placement of the flap and implant until initiation of radiation therapy should be at least 6 weeks. The time between initiation of radiation therapy and the onset of deleterious effects on the bone is also 6 weeks. Therefore, when the bone surrounding the implant experiences the effects of radiation therapy, we can say that osseointegration has occurred.
- The success rate of osseointegration increases if the implant has no abnormalities of vascularization or capacity for regeneration.
- The morbidity of a second procedure can be avoided, as can potential complications of soft tissue and bone (risk of osteonecrosis).
- Functional rehabilitation is faster: patients can benefit from dental rehabilitation within the first year after surgery and thus enjoy a better quality of life sooner.
- Costs are reduced by obviating the need for hyperbaric oxygen.

However, primary implants also have disadvantages. Authors who do not favor primary implants warn of the following drawbacks [46]:

- Better long-term assessment of postsurgical function and, therefore, better selection of candidates who can genuinely benefit from prostheses fitted on implants
- Intraoperative difficulty deciding on the optimal position of the implants depending on the prostheses
- Problems with the thickness of the soft tissue and possible complications of osseointegration in the case of dehiscence, delays in scarring, and postsurgical infection
- Implants that will not be functional because of early recurrence. We know that 80 % of locoregional recurrences occur during the first 2–4 years of survival.
- Similarly, despite appropriate osseointegration and survival, some implants will not support a prosthesis owing to comorbidity or the fact that anatomic and functional abnormalities are so severe (minimum tongue mobility, lip incompetence,

velopharyngeal insufficiency) that, even in cases with successful occlusal rehabilitation, chewing and swallowing are impossible.

In general, our experience with primary implants is very useful, but if we are unsure of the correct position for an implant, we do not place it. However, this situation becomes increasingly rare as the surgeon gains experience. Very thick or very scant soft tissue was once problematic for rehabilitation. However, we can now use a series of procedures to refine this tissue and thus overcome associated difficulties.

Cost is one of the main reasons against primary implants; however, we defend this approach, even if medium-term expectations are limited. In advanced stages III and IV in the oral cavity, 5-year survival is 40–50 %, (Blanchard et al. [47]); however, in the literature, the need for immediate reconstruction is accepted in the vast majority of cases [47], even though we know that one of every two patients will die within the first 5 years after surgery. The same could be said of dental rehabilitation, which is yet another phase of reconstructive treatment and one that provides patients with a clearly improved quality of life, albeit for a short period.

Schoen et al. [48] report that in advanced stages, the disadvantages are less important. Therefore, they recommend immediate placement of implants in all patients treated with curative intent.

In their 7-year retrospective study, Schepers et al. [22] analyzed 139 implants in the intraforaminal region of the mandible during ablative surgery. In 61 cases, the patient received complementary radiation therapy. Osseointegration was successful in 97 % of implants that were subsequently irradiated and 100 % in those that were not. The success rate for prostheses was 75 %; the remaining 25 % of implants failed owing to recurrence, early metastasis, or other causes.

In their 2011 systematic review, Barber et al. [46] found the success rate for primary implants to range between 96 and 100 %. In 2008, Schoen et al. [48] carried out a prospective quality of life study in 50 cancer patients undergoing rehabilitation with primary implants in the remnant interforaminal region of the mandible. Only 35 received overdentures. Twelve of those who did not receive implants died within 12 months of surgery. No complications were reported, and osseointegration was successful in 97 % of cases, irrespective of whether the patient received adjuvant radiation therapy. Quality of life is generally better in patients who undergo surgery without radiation therapy than in those who receive radiation therapy, and the functional improvement gained with implants is also better in patients who have not undergone radiotherapy. Therefore, the key factor for quality of life is the complications arising from radiation therapy and not primary placement of implants, for which osseointegration rates are almost normal. The authors defend primary placement, since even patients who have received radiation therapy benefit from rehabilitation with implants 10 months after surgery; if implants are placed in a secondary procedure, this interval at least doubles. They conclude that in any cancer treatment administered with curative intent, placement of implants should be evaluated, and if these are chosen, they should be fitted in a primary procedure where possible.

As for secondary placement, Visch et al. [23] concluded that 6 months after radiation therapy, there are no differences in implant survival, regardless of whether they are fitted at 1 year or at 4 years. In a systematic review, Colella et al. [49] found no statistically significant differences between primary and secondary implants and concluded that placement of implants should be based on other variables. In 2013, Mizbah et al. [50] presented the results of a retrospective study with two groups of patients who differed according to whether their implants were fitted in a primary or secondary procedure. No significant differences in implant survival were found between the groups (9 % failure of osseointegration for both groups). In the case of primary implants, 82 % could support prostheses; in secondary implants, this percentage increased to 93 %, perhaps because implantation was more accurate. Nevertheless, patients treated with primary implants benefit from prostheses at least 20 months before those treated with secondary implants (7 months compared with 27). Furthermore, 17 % of primary implants and 4 % of secondary implants are never used owing to early recurrence, soft tissue complications, or trismus. The authors conclude that the 20-month advantage in rehabilitation compensates for the expense of new procedures and the 17 % of primary implants that are not functional.

In 2006, Garrett et al. [15] defended the use of secondary implants on a cost basis: in their prospective study, 44 % of cancer patients were unable to receive prostheses owing to early recurrence, lack of cooperation, or satisfaction with conventional prostheses. In 2010, Korfage et al. [51] adopted a different focus. In their study, 50 patients were treated with primary implants and followed for 5 years. After 1 year, 12 patients had died; after 5 years 26 patients had died (11 of tumor-related causes and 15 of other causes). However, among the patients who survived, 92 % benefited from their prosthesis at 1 year and 83 % at 5 years, thus demonstrating a clear and early improvement in quality of life. According to the authors, these findings justify primary implantation within the framework of a reasonable prognosis for the tumor.

With respect to extraoral implants for retention of facial epithesis, Dings et al. [52] performed a retrospective study in 2011 and found that implants placed in previously irradiated facial bone failed in 18 % of cases, whereas in those placed in nonirradiated bone or in a primary procedure in bone that was subsequently to be irradiated, the osseointegration failure rate fell to 9 %. The authors concluded that the extraoral implants placed during ablation had a 90 % survival rate at 5 years, whereas in those placed after ablation, the survival rate fell to 65 %.

In the 2013 literature review by Nooh [24], the success rate for primary implants was 92.2 %, whereas that of the secondary implants was 88.9 %. The difference was not statistically significant.

Esposito and Worthington [53] reported on the use of hyperbaric oxygen in patients who had received radiation therapy. The authors stated that despite the scant research in this area and the high risk of bias, the evidence obtained shows no clinical benefit for hyperbaric oxygen in patients who have undergone radiation therapy and are to receive implants.

Based on experience in our department until 2006 [54–56], we concluded that primary implants osseointegrate better than secondary implants in irradiated bone. However, since a primary procedure requires placement of an implant in a position that is not optimal for the prostheses, the number of osseointegrated implants increases, although occasionally, some implants cannot support prostheses (sleepers). Since 2006, we have used primary and secondary implants with equal frequency; therefore, in case of doubt or when it is likely that the outcome of the primary procedure will not be optimal, we defer implantation until at least 1 year after radiotherapy. With the currently available moderately rough RBM implants, rates of osseointegration are almost equal for primary and secondary implants; therefore, the speed of rehabilitation is no longer an argument in favor of primary placement. For us, the major advantage of primary placement is the full functional rehabilitation achieved during the first year after cancer treatment. With a secondary procedure, this process takes much longer.

We agree with Schoen et al. [3] that, in secondary placement, there is a need for surgery with appropriate antibiotic coverage. The approach should be as conservative as possible to ensure an appropriate blood supply to the bone, minimum detachment of periosteum, abundant irrigation, and low-speed drilling.

Schoen et al. [48] showed that prostheses placed on implants improve quality of life in terms of oral function and the degree of satisfaction provided by the teeth. Therefore, dental implants should be considered in any cancer patient treated with curative intent, especially if the patient is edentulous.

Clinical Cases 1 (Figs. 6.1–6.7)

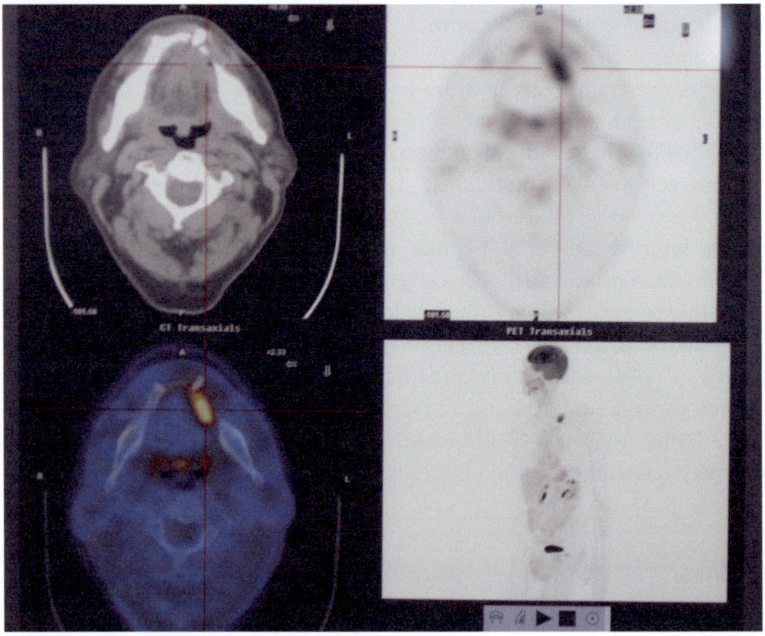

Fig. 6.1 Left floor of the mouth squamous cell carcinoma

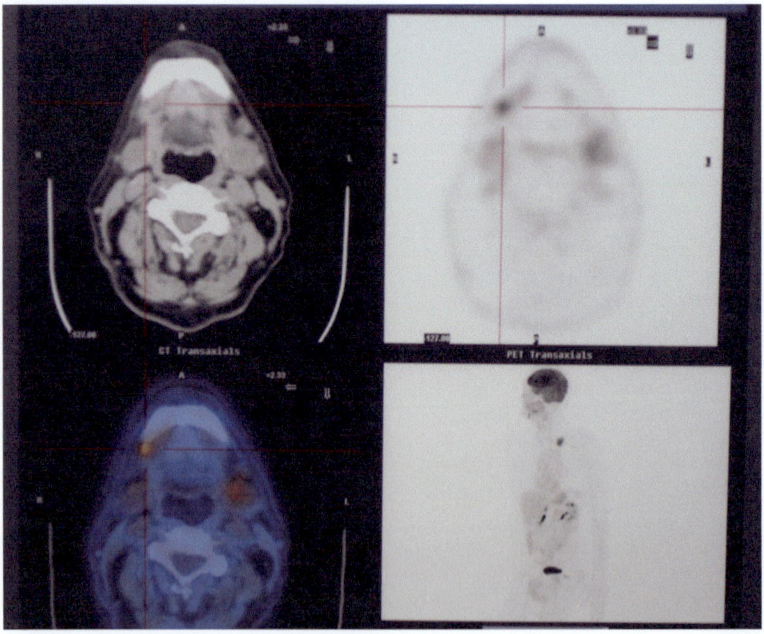

Fig. 6.2 PET/TC bilateral positive cervical node hipercaptation

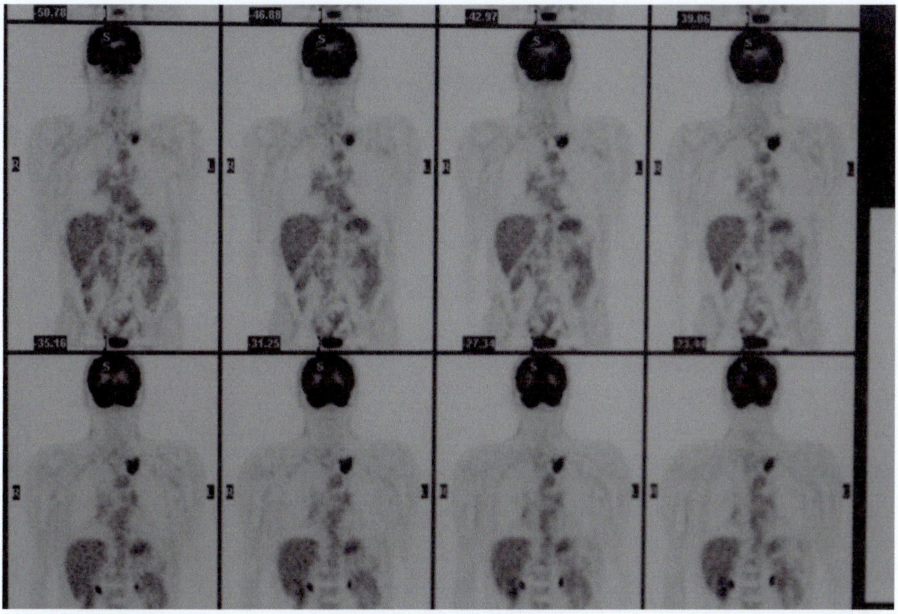

Fig. 6.3 Preoperative PET/CT positive image in left lung apex suggesting a lung metastasis

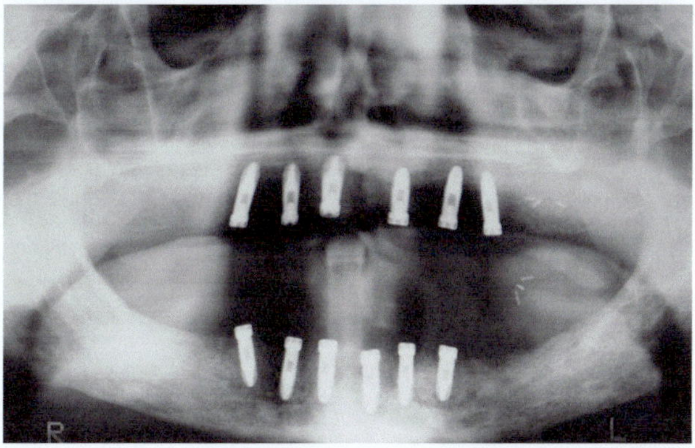

Fig. 6.4 The patient underwent a floor of the mouth resection with clear margins and bilateral neck dissection. Lung surgery with clear margins confirms squamous cell carcinoma. Adjuvant locoregional radiotherapy due to bilateral cervical lymph node infiltration. pT2N2CM1. One year after the end of the radiotherapy under local anesthesia secondary implant placement

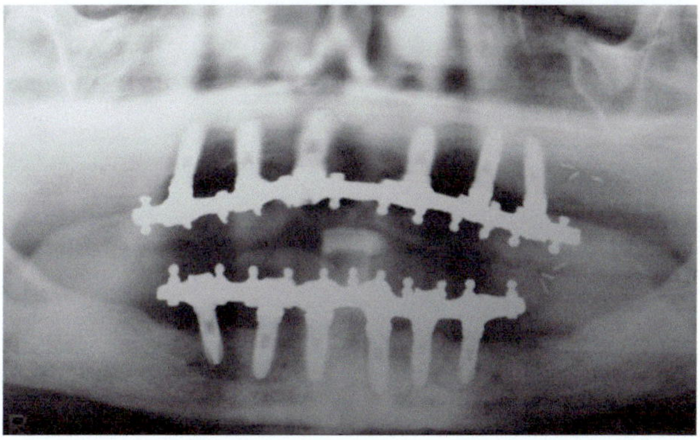

Fig. 6.5 Final orthopantomogram with two fix screw-retained hybrid prosthesis

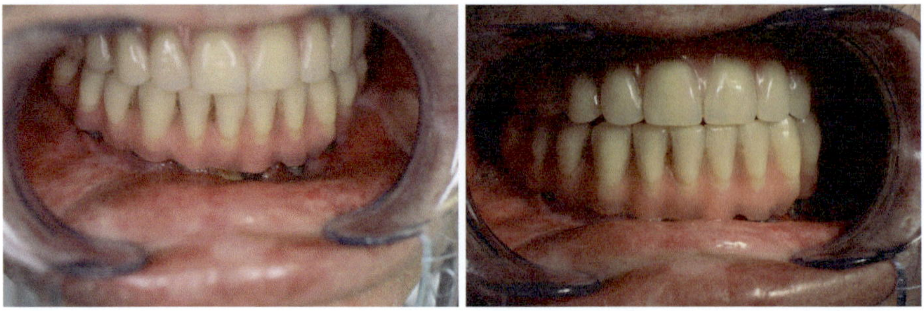

Fig. 6.6 Hybrid fix screw-retained "ad modum Bránemark" final occlusion with small flanges. Notice the left nasolabial skin paddle. Patient survives more than 6 years after the dental rehabilitation and pass away due to a secondary lung tumor

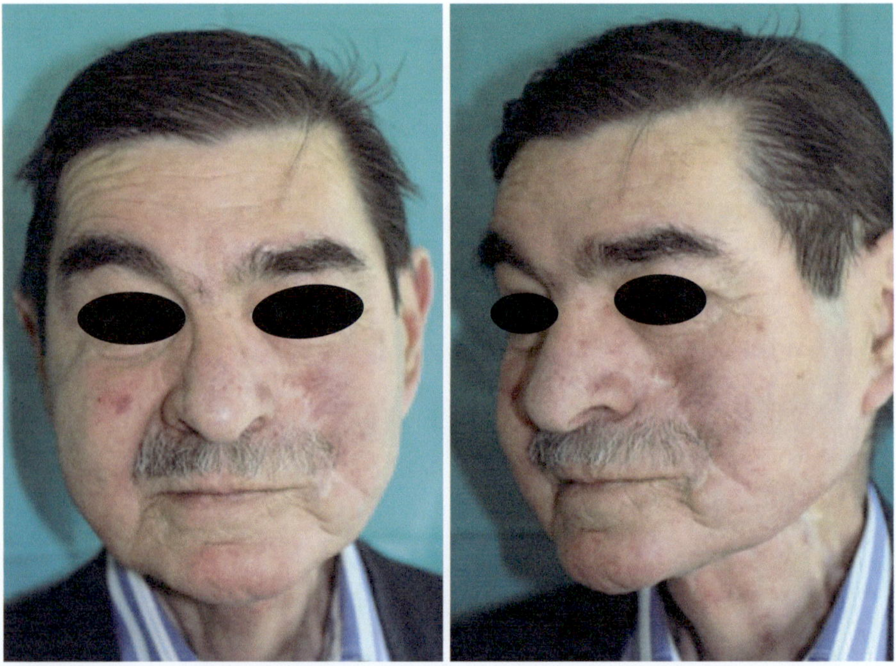

Fig. 6.7 Prosthesis in place and the patient showing the left nasolabial flap scar

Clinical Cases 2 (Figs. 6.8–6.18)

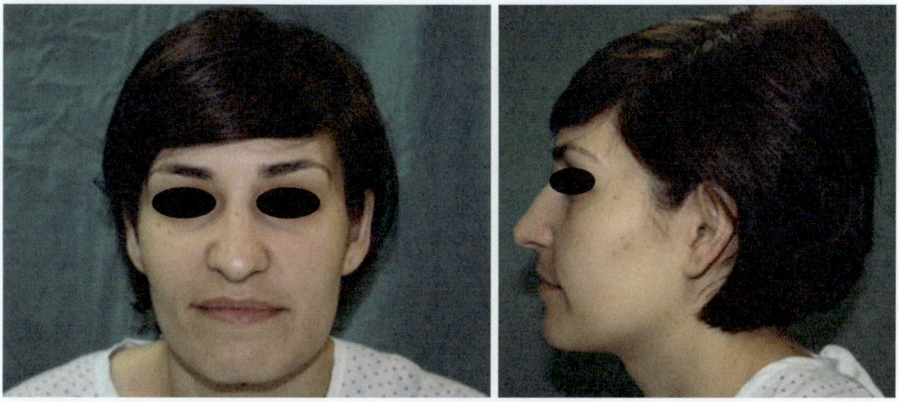

Fig. 6.8 A 28-year-old patient with a left mandibular ameloblastoma, preoperative frontal and lateral views

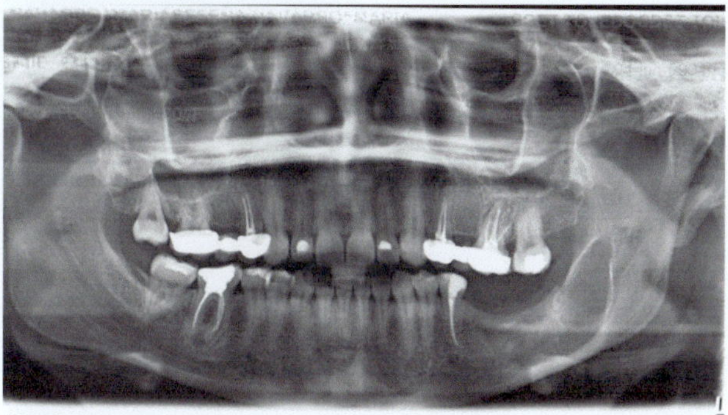

Fig. 6.9 Ameloblastoma involving left body, angle and ascending mandibular ramus

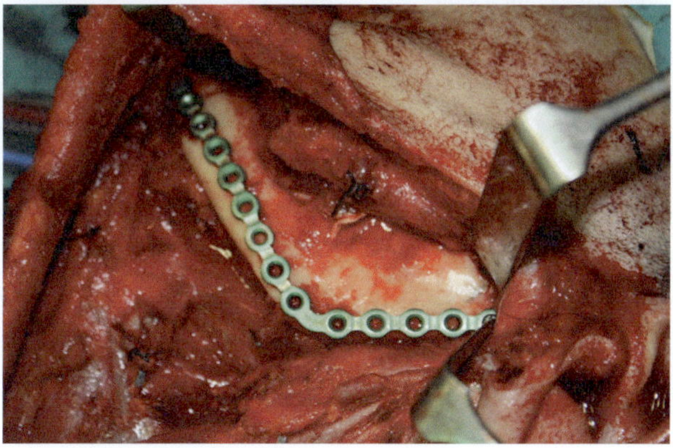

Fig. 6.10 Intraoperative view: reconstructive plate prebending

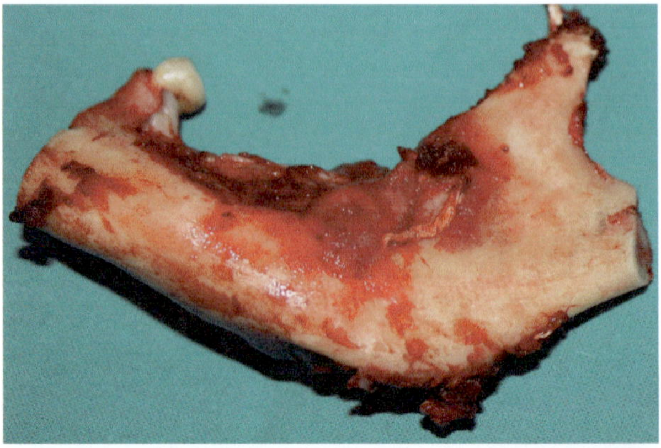

Fig. 6.11 Specimen after the resection

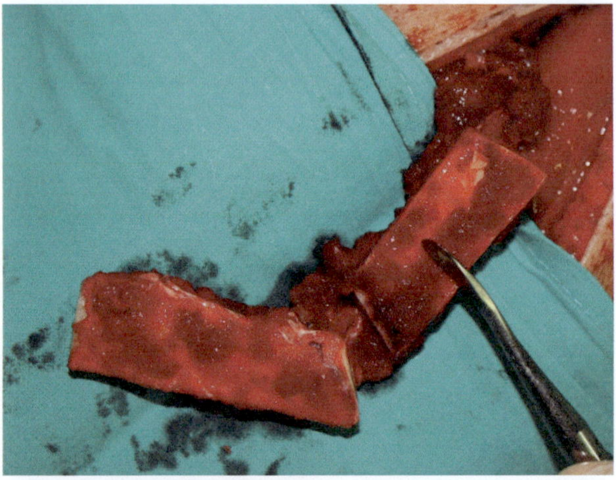

Fig. 6.12 Fibula flap with a sagittal split osteotomy for accurate reconstruction of the mandibular angle

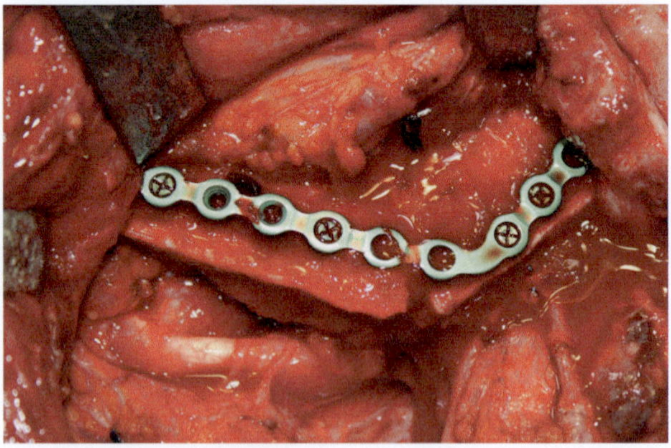

Fig. 6.13 Fibula flap in place with sagittal split osteotomy

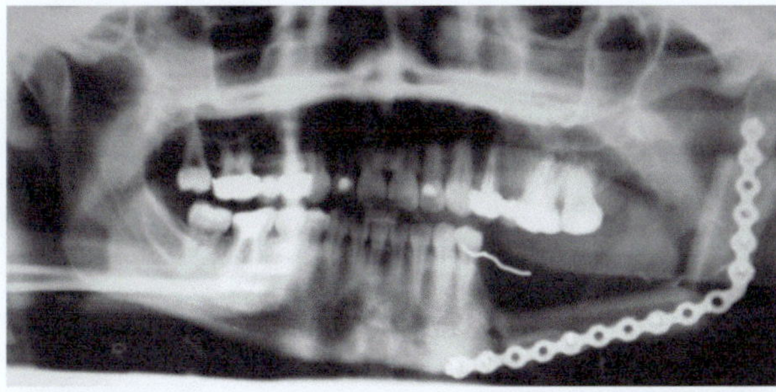

Fig. 6.14 Postoperative view with a conventional acrylic removable prosthesis

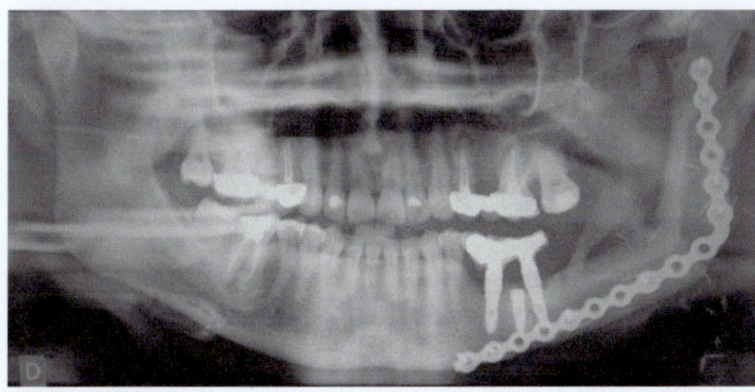

Fig. 6.15 Final orthopantomogram, one sleeper and the fixed screw-retained ceramometalic bridge

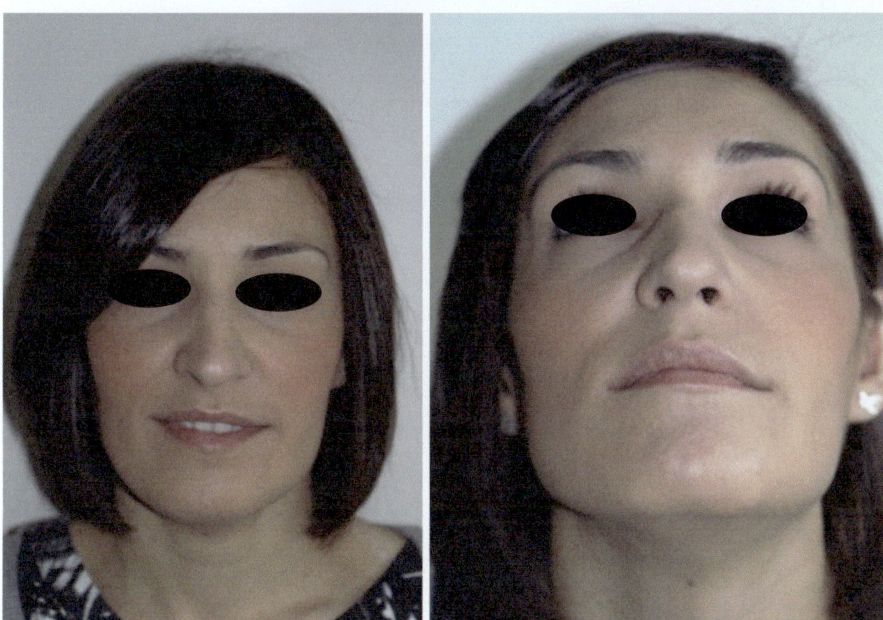

Fig. 6.16 Final frontal view and detail of the goniac angle symmetry

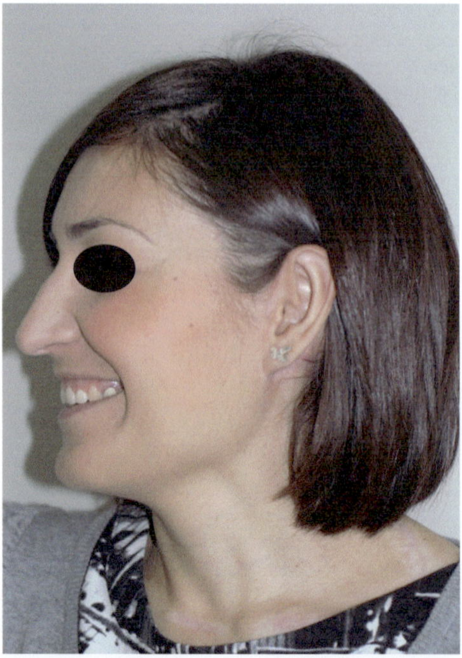

Fig. 6.17 Final lateral view

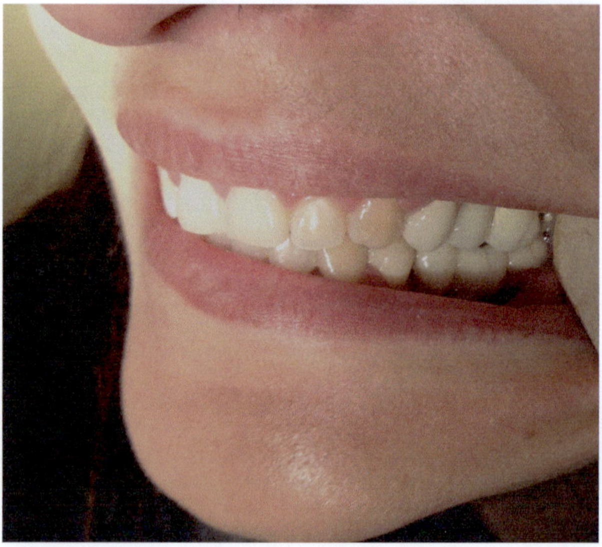

Fig. 6.18 Detail of the occlusion

Clinical Cases 3 (Figs. 6.19–6.35)

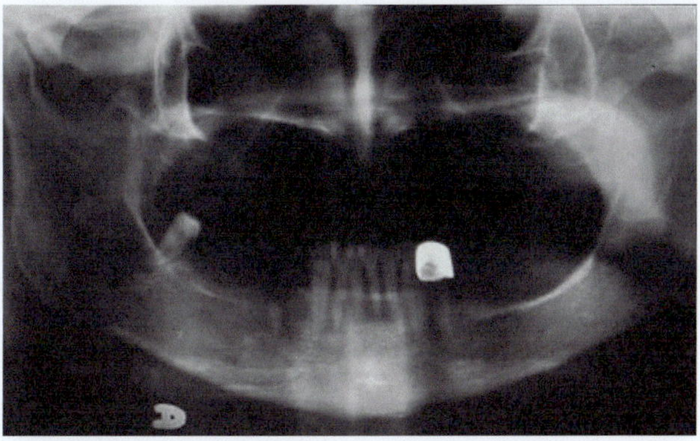

Fig. 6.19 1996: floor of the mouth squamous cell carcinoma, resection with clear margins, bilateral neck dissection, and reconstruction with radial forearm flap. Adjuvant radiotherapy

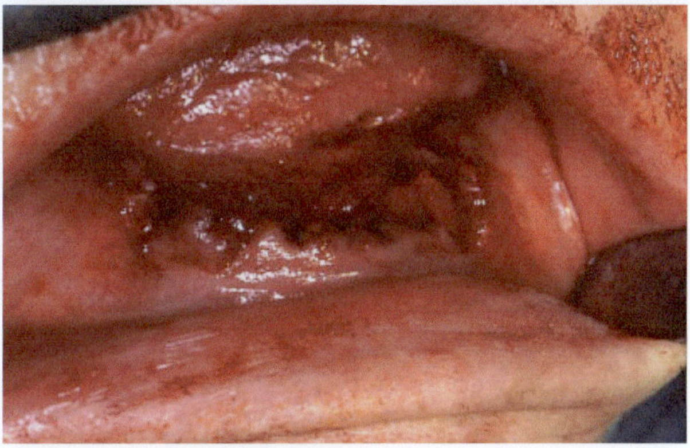

Fig. 6.20 One year after the end of radiotherapy tooth extraction under general anesthesia

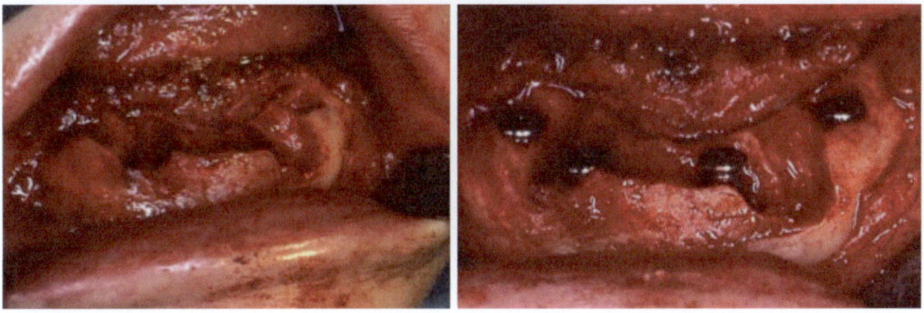

Fig. 6.21 Despite bone defects implants achieved satisfactory primary stability

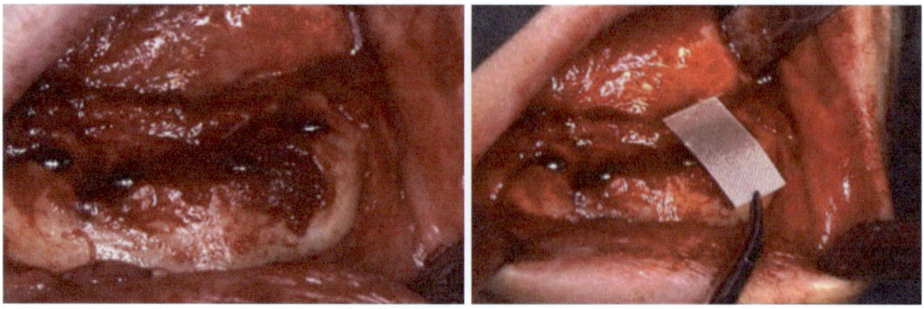

Fig. 6.22 The bone defects surrounding the implants were treated using bone-guided regeneration with bone grafts and resorbable membranes

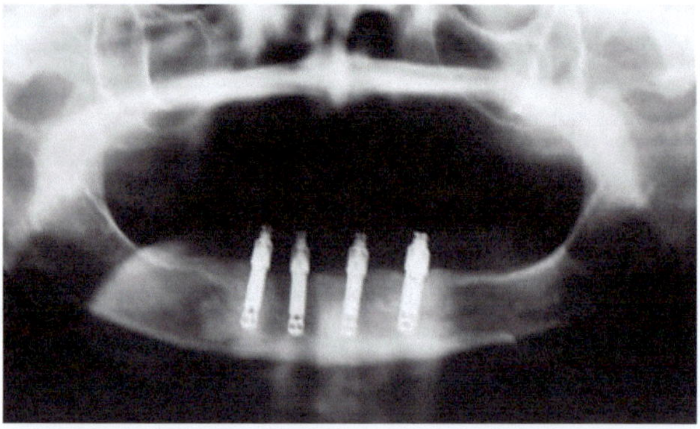

Fig. 6.23 Healing period was uneventful, orthopantomogram taken at the second stage surgery

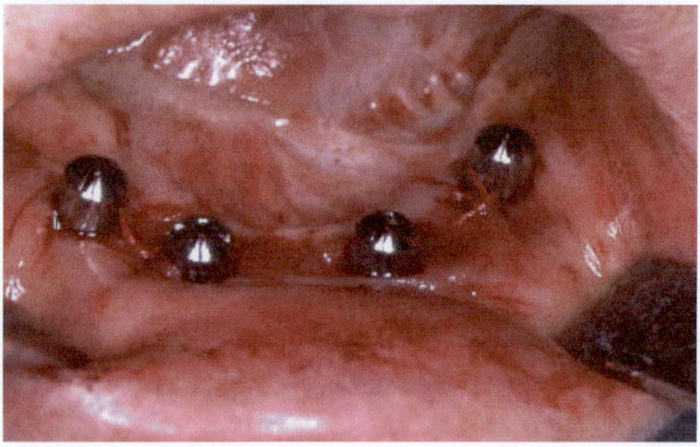

Fig. 6.24 Atraumatic second stage surgery

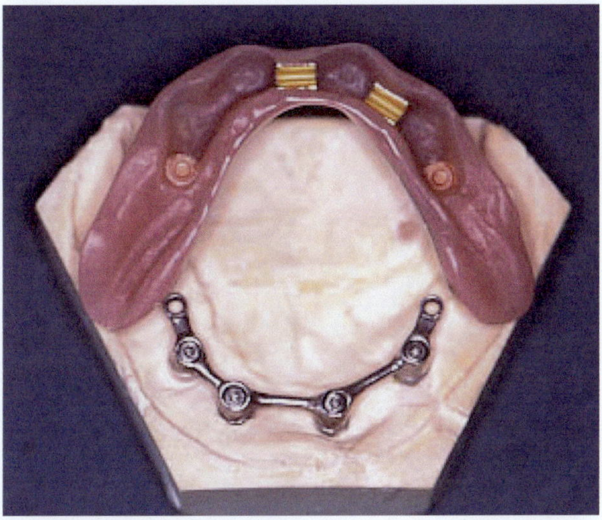

Fig. 6.25 Implant retained and supported overdenture

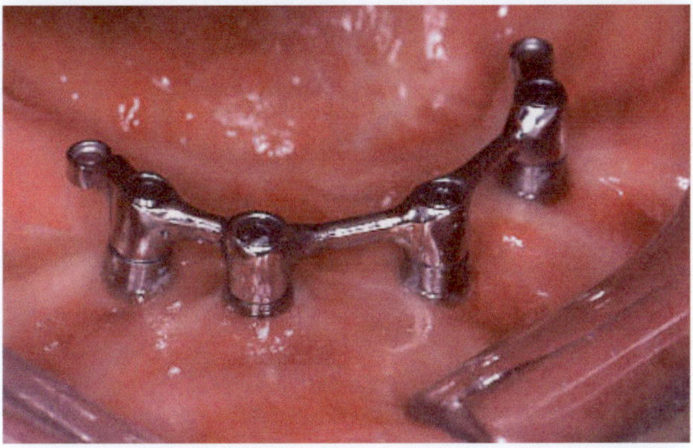

Fig. 6.26 1997 Behavior of this heavily irradiated peri-implant mucosa

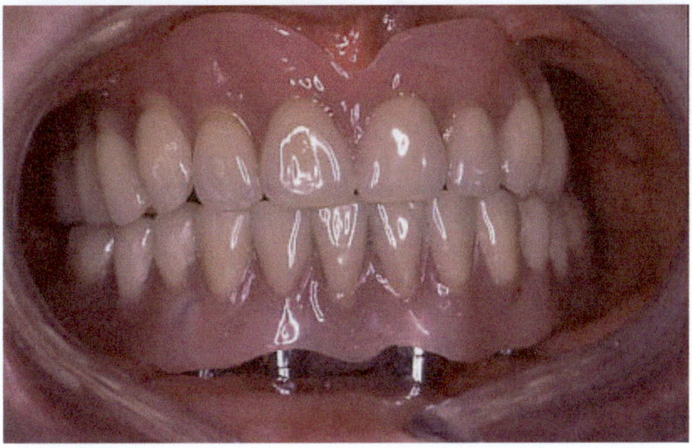

Fig. 6.27 Final occlusion 1997

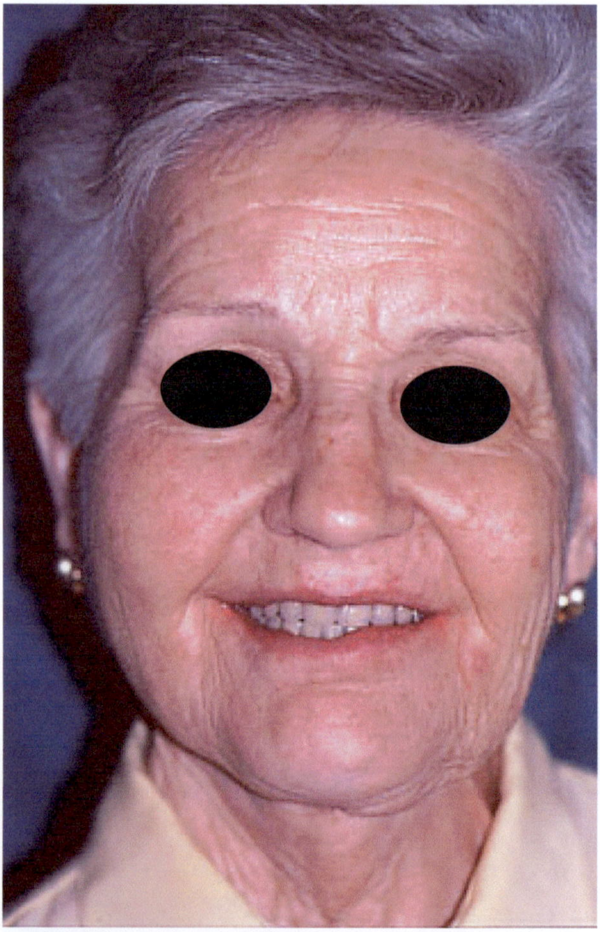

Fig. 6.28 1997 final picture

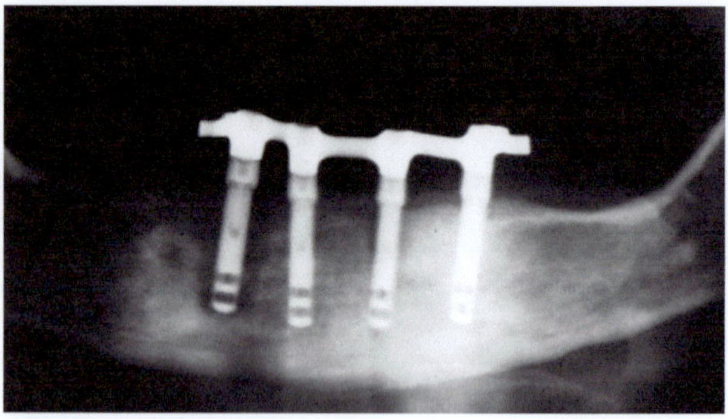

Fig. 6.29 Peri-implant bone loss after 14 years of loading

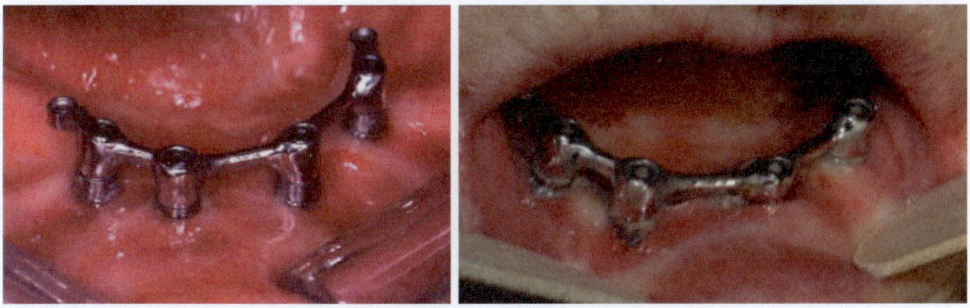

Fig. 6.30 Soft tissues around the framework in 1997 and after 14 years of loading

Fig. 6.31 Retrieving implants in radiated bone 14 years later

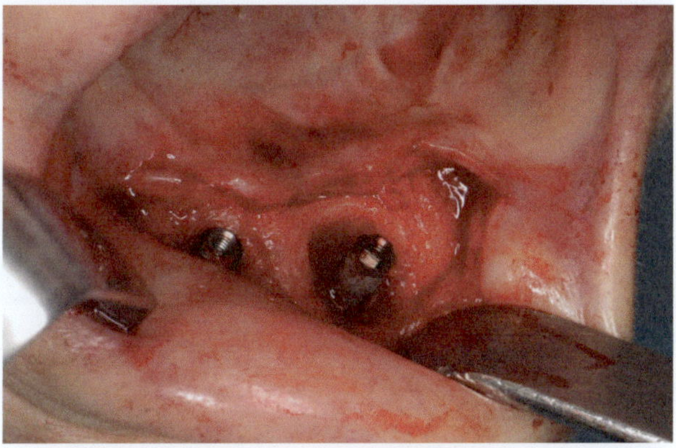

Fig. 6.32 After 8 months period for healing mild bone regeneration in the irradiated mandible without hyperbaric oxygen treatment

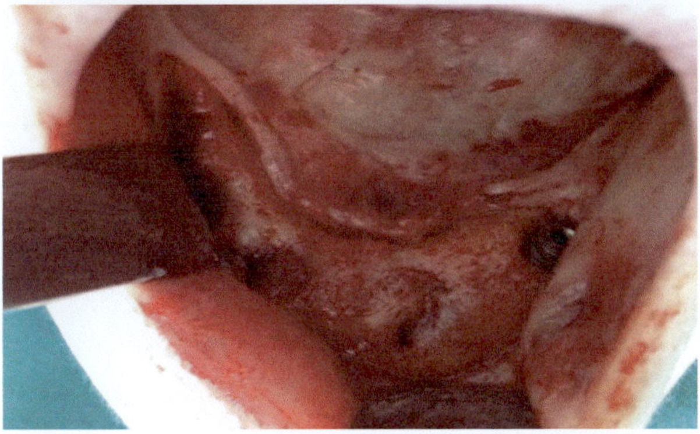

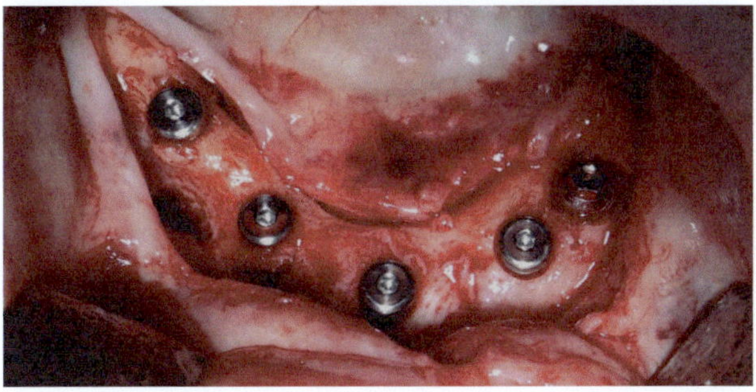

Fig. 6.33 New first stage surgery placing four RBM external hexagon implants MG osseous

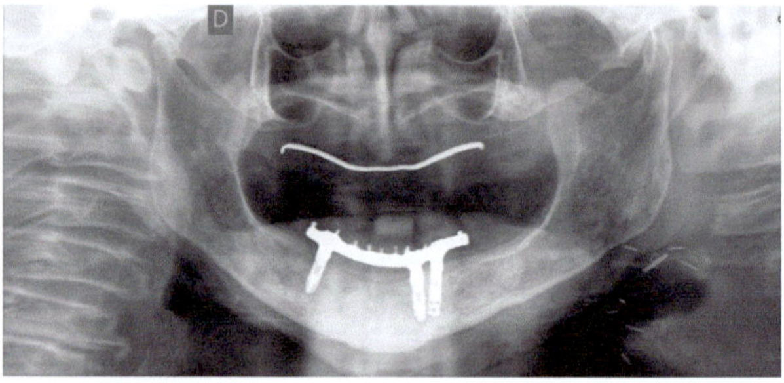

Fig. 6.34 Regarding new implants, two did not achieve adequate osseointegration, but the remaining are able to support a new fixed screw-retained prosthesis

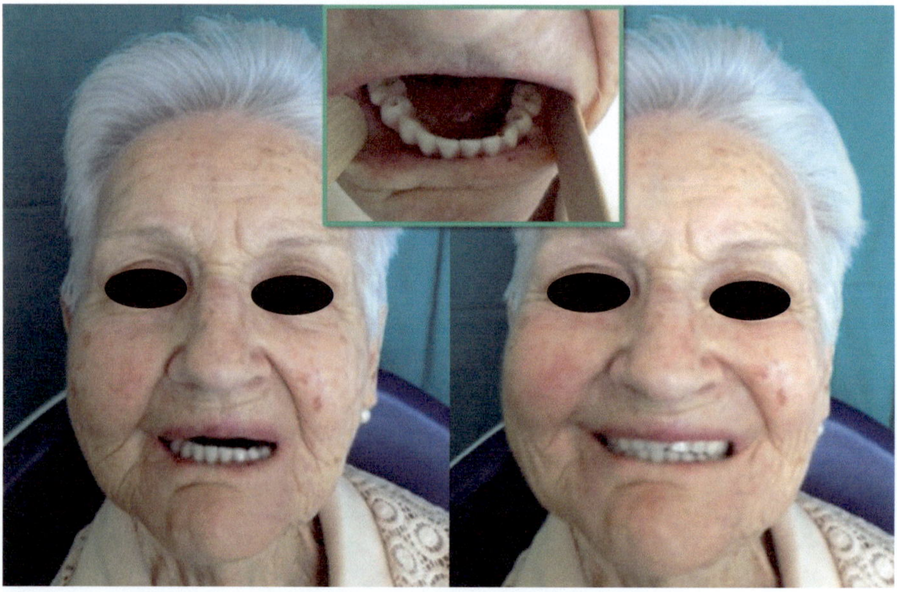

Fig. 6.35 Fixed screw-retained hybrid prosthesis in the mandible 14 years after the initial implant treatment

Clinical Cases 4 (Figs. 6.36–6.42)

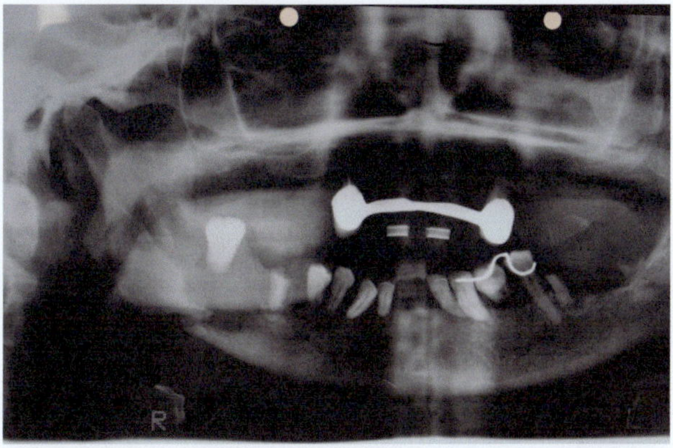

Fig. 6.36 Mandibular fracture due to right retromolar trigone squamous cell carcinoma bone infiltration

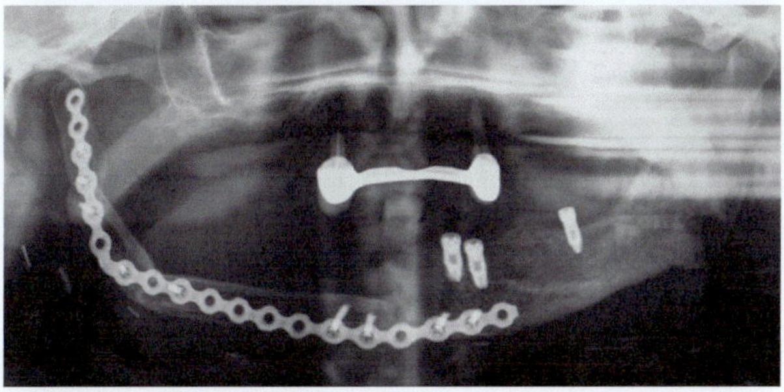

Fig. 6.37 Bilateral neck dissection, resection with clear margins an immediate reconstruction by means of a fibula osteomyocutaneous flap. Immediate implant placement in the remnant mandible not in the flap. The patient underwent postoperative radiotherapy

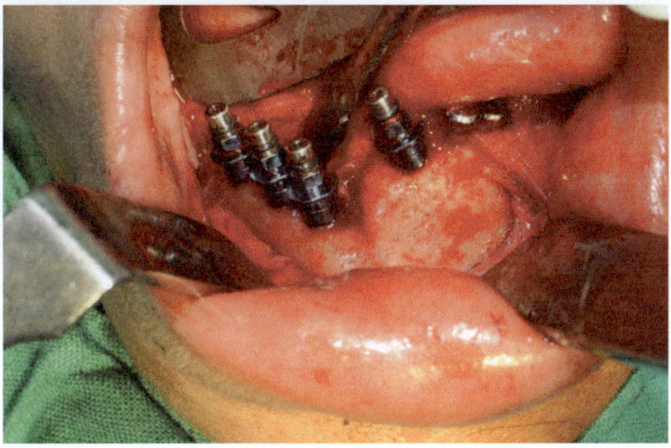

Fig. 6.38 One year after the end of the radiotherapy, secondary implant MG osseous placement in the fibula flap

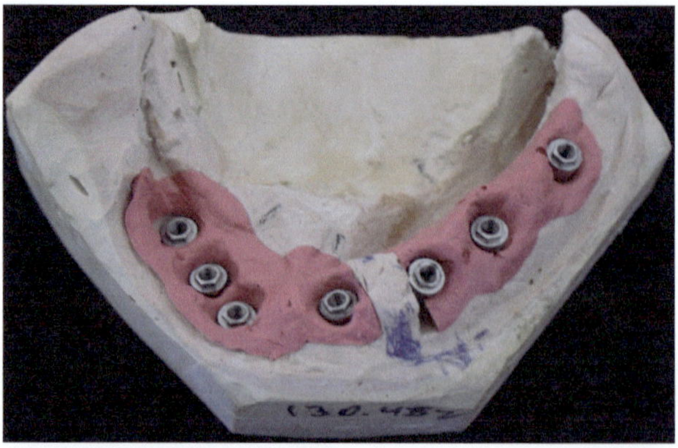

Fig. 6.39 Master cast demonstrating proper osseointegration of the primary and secondary implants

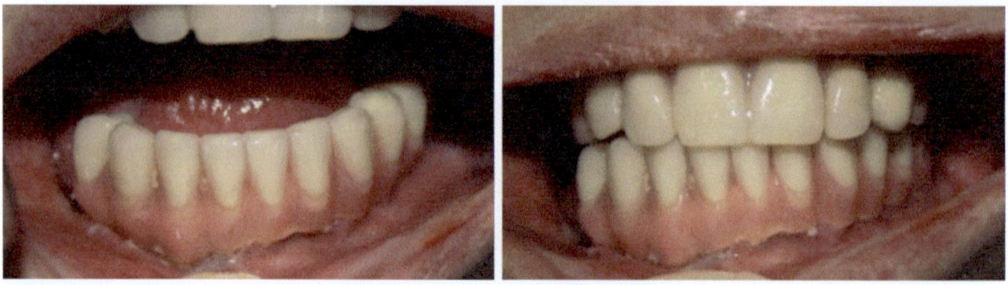

Fig. 6.40 Mandibular fixed screw-retained hybrid prosthesis with small acrylic flanges

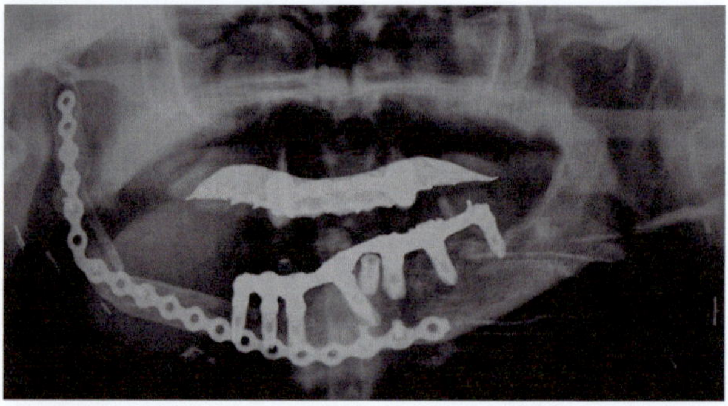

Fig. 6.41 Final orthopantomography showing one “sleeper,” a fully osseointegrated implant that does not support the prosthesis

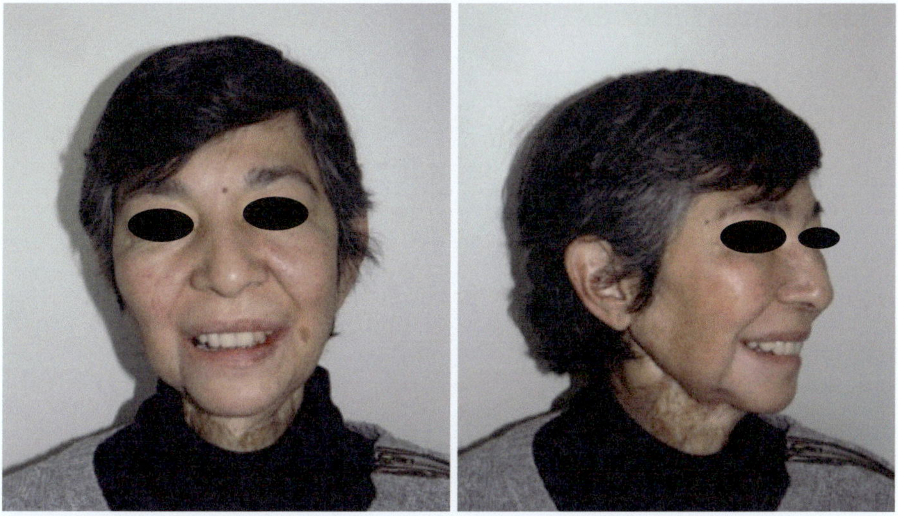

Fig. 6.42 Final view of the patient with the prosthesis in place

Clinical Cases 5 (Figs. 6.43–6.48)

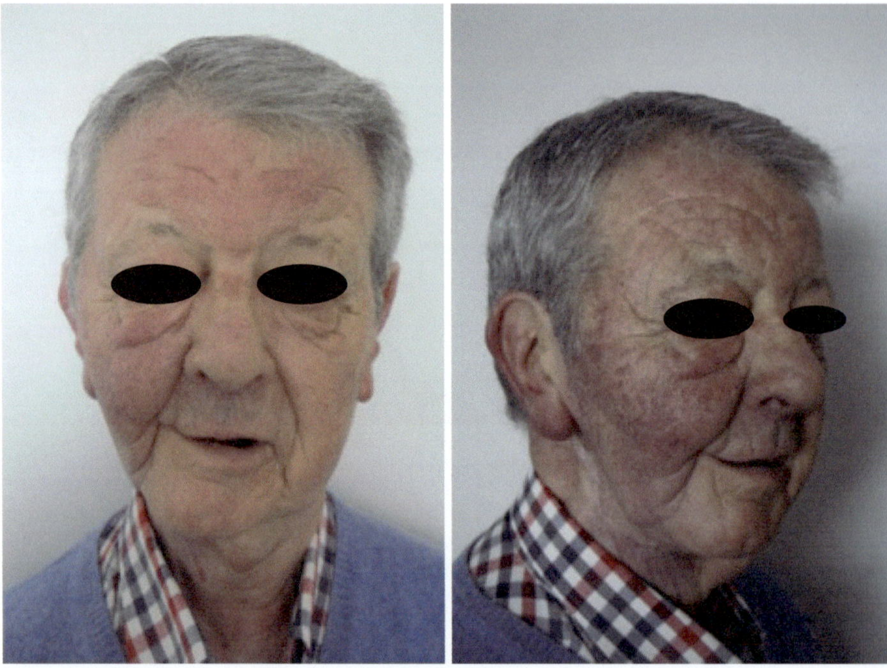

Fig. 6.43 A 72-year-old patient who suffer two different tumors in the right mandibular area. Right neck dissection, right mandibulectomy and adjuvant radiotherapy, The patient was not reconstructed due to different comorbid conditions. He presents deviation of the chin and mandible towards the affected side with the movements based on one single TMJ. Severe imitation of the lateral and protrusive movements with a preserved opening (the so-called "cocodrile occlusion")

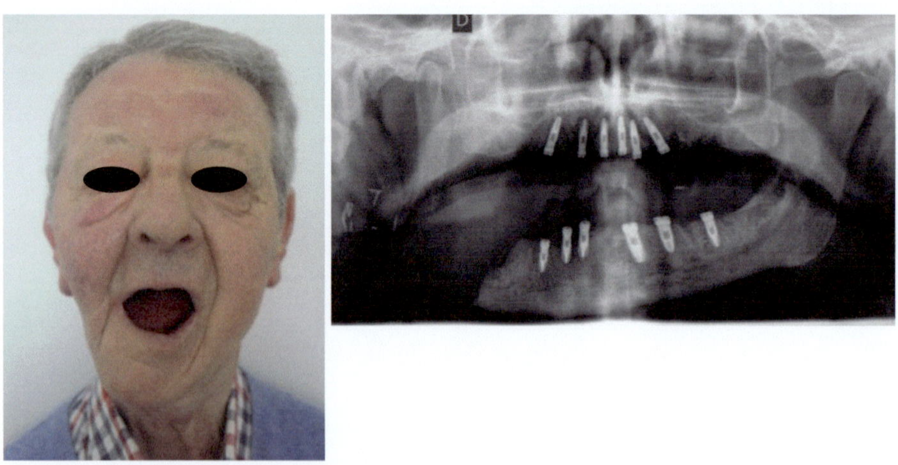

Fig. 6.44 An implant supported and retained prosthesis is the only hope for a dental rehabilitation in these lateral non reconstructed mandibular defects

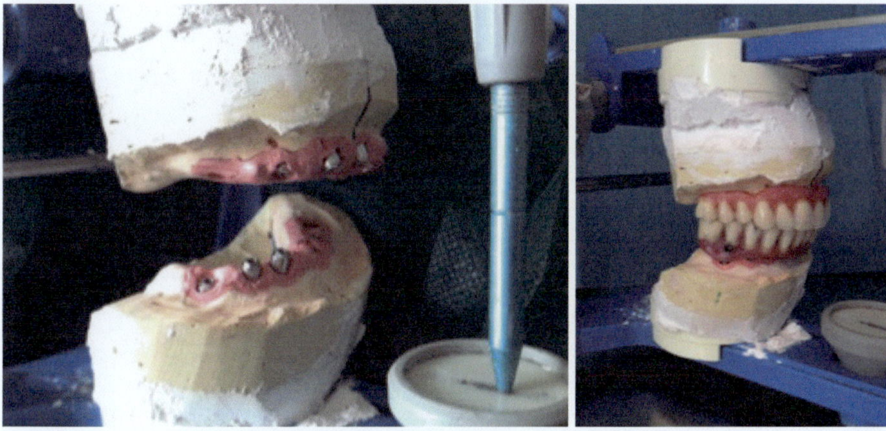

Fig. 6.45 The prosthesis and master casts mounted in an semiadjustable articulator showing the mandibular deviation and the discrepancies between both jaws

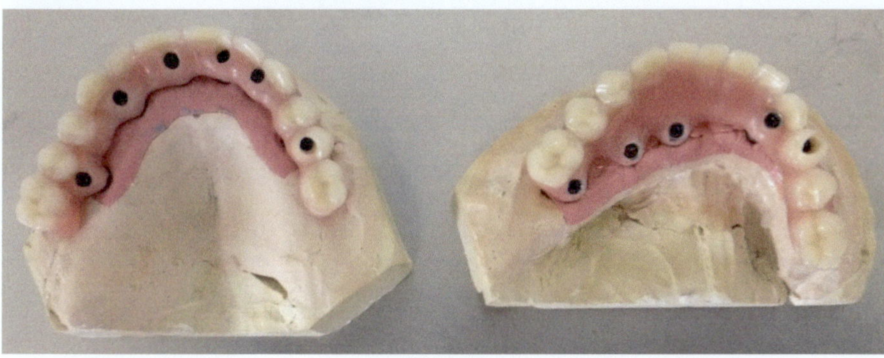

Fig. 6.46 Notice the distance between implant position and the ideal mandibular teeth location due to the bone shift towards the affected side

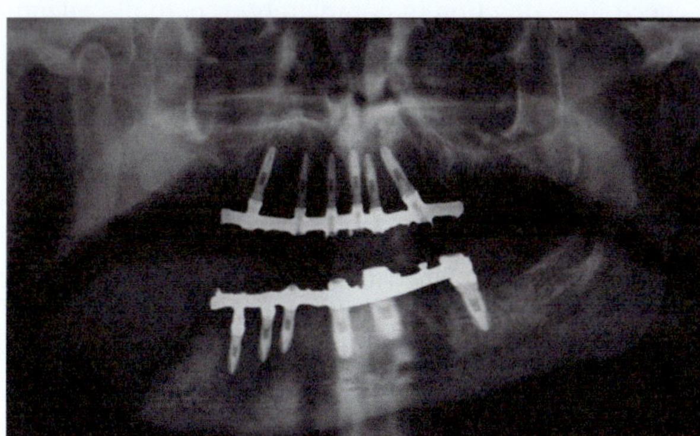

Fig. 6.47 Final orthopantomogram demonstrating the metallic framework passive fixation

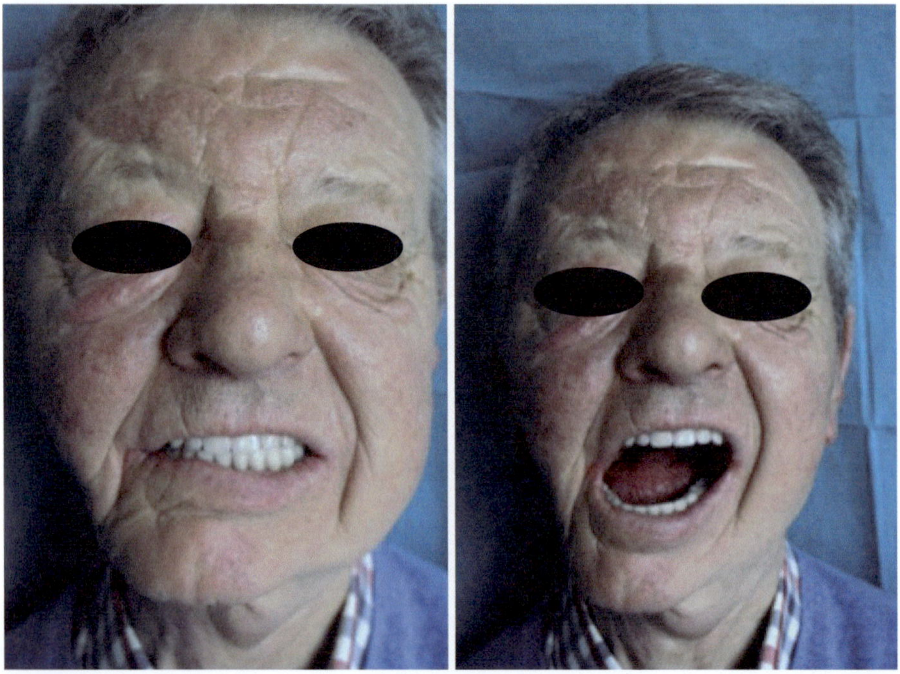

Fig. 6.48 Final occlusion in a radiated nonreconstructed patient after two different squamous cell carcinoma primaries

Conclusions

The most appropriate treatment for the patient is decided by the head and neck cancer team based on tumor characteristics (clinical classification, histopathology, results of imaging tests), the estimated size and location of the defect, the reconstruction method, and the predicted need for complementary radiation therapy. Our surgical team analyzes the situation of each patient and assesses the need for extraction in completely or partially edentulous patients, the indication for implants to support prostheses, and the placement of implants in a primary or secondary procedure.

Our working method can be summarized in the following conclusions:

1. We use RBM screw implants with intermediate surface roughness (1.2–1.56 Ra/μm depending on the area measured, MG Osseous®, Mozo-Grau®) and an external connection because of their versatility in the restoration process.
2. We place implants in a primary procedure if we can achieve the ideal position for supporting the prostheses. If we feel this is not possible, we delay placement until the second procedure. Furthermore, if the implants interfere with the viability of the reconstruction method (e.g., excessive detachment of the periosteum of the fibula flap), we delay the procedure.
3. We prefer to place implants during ablative and reconstructive procedures because it ensures much quicker functional rehabilitation for the patient.

4. In the case of secondary implants, we prefer to wait 1 year after radiation therapy before placing the implants.
5. In our series, we found no significant differences in the success rates for osseointegration between primary and secondary implants. We did not use hyperbaric oxygen. The risk of osteoradionecrosis associated with secondary implant surgery is minimal.
6. In patients who have not undergone radiation therapy, the second phase is the same as for noncancer patients; in patients who have undergone radiation therapy, we allow twice as long for osseointegration and use minimally aggressive surgery, almost always under local anesthesia.
7. Our first choice for prostheses is implant-supported, implant-retained screwed fixed rehabilitation with no mucosal support.
8. The ideal number of implants is that which enables us to use a fixed prosthesis, i.e., normally 4–6 per arch in completely edentulous patients.
9. The main reasons that placed implants are not used with prostheses are death from locoregional recurrence, second primary cancer or distant metastasis, death not related to the tumor, and lack of patient cooperation.
10. We recommend overdentures in cases with three or fewer implants on an edentulous arch or when there are major soft tissue limitations, a marked increase in interarch distance, major limitations of tongue movement, and deviated mandible.
11. Follow-up of cancer patients who undergo rehabilitation with implants should be rigorous owing to the complications and problems associated with prostheses.
12. We recommend complete functional rehabilitation in all cancer patients whose surgery is performed with curative intent. Therefore, we recommend implant-supported dental rehabilitation because of the clear improvement in quality of life.

References

1. Urken ML, Moscoso JF, Lawson W, et al. Systematic approach to functional reconstruction of the oral cavity following partial and total glossectomy. Arch Otolaryngol Head Neck Surg. 1994;120(89):589–601.
2. Komisar A, editor. Mandibular reconstruction. New York: Thieme; 1997. p. 1–9.
3. Schoen PJ, Reintsema H, Raghoebar GM, Vissink A, Roodenburg JLN. The use of implant retained mandibular prostheses in the oral rehabilitation of head and neck cancer patients. A review and rationale for treatment planning. Oral Oncol. 2004;40:862–71.
4. Urken M. Composite free flaps in oromandibular reconstruction. Review of the literature. Arch Otolaryngol Head Neck Surg. 1991;117:724–31.
5. Roumanas ED, Garrett N, Blackwell KE, Freymiller E, Abemayor E, Wong WK, Beumer 3rd J, Fueki K, Fueki W, Kapur KK. Masticatory and swallowing threshold performances with conventional and implant-supported prostheses after mandibular fibula free-flap reconstruction. J Prosthet Dent. 2006;96(4):289–97.
6. Kramer DC. The radiation therapy patient: treatment planning and postreatment care. In: Taylor TD, editor. Clinical maxillofacial prosthesis. Chicago: Quintessence; 2000.

7. Nelson K, Heberer S, Glatzer C. Survival analysis and clinical evaluation of implant-retained prostheses in oral cancer resection patients over a mean follow-up period of 10 years. J Prosthet Dent. 2007;98:405–10.
8. Heberer S, Kilic S, Hossamo J, Raguse JD, Nelson K. Rehabilitation of irradiated patients with modified and conventional sandblasted acid-etched implants: preliminary results of a split-mouth study. Clin Oral Implants Res. 2011;22:546–51.
9. Buddula A, Assad DA, Salinas TJ, Garces YI, Volz JE, Weaver AL. Survival of turned and roughened dental implants in irradiated head and neck cancer patients: a retrospective análysis. J Prosthet Dent. 2011;106:290–6.
10. Fenlon MR, Lyons A, Farrell S, Bavisha K, Banerjee A, Palmer RM. Factors affecting survival and usefulness of implants placed in vascularized free composite grafts used in post-head and neck cancer reconstruction. Clin Implant Dent Relat Res. 2012;14:266–72.
11. Gander T, Studer S, Studer G, Grätz KW, Bredell M. Medium-term outcome of Astra Tech implants in head and neck oncology patients. Int J Oral Maxillofac Surg. 2014;43:1381–5.
12. Albrektsson T. Hydroxyapatite-coated implants: a case against their use. J Oral Maxillofac Surg. 1998;56:1312–26.
13. Smölka K, Krehenbuehl M, Eggensperger N, Hallermann W, Thoren H, Lizuka T, et al. Fibula free flap reconstruction of the mandible in cancer patients. Evaluation of a combined surgical and prosthodontic treatment concept. Oral Oncol. 2008;44:1861–5.
14. Weischer T, Mohr C. Ten-year experience in oral implant rehabilitation of cancer patients: treatment concept and proposed criteria for success. Int J Oral Maxillofac Implants. 1999;14:521–8.
15. Garrett N, Roumanas ED, Blackwell KE, Freymiller E, Abemayor E, Wong WK, Gerratt B, Berke G, Beumer 3rd J, Kapur KK. Efficacy of conventional and implant-supported mandibular resection prostheses: study overview and treatment outcomes. J Prosthet Dent. 2006;96:13–24.
16. Kovacs AF. Clinical analysis of implant losses in oral tumor and defect patients. Clin Oral Implants Res. 2000;11:494–504.
17. Linsen S, Martini M, Stark H. Long-term results of endosteal implants following radical oral cancer surgery with and without adjuvant radiation therapy. Clin Implant Dent Relat Res. 2012;14:250–8.
18. Mancha de la Plata M, Gías LN, Díez PM, Muñoz-Guerra M, González-García R, Lee GY, Castrejón-Castrejón S, Rodríguez-Campo FJ. Osseointegrated implant rehabilitation of irradiated oral cancer patients. J Oral Maxillofac Surg. 2012;70:1052–63.
19. Fang W, Liu YP, Ma Q, Liu BL, Zhao Y. Long-term results of mandibular reconstruction of continuity defects with fibula free flap and implant-borne dental rehabilitation. Int J Oral Maxillofac Implants. 2015;30:169–78.
20. Roumanas ED, Markowitz BL, Lorant JA, Calcaterra TC, Jones NF, Beumer 3rd J. Reconstructed mandibular defects: fibula free flaps and osseointegrated implants. Plast Reconstr Surg. 1997;99:356–65.
21. Weischer T, Schettler D, Mohr C. Concept of surgical and implant-supported prostheses in the rehabilitation of patients with oral cancer. Int J Oral Maxillofac Implants. 1996;11:775–81.
22. Schepers RH, Slagter AP, Kaanders JHAM, Van den Hoogen FJA, Merkx MAW. Effect of postoperative radiotherapy on the functional result of implants placed Turing ablative surgery for oral cancer. Int J Oral Maxillofac Surg. 2006;35:803–8.
23. Visch LL, Van Waas MA, Schmitz PI, Levendag PC. A clinical evaluation of implants in irradiated oral cancer patients. J Dent Res. 2002;81:856–9.
24. Nooh N. Dental implant survival in irradiated oral cancer patients: a systematic review of the literature. Int J Oral Maxillofac Implants. 2013;28:1233–42.
25. Tanaka TI, Chan HL, Tindel DI, MAceachern M, Oh TJ. Updated clinical considerations for dental implant therapy in irradiated head and neck cancer patients. J Prosthodont. 2013;22:432–8.
26. Dental Implants. National Institutes of Health consensus development conference statement. 1988; 7:3.

27. Nabil S, Samman N. Risk factors for osteoradionecrosis after head and neck radiation: a systematic review. Oral Surg Oral Med Oral Pathol Oral Radiol. 2012;113:54–69.
28. Nabil S, Samman N. Incidence and prevention of osteoradionecrosis after dental extraction in irradiated patients: a systematic review. Int J Oral Maxillofac Surg. 2011;40:229–43.
29. Arnold M, Stas P, Kummermehr J, Schultz-Hector S, Trott KR. Radiation induced impairment of bone healing in the rat femur: effects of radiation dose, sequence and interval between surgery and irradiation. Radiother Oncol. 1998;48:259–65.
30. Brasseur M, Brogniez V, Gregoire H, Reychler H, Lengelé B, D'Hoore W, Nyssen-Behets C. Effects of irradiation on bone remodelling around mandibular implants: an experimental study in dogs. Int J Oral Maxillofac Surg. 2006;35:850–5.
31. Schweiger J. Titanium implants in irradiated dog mandibles. J Prosthet Dent. 1988;60:75–84.
32. Larsen PE, Stronczek MJ, Beck FM, Rohrer M. Osteointegration of implants in irradiated bone with and without adjunctive hyperbaric oxygen. J Oral Maxillofac Surg. 1993;51:280–7.
33. Bolind P, Johansson CB, Johansson P, Granstrom G, Albrektsson T. Retrieved implants from irradiated sites in humans: a histological/histomorphometric investigations of oral and craneofacial implants. Clin Implant Dent Relat Res. 2006;8:142–50.
34. Ihde S, Kopp S, Gundlach K, Konstantinović VS. Effects of radiation therapy on craniofacial and dental implants: a review of the literature. Oral Surg Oral Med Oral Pathol Oral Radiol Endod. 2009;107:56–65.
35. Marx RE, Morales MJ. El uso de implantes en la reconstrucción de pacientes con neoplasias orales. Clin Odont North Am. 1998;1:189.
36. Marx RE. A new concept in the treatment of osteoradionecrosis. J Oral Maxillofac Surg. 1982;41:351.
37. Taylor TD, Worthington P. Osseointegrated implant rehabilitation of the previously irradiated mandible: results of a limited trial at 3 to 7 years. J Prosthet Dent. 1993;69:60.
38. Niimi A, Ueda M, Keller E, et al. Experience with osseointegrated implants placed in irradiated tissues in Japan and the United States. Int J Oral Maxillofac Implants. 1998;13:407.
39. Ali A, Patton DW, El Sharkawi AM, et al. Implant rehabilitation of irradiated jaw: a preliminary report. Int J Oral Maxillofac Implants. 1997;12:523.
40. Eckert SE, Desjardins RP, Keller EE, Tolman DE. Endosseous implants in an irradiated tissue bed. J Prosthet Dent. 1996;76:45–9.
41. Buddula A, Assad DA, Salinas TJ, Garces Y, Volz JE, Weaver AL. Survival of dental implants in irradiated head and neck cancer patients: a retrospective analysis. Clin Implant Dent Relat Res. 2012;5:716–22.
42. Chambrone L, Mandia J, Shibli JA, Romito GA, Abrahao M. Dental implants installed in irradiated jaws: a systematic review. J Dent Res Clin Res. 2013;92(suppl2):119–30.
43. Zheng M, Li L, Tang Y, Liang XH. How to improbé the survival rate of implants after radiotherapy for head and neck cancer? J Periodontol Implant Sci. 2014;44:2–7.
44. Sclaroff A, Haughey B, Gay WD, Paniello R. Immediate mandibular reconstruction and placement of dental implants at the time of ablative surgery. Oral Surg Oral Med Oral Pathol. 1994;78:711–77.
45. Urken ML, Buchbinder D, et al. Functional evaluation following microvascular oromandibular reconstruction of the oral cancer patient: a comparative study of reconstructed and nonreconstructed patients. Laryngoscope. 1991;101:935–50.
46. Barber AJ, Butterworth CJ, Rogers SN. Systematic review of primary osseointegrated dental implants in head and neck oncology. Br J Oral Maxillofac Surg. 2011;49:29–36.
47. Blanchard P, Baujat B, Holostenco V, Bourredjem A, Baey C, Bourhis J, Pignon JP, MACH-CH Collaborative Group. Meta-analysis of chemotherapy in head and neck cancer (MACH-NC): a comprehensive analysis by tumour site. Radiother Oncol. 2011;100:33–40.
48. Schoen PJ, Raghoebar GM, Bouma J, Reintsema H, Burlage FR, Roodenburg JLN, Vissink A. Prosthodontic rehabilitation of oral function in head–neck cancer patients with dental implants placed simultaneously during ablative tumour surgery: an assessment of treatment outcomes and quality of life. Int J Oral Maxillofac Surg. 2008;37:8–16.

49. Colella G, Cannavale R, Pentenero M, Gandolfo S. Oral implants in radiated patients: a systematic review. Int J Oral Maxillofac Implants. 2007;22:616–22.
50. Mizbah JP, Dings JHAM, Kaanders FJA, Van den Hoogen R, Koole GJ, Meijer MAW. Merkx: Interforaminal implant placement in oral cancer patients: during ablative surgery or delayed? A 5-year retrospective study. Int J Oral Maxillofac Surg. 2013;42:651–5.
51. Korfage A, Schoen PJ, Raghoebar GM, Roodenburg JL, Vissink A, Reintsema H. Benefits of dental implants installed during ablative tumour surgery in oral cancer patients: a prospective 5-year clinical trial. Clin Oral Implants Res. 2010;21:971–9.
52. Dings JPJ, Maal TJ, Muradin KJ, Ingels BJ, Klevering BJ, Koole MA, Merkx MA, Meijer GJ. Extraoral implants: insertion per or postablation? Oral Oncol. 2011;47:1074–8.
53. Esposito M, Worthington HV. Intervention for replacing messing teeth: hyperbaric oxygen therapy for irradiated patients who require dental implants. Cochrane Database Syst Rev. 2013;9:1–19.
54. Cuesta-Gil M, Ochandiano Caicoya S, Riba García F, Duarte Ruiz B, Navarro Cuéllar C, Navarro Vila C. Oral rehabilitation with osseointegrated implants in oncologic patients. J Oral Maxillofac Surg. 2009;67(11):2485–96.
55. Cuellar CN, Caicoya SJO, Sanz JJA, Cuéllar IN, MazaMuela C, Vila CN. Mandibular reconstruction with iliac crest free flap, nasolabial flap and osseointegrated implants. J Oral Maxillofac Surg. 2014;72(6):1226.e1–15.
56. Navarro-Vila C, Borja-Morant A, Cuesta M, López-de-Atalaya F, Salmerón JI, Barrios JM. Aesthetic and functional reconstruction with the trapezius osseomyocutaneous flap and dental implants in oral cavity cancer patients. J Craniomaxillofac Surg. 1996;24:322–9.

Reconstruction in Facial Paralysis

7

Teresa González Otero and Ignacio Navarro Cuellar

Abstract

The objective of reconstructive procedures in the patient affected by facial paralysis is to achieve symmetry both at rest and in movement, with as natural a facial expression as possible. Diagnosis of facial paralysis is based mainly on clinical findings, although electromyographic data are also frequently used. Once facial paralysis has been diagnosed, it is important to establish the degree of motor function involvement. Treatment of facial paralysis should be planned on an individual basis and should be carried out at specialized centers with a facial paralysis unit staffed by appropriately trained health professionals.

7.1 Introduction

The facial nerve is responsible for facial expression. The devastating consequences of damage to the facial nerve can have a huge clinical and psychological impact on a patient's quality of life. The objective of reconstructive procedures in the patient affected by facial paralysis is to achieve symmetry both at rest and in movement, with as natural a facial expression as possible, bearing in mind that the return to completely normal facial function is impossible. Other key objectives are to

T. González Otero, MD, PhD, FEBOMS (✉)
Consultant at Oral and Maxillofacial Surgery Department,
La Paz University Hospital, Madrid, Spain
e-mail: gusarapillo2003@yahoo.es

I. Navarro Cuellar, MD, DDS, FEBOMS
Consultant at Oral and Maxillofacial Surgery Department,
Virgen de la Salud Hospital, Toledo, Spain
e-mail: nnavcu@hotmail.com

C. Navarro Vila (ed.), *Reconstructive Oral and Maxillofacial Surgery*,
DOI 10.1007/978-3-319-20487-1_7

minimize spasm and synkinesis and to ensure that facial expression is as emotional as possible. The role of rehabilitation is essential in this process.

In addition to facial asymmetry and lack of expression, the patient with facial paralysis is also severely affected by ophthalmic problems that leave the eyeball unprotected, such as lagophthalmos. The patient is unable to close the upper eyelid owing to failure of the orbicularis oculi, although it is possible to open the eyelid because the levator muscles, which are innervated by the third cranial pair, continue to function. In addition, the loss of tone in the lower eyelid leads to ectropion, which also exposes the eyeball. This exposure frequently leads to conjunctivitis, corneal ulceration, increased sensitivity, and even reduced visual acuity. Nighttime occlusion with patches is often necessary, as is application of artificial tears and ointments.

Therefore, surgical treatment of facial paralysis should be carried out at specialized centers with a facial paralysis unit staffed by appropriately trained health professionals. Centers of this type have the necessary resources to ensure that each case is addressed on an individual basis.

7.2 Etiology

Facial paralysis has several causes and can be classified into various types. However, facial paralysis that requires surgery can leave permanent sequelae and is usually due to injury and iatrogenic lesions. Surgery to treat tumors of the cerebellopontine angle and surgery of the parotid gland are the most frequent causes of facial paralysis. However, we must not forget that the few cases of conditions such as Bell's palsy and Ramsay Hunt syndrome that progress poorly can benefit from specific reconstructive techniques. Congenital facial paralysis can also benefit from facial surgery.

Iatrogenic lesions of the facial nerve (which can occur during otologic surgery, such as surgery of the cerebellopontine angle and of the parotid gland) can be avoided or minimized through a sound knowledge of the anatomy of the nerve, a meticulous surgical technique, and the use of the intraoperative facial nerve stimulator. Injuries to the facial nerve should be repaired immediately if possible. Another very typical situation in clinical practice is excessive stimulation and manipulation of the nerve during cranial base surgery. This does not produce loss of continuity of the nerve, although it does generate the most doubts over whether and when to perform surgery. In principle, it is recommended to wait, since the best facial function is achieved with the nerve itself, although there may be cases in which reinnervation techniques are sometimes performed during the first year, depending on clinical progress during the first months, electromyographic data, age, and patient expectations.

7.3 Factors to Be Taken into Account When Deciding on a Surgical Approach

Clinical presentation of facial paralysis depends on the location of the lesion. Central paralysis, which is caused by cerebrovascular accidents or tumors above the facial nucleus (in the protuberance), is characterized by the fact that it supplies the upper third, which has a crossed cerebral pattern. Therefore, unlike peripheral facial paralysis, only the lower part of the face is affected, leaving frontal and eyelid function unaltered. Peripheral facial paralysis is caused by lesions of the motor fibers of the seventh cranial pair along its course from the facial nucleus in the brain stem to the point where the nerve exits the stylomastoid foramen. In such cases, all those muscles supplied by the facial nerve on the corresponding half of the face are affected to differing degrees depending on the intensity of the lesion. Involvement of the orbicularis oculi leads to Bell's phenomenon (exposure of the sclera due to rotation of the eye in order to prevent closure of the eyelid).

Interruption of nerve impulses to the facial muscles triggers a series of pathologic reactions. The first event is a progressive loss of muscle fiber, which can decrease muscle size to half in only 2 weeks. The fibers gradually decrease in size until approximately 120 days after denervation, at which time the process of atrophy seems to slow down and stabilize. Hyalinosis and total degeneration are observed after 2–3 years. The time during which muscle fibers can be recovered is paramount, since it sets a limit for reinnervation techniques. Current consensus indicates intervention before 18 months have passed in order to ensure that a large number of motor end plates can respond satisfactorily to new axons. In any case, serial electromyographic studies should be performed to monitor the progress of paralysis and the status of denervated muscles. The ideal scenario for the reinnervation techniques that we comment on below would be stable fibrillation potentials over time, which indicate denervation but conserved muscle tone.

Diagnosis of facial paralysis is based mainly on clinical findings, although electromyographic data are also frequently used. Once facial paralysis has been diagnosed, it is important to establish the degree of motor function involvement. A common approach is the House–Brackmann score, which divides facial paralysis into six grades (I is normal function and VI total paralysis). Cases requiring surgery tend to be the most severe (grades IV, V, and VI), although milder cases can often benefit from complementary techniques (see below).

A key element of reconstructive surgery to treat facial paralysis is the availability of easily interpreted visual scales that enable us to evaluate the results of the reconstruction and compare outcomes with those recorded by other centers. Therefore, appropriate video recording is an essential aspect of patient progress [1].

Treatment of facial paralysis should be planned on an individual basis, taking into account a series of basic data, as follows: origin of the lesion; differentiation between whether the lesion has resulted from a failure in the generation or transmission of the impulse; time since onset and, therefore, status of facial muscle; and involvement of other cranial pairs. It is also very important to consider patient-dependent factors, such as comorbidity, age, cooperation, and expectations. Taken together, these factors enable us to establish three main treatment groups:

1. Less than 18 months since onset with preserved impulse. These cases involve damage to and lesions of the trunk of the facial nerve or its main branches at the point where it exits the stylomastoid foramen, for example, lesions caused by open trauma that section the nerve and damage resulting from surgery to treat

malignant tumors of the parotid. We can resolve the interruption of the stimulus by direct surgery or placement of a graft if direct suture is too tight. The sural nerve or the auricular nerve can be used in these cases. The sooner neurorrhaphy is performed, the better the outcome will be. It is necessary to record the time between anastomosis and appearance of the impulse in the paralyzed muscle. Surgery is usually performed at the time the lesion is caused and, if this is not possible, within the first few months.

2. Less than 18 months with failed impulse. The most common lesions are those resulting from the progress or removal of schwannoma of the eighth nerve and other types of intracerebral tumors or lesions. In these cases, the proximal nervous impulse is not generated despite the fact that the facial nerve is undamaged throughout its course along the petrous portion of the temporal bone, as is the extracranial facial nerve and its branches. In these cases, and provided that the facial muscles are shown to be viable using electromyography, we can use the nerve impulse generated by the other cranial pair by directing it across the facial nerve and its intact branches. The three options are as follows: (a) using the contralateral facial nerve impulse by means of cross-graft(s) of the sural nerve within 3 months of onset, that is, when we are completely sure that the lesion of the facial nerve is incurable; (b) end-to-end anastomosis of XII–VII after sacrificing the hypoglossal nerve or semi-end-to-end anastomosis [2] without sacrificing the seventh nerve; and (c) direct masseter–facial nerve anastomosis by dissecting the facial nerve from the ear or by placement of an auricular nerve graft between the facial nerve and the masseteric nerve [3]. When the source of the nerve impulse is a nerve other than the facial nerve and even though the graft can be performed in a single procedure, cross-facial nerve grafting is usually performed during the same procedure in order to achieve an emotional smile in the long term.
3. More than 18 months with established muscle atrophy. This category includes all types of long-term established facial paralysis, regardless of etiology, that is,

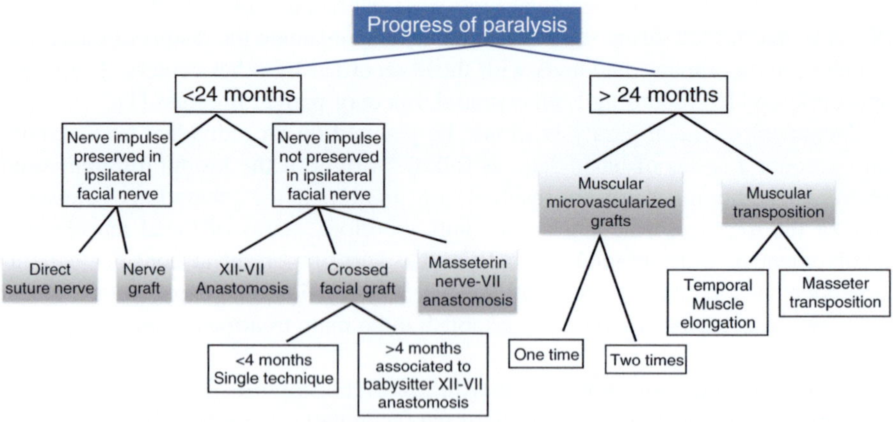

Fig. 7.1 Treatment algorithm used in the facial palsy unit of La Paz University Hospital

regardless of whether or not the impulse had failed. In cases of this type, facial muscle function cannot be recovered, and other muscles must be used. We can perform static techniques, such as elongation of the temporal muscle, or dynamic techniques based on microvascular muscle flaps, such as the gracilis flap or latissimus dorsi flap combined (or not) with a previous cross-graft (Fig. 7.1).

Below we analyze some of the most common surgical techniques, with emphasis on the main features of surgery and the latest approaches.

7.4 Direct Suture with or Without Interposition Graft

Successful outcome depends mainly on tension at the site of anastomosis [4] and the time since the lesion occurred [5]. Therefore, when feasible, neurorrhaphy should be performed when the lesion occurs. If the suture is tense or it is necessary to bridge a nerve defect, we can use a sural nerve or auricular nerve graft. The great auricular nerve is ideal because it is in the same surgical field and, anatomically, gives off several branches that enable us to reconstruct several branches of the facial nerve when necessary. The sural nerve can be used in cases requiring a very long graft (Figs. 7.2 and 7.3).

Every attempt should be made to reconstruct all the nerve branches to the limit set by the mid-pupillary line. At more anterior sites, it is practically impossible to find a branch for anastomosis.

The surgical technique we use for neurorrhaphy involves several epineural stitches, enough to provide stability to the nerve and prevent the loss of axonal white matter, but not so many that the suture material itself interferes with reinnervation. When suturing is intrapetrous, only two stitches are made on the anterior surface; the posterior surface provides a stable point owing to the location of the nerve in the bony canal. Microsurgical suturing is completed with fibrin sealant (Tissucol®).

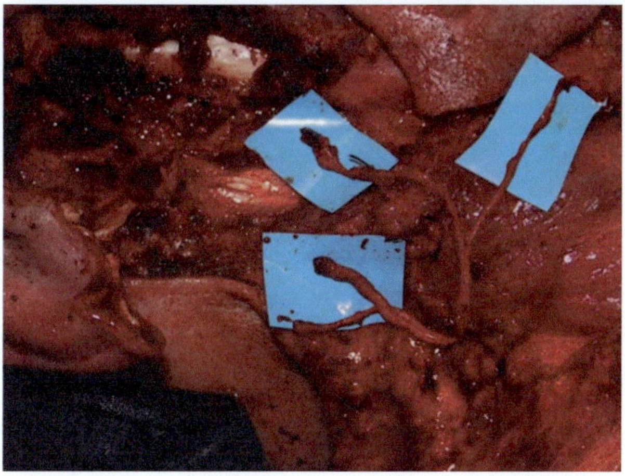

Fig. 7.2 Parotid gland carcinoma. Facial nerve reconstruction from the intramastoid area (facial nerve trunk) to the anterior facial nerve branches

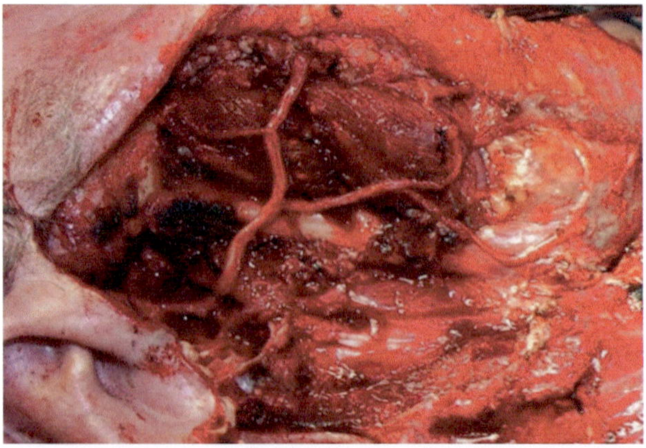

Fig. 7.3 The major auricular nerve is used as a graft with its four branches

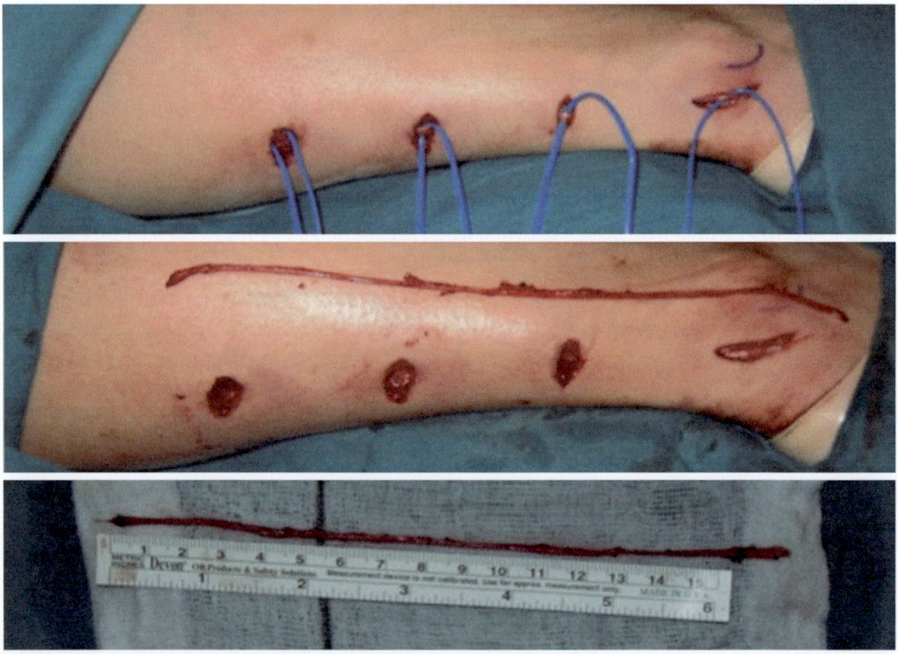

Fig. 7.4 Sural nerve dissection through small transversal incisions

The best functional results with this technique are achieved if reconstruction is early. Results can even be evaluated as early as the first months after surgery (Fig. 7.4).

In specific situations where it is necessary to bridge major defects of the facial nerve in patients with poorly vascularized tissue (e.g., those undergoing massive ablation, chemotherapy, and radiation therapy), the free vascularized nerve graft seems superior to the nonvascularized graft [6, 7].

7.5 Hypoglossal–Facial Nerve Anastomosis

In this approach, the hypoglossal nerve is sectioned beyond the descending branch, and end-to-end anastomosis is performed at the distal end of the facial nerve. Sacrificing the hypoglossal nerve leads to hemitongue atrophy, which causes some discomfort. The main advance in recent years has been hypoglossal–facial nerve semi-end-to-end anastomosis, which is performed by dissecting the facial nerve along its intrapetrous course and bringing it down to the level of the hypoglossal nerve, to which it is joined without having to completely section the nerve [8].

Hypoglossal–facial nerve anastomosis is a simple, quick technique with very good results. The first signs of reinnervation generally appear 5–6 months after surgery and include reappearance of expression wrinkles and folds, especially in the nasolabial fold, and a return to facial symmetry at rest. The patient will subsequently be able to develop the first voluntary contractions with the help of rehabilitation and retraining.

This technique is used both as definitive treatment and "babysitter" treatment for maintaining facial muscle tone while waiting for the impulse in the cross-graft performed during surgery [9, 10].

During rehabilitation, the patient is taught to smile using the impulse in the hypoglossal nerve, that is, with tongue movements, despite the limitations, this imposes on the ability to achieve a spontaneous and emotional smile. If the patient has undergone cross-facial nerve grafting, a specific rehabilitation program must be designed to achieve emotional smiling once the electromyographic data show that the impulse has reached the muscles on the paralyzed side from the contralateral facial nerve.

If only one surgical procedure is performed (hypoglossal–facial nerve anastomosis combined with cross-grafting, the microsurgical sutures are end-to-side between the sural nerve and facial nerve grafts on the affected side. Monitoring with electromyography is performed at approximately 12 months. If a contralateral facial nerve impulse is detected in the muscles of the affected side, specific rehabilitation must be started. If surgery is to be performed in two procedures (hypoglossal–facial nerve anastomosis combined with cross-grafting without anastomosing the distal end to the damaged facial nerve), the second procedure will be at approximately 8–10 months in order to anastomose end-to-end the ends of the sural nerve to the facial nerve of the affected side. At 6–8 months after the second procedure, electromyography can show whether the impulse has arrived and, thus, rehabilitation can start.

Both options are feasible. Our series show that long-term results are slightly better in patients who underwent two procedures, probably owing to the better conservation of the facial muscles when the contralateral facial nerve impulse arrives, since it receives a stronger impulse from the hypoglossal nerve. Nevertheless, most interventions involve only one procedure since the results are also good and general anesthesia is used. In addition, the second procedure is often complicated, even though the end of the nerve is marked with synthetic material. It is important to evaluate each patient on an individual basis and take his or her preferences into account (Figs. 7.5, 7.6, 7.7, and 7.8).

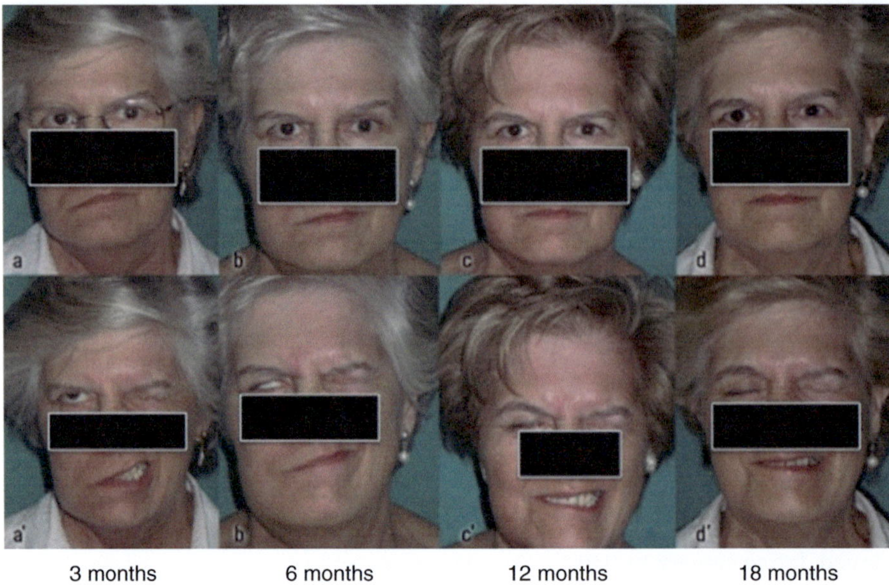

Fig. 7.5 Clinical evolution of a facial nerve reconstruction (orbicularis oris, orbicularis oculi, and zygomaticus muscle branches) using a major auricular nerve graft. The frontal and marginal branches palsy are camouflaged with botulinum toxin

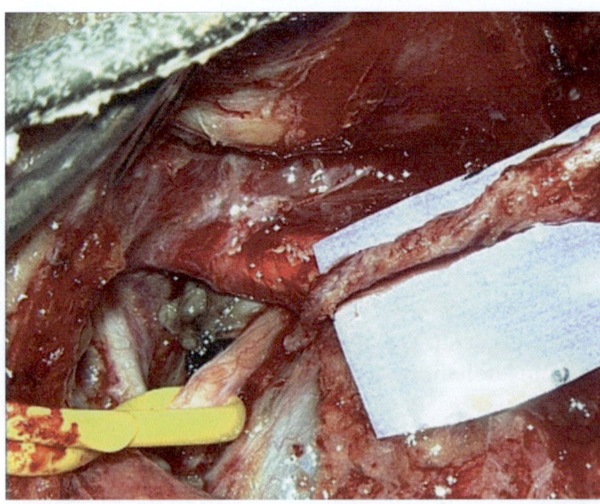

Fig. 7.6 Facial nerve dissected and descended from its temporal location to the hypoglossal nerve

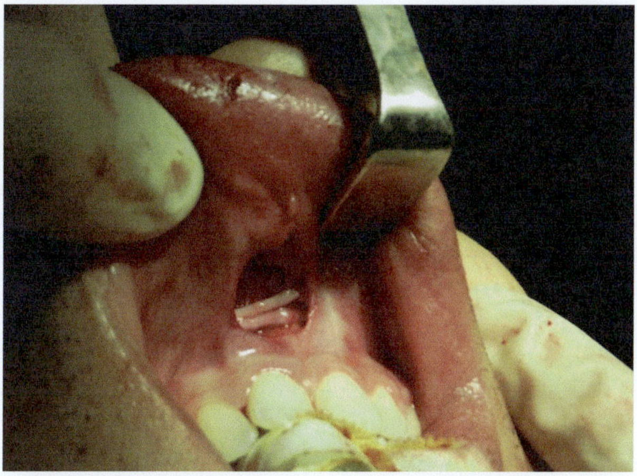

Fig. 7.7 Small superior lip vestibular incision used to tunnel sural nerve grafts

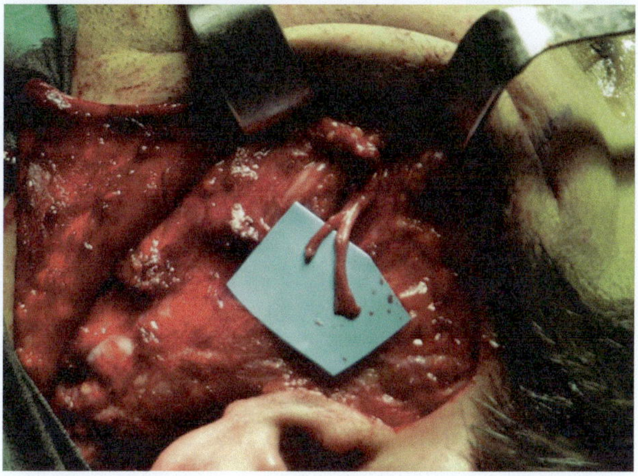

Fig. 7.8 Sural nerve graft ready to be anastomosed on hemifacial palsy side

7.6 Masseteric–Facial Nerve Anastomosis

Facial reinnervation can also be achieved using the masseteric nerve, the motor branch of the trigeminal nerve. The masseteric nerve is easy to locate within the masseter using appropriate references. Sacrifice produces no major sequelae, except for a slight loss of strength when chewing in some cases [11].

The facial nerve can be reinnervated using an auricular nerve graft from the masseteric nerve to the damaged trunk of the facial nerve at the point where it exits the stylomastoid foramen. The procedure can also be performed directly without a graft by dissecting the facial nerve from the ear, especially in totally deaf patients who undergo surgery for tumors of the cerebellopontine angle, and placing it beside the masseteric nerve, as in semi-end-to-end hypoglossal–facial nerve anastomosis. The axons do not have to cross another microsurgical suture, thus facilitating reinnervation and sacrifice of the auricular nerve.

During the rehabilitation process, the patient is taught to smile by using the stimulus from the masseter and instructing him or her to bite down. In principle, this seems to be a more natural way of generating a smile than moving the tongue.

7.7 Cross-Facial Nerve Grafting from the Healthy Side

The most common graft is the sural nerve graft, which is obtained from the leg via 2 or 3 small transverse incisions measuring approximately 1 cm and a retromalleolar incision. Fewer incisions may be necessary if the procedure is based on endoscopy and a headlight. Longitudinal incisions should not be made for cosmetic reasons (Fig. 7.9).

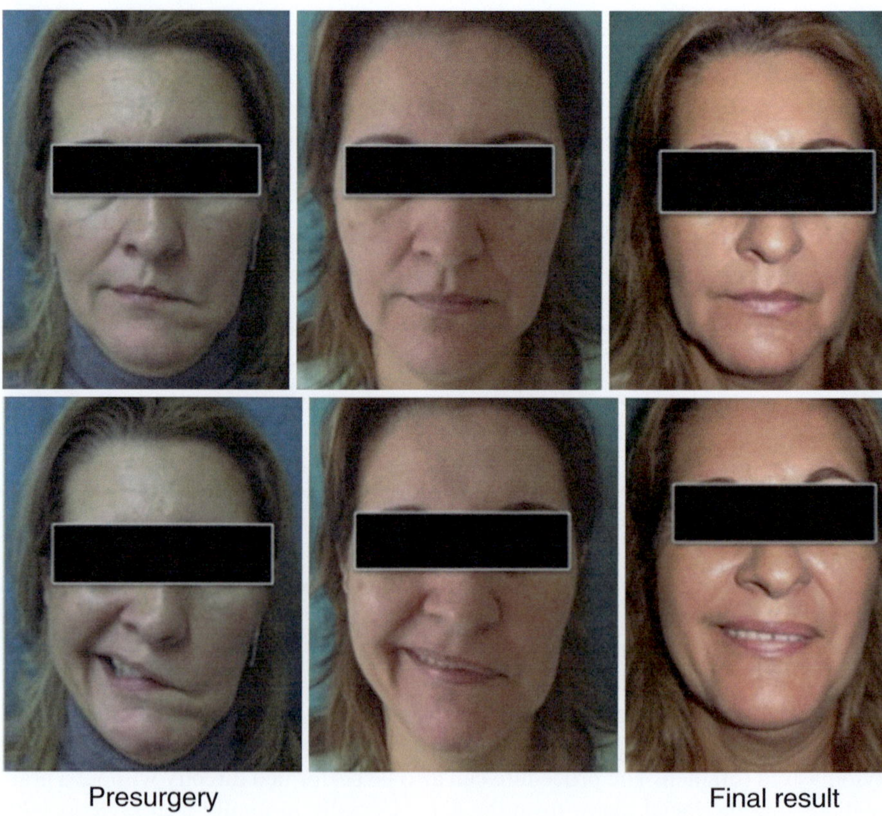

Fig. 7.9 Facial nerve orbicularis oris branch reconstruction using a facial–hypoglossal nerve and cross-face graft anastomoses. At the final result, the cross-face graft is working properly showing a better emotional smile

The facial incisions should be of the facelift type in order to avoid unnecessary scarring. We generally use a ventriculoperitoneal shunt to transfer the graft to the paralyzed side. If two procedures are performed, the graft must be marked with a piece of silicone joined to the distal end with non-resorbable suture, which enables the end to be located easily during the second procedure and prevents damage to the nerve during surgery.

The branch chosen is always that which is to be sacrificed on the unaffected side, ensuring that it has sufficient contractile strength and can perform the desired function without its sacrifice entailing an irreparable loss of function on the healthy side. Several branches from the same area can be used; these are stimulated electrically before choosing which one to sacrifice.

The outcome of this technique is more natural and emotional than that of hypoglossal–facial nerve anastomosis, since the stimulus originates in the facial nerve on the unaffected side, although for the technique to be successful, appropriate rehabilitation is necessary. At the same time, the result could be less predictable than in hypoglossal–facial nerve anastomosis since the growing axons have to overcome a long graft and two anastomoses. Furthermore, as the branches of the facial nerve provide a weak impulse, this technique may not provide completely satisfactory results for the patient or for the surgeon, unless it is performed within 3 months of the onset of paralysis and the patient is young.

In cases of partial paralysis that affects smiling, a cross-graft can be performed with end-to-end neurorrhaphy to a branch of the unaffected side and end-to-side neurorrhaphy to the affected branch, which provides some stimulus (and should not therefore be sacrificed), yet insufficient stimulus for a normal expression [12].

Prophylactic cross-facial nerve grafting can also be used in patients whose surgery is not urgent and in whom the facial nerve is to be sacrificed. A cross-facial nerve graft is performed before sacrificing the facial nerve. Thus, the muscles will maintain their function to the detriment of the stimulus from the contralateral facial nerve, outcome is better, and the psychological impact of complete facial paralysis is considerably diminished [13].

7.8 Temporalis Muscle Transfer Muscle for Dynamic Smile Reconstruction

The temporalis muscle has been used for some time to rehabilitate the smile of patients with facial paralysis. This approach has advanced considerably during the last 10 years with the move from transfer to elongation of the muscle, as made popular by Labbé. In the transfer procedure, the temporalis muscle was twisted above the zygomatic arch with the subsequent cosmetic defect in the temporal area due to the lack of muscle accompanied by bulging over the arch even when the arch is cut. In elongations, the tendon of the temporalis muscle is disinserted, and with the latest innovations introduced by Labbé, it is not even necessary to cut the zygomatic arch [14, 15].

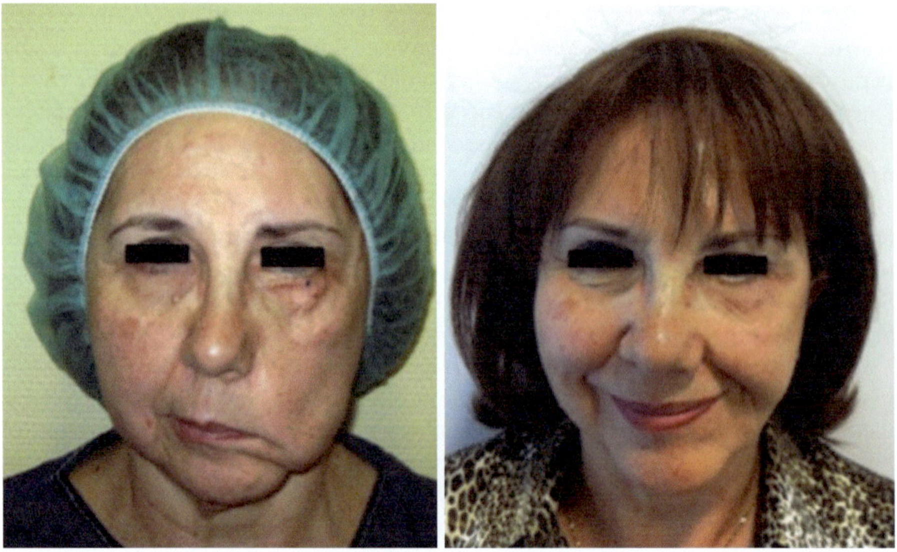

Fig. 7.10 Thirty years facial palsy evolution. Final result after temporal muscle elongation

The key of the technique lies in using the posterior half of the temporalis muscle for lengthening and anchoring to the orbicularis muscle of the upper lip. Two incisions are made: a hemicoronal zigzag incision and another in the nasolabial fold. The latter should be designed before surgery with the patient standing and following the contralateral fold as a guide. After a subgaleal brow lift, the temporalis muscle is exposed, and the aponeurosis is opened only in the posterior half, leaving a 5-mm band of temporal aponeurosis; the muscle is detached deep in the anterior half and the insertions released in the temporal region and zygomatic arch without detaching from the lateral wall of the orbit or the temporal crest. The sphenotemporal crest must be detached with great caution, because this part of the procedure is performed blind and this area is where the pedicles are obtained. The incision in the nasolabial fold gives us access to the coronoid process, which we cut after following the Bichat fat pad. In order to bring the temporalis muscle down so that it reaches the orbicularis oris, it is necessary to detach all the fibers with the pterygoid and the masseter. Once the coronoid fragment has been withdrawn, the tendon of the temporalis muscle is fixed to the modiolus and superior orbicularis oris depending on the type of smile. In this technique, it is very important to begin rehabilitation within 2–3 weeks after surgery. Even though the movement of the commissure of the mouth is based in principle on the movements of chewing, over time, and in very specific cases, a more emotional smile can be achieved. However, the result will never be as good as that obtained using the microsurgical techniques described below, which are the approach of choice in patients affected facial paralysis for longer periods (Fig. 7.10).

7.9 Microvascular Muscle Flaps

Microvascular muscle flaps can be harvested in one or two surgical procedures, depending on whether the graft is sufficiently long to reach the contralateral side or whether it is necessary to perform a previous cross-facial nerve graft. If two procedures are performed, then these should be separated by approximately 10 months to enable the axons to grow via the nerve graft. A positive Tinel sign shows that this growth has been successful.

The most frequently used muscle in these reconstructions is the gracilis, which is easy to harvest and has constant anatomic references. In addition, since the role of this muscle is covered by other adductors in the area, there are no functional consequences. The vascular pedicle is located between the long adductor above and the short adductor below. It is relatively short (approximately 6 cm) because it finishes in the femoral vessels, although it is sufficiently long to reach the facial or temporal vessels. The vascular pedicle is located on the deep aspect of the muscle and enters the muscle perpendicularly at 8–10 cm below the pubic tubercle.

Motor nerve supply is via the anterior branch of the obturator nerve, which enters the muscle obliquely 2–3 cm above the vascular pedicle and is easily distinguished between the long and short adductors for some 6–8 cm. The truly interesting feature of this nerve is that we can follow it to the obturator foramen (i.e., it can reach–12 cm in length), thus enabling us to perform reconstruction in a single procedure. Therefore, it is necessary to follow the nerve in its second anatomic region, from where it enters the deep part of the short adductor and exits to course between the external obturator muscle below and the pectineus muscle above. Intraneural dissection is performed in this last section by lengthening the initial incision along the inguinal fold or using an endoscope [16].

Innervation of the gracilis muscle is via the fascicles, thus making it possible to select the exact fragment of muscle to be harvested, of appropriate size and contractile force, using intraoperative electrical stimulation of the nerve fascicle selected. Nevertheless, we sometimes remove the Bichat fat pad to prevent bulging when the flap is placed on the face (Fig. 7.11).

The microvascular gracilis muscle flap can also be harvested in a single procedure by obtaining the supply from the masseter nerve. This is the most common technique to treat bilateral facial paralysis in patients with Moebius syndrome, in whom the contralateral facial nerve cannot be used. However, in such cases, it is impossible to obtain an emotional smile [17]. An additional option involves using the gracilis muscle in a single procedure to obtain an emotional smile by combining reinnervations of the muscle using the ipsilateral masseter nerve with a cross-facial graft of the sural nerve anastomosed end-to-side to the obturator nerve, which acts as a trigger and thus enables a spontaneous smile (Figs. 7.9 and 7.12) [18].

Other muscles with a motor nerve that is sufficiently long to perform reconstruction in a single procedure include the latissimus dorsi [19], the rectus abdominis [20], and the short head of the biceps femoris [21].

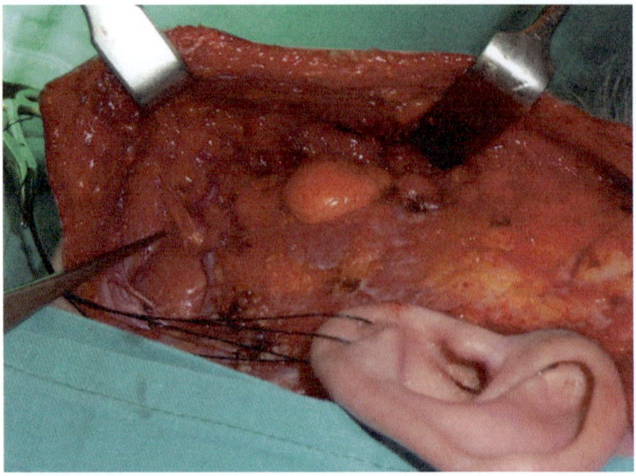

Fig. 7.11 Sometimes Bichat adipose pad can be removed to avoid gracilis muscle flap excessive bulging

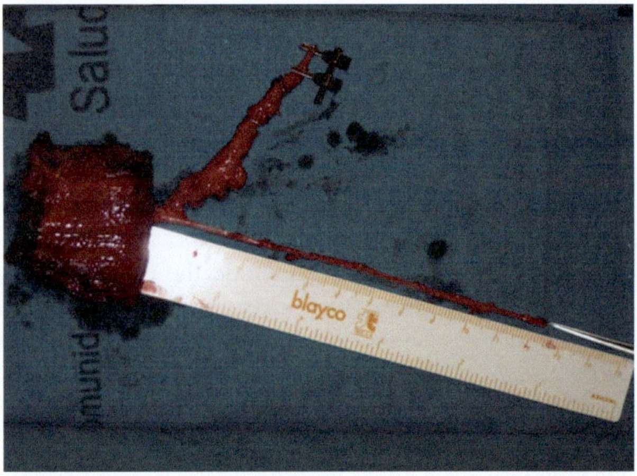

Fig. 7.12 Latissimus dorsi muscle flap. The nerve length allows a one-stage surgery

This surgical technique provides the best functional outcome in patients with prolonged facial paralysis. More than half of the patients achieve voluntary contractions of the graft without dyskinesia, and with good rehabilitation, many can achieve an emotional smile, especially children and young people, whose brain plasticity is much greater. If the technique is performed in a single procedure, there is less time to wait before seeing the results, a second procedure is avoided, and morbidity is reduced. However, facial symmetry seems to improve if the technique is performed in two procedures, although larger series are necessary before this hypothesis can confirmed (Fig. 7.13 and 7.14) [22].

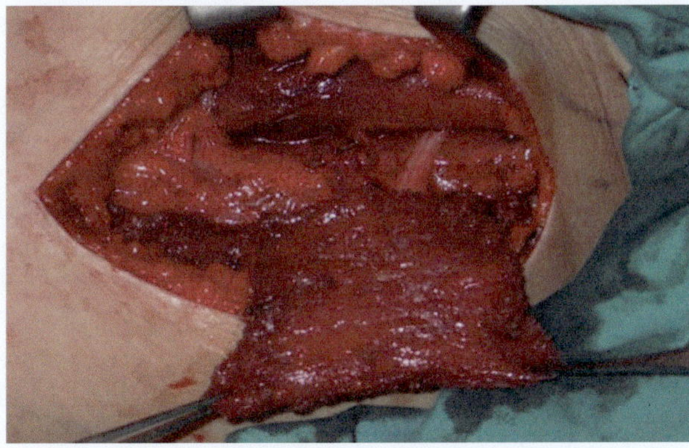

Fig. 7.13 Gracilis muscle flap with its vascular pedicle and obturator nerve

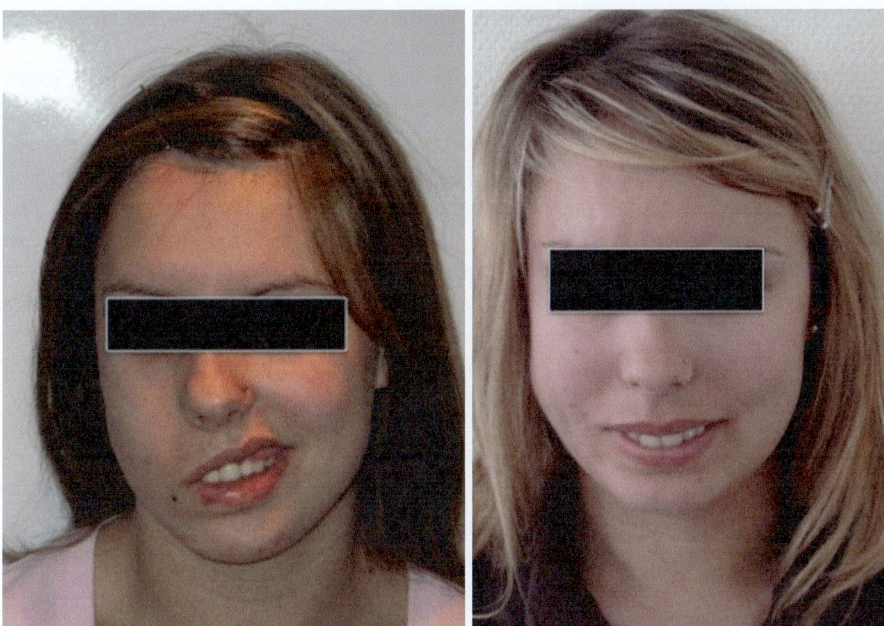

Fig. 7.14 Right facial palsy after pontocerebellar angle tumor. It was reconstructed with a two-stage gracilis flap surgery

7.10 Complementary Surgical Approaches

Facial paralysis can be treated using a wide variety of complementary surgical procedures. Below we describe some of the most common:

Upper eyelid weights: Weight implants in the upper eyelid enable the eye to close with gravity. These weights replace the function of the orbicularis oculi and take over that of the levator muscles. The objective is to achieve complete closure of the eyelid with minimal ptosis on opening (<2 mm). We place a flexible platinum chain implant [23] using a retrograde post-levator approach [24, 25]. The probability of complications is markedly reduced by an appropriate choice of weight, accurate placement of the weight (maximum lagophthalmos in voluntary closure), and careful surgery.

Canthopexy and canthoplasty: The difference between these techniques lies in cutting or merely suspending the lateral canthal tendon. Each technique can be performed using a number of approaches. We mostly use external canthoplasty with a tarsal strip. These techniques are often combined with static lower eyelid suspension with a tarsal strip.

Auricular cartilage grafts in the lower eyelid: External lateral canthoplasty is not sufficient to correct deformity of the lower eyelid in very severe cases of ectropion and laxity. An alternative to the tarsal strip is placement of an auricular graft according the technique of Krastinova et al. [26]. The auricular cartilage graft acts as a splint that strengthens the lower eyelid and gives it the ability to resist gravity. The effects of dry eye, epiphora, keratitis, and conjunctivitis are reduced, and there have been no reports of graft resorption, infection, or extrusion. The main drawbacks are possible partial lower visual field loss due to the reduced range and mobility of the grafted lower eyelid and the potentially poor long-term resulting from the curvature of the graft, especially in patients with very thin skin. Consequently, we only use this approach in very specific cases.

Facelifting and blepharoplasty: Both are used to correct ptosis associated with muscular inactivity.

- Lower lip plasty, oral commissuroplasty, myectomy of the lower lip muscles on the unaffected side, and selective marginal mandibular neurectomy on the unaffected side to correct the deformity caused by mandibular nerve palsy [27].
- In addition to complementary surgical approaches, botulinum toxin plays a key role in the treatment of facial paralysis, both during the rehabilitation process and in cosmetic outcome, especially in the treatment of dyskinesia and muscle spasm.

References

1. Tomat LR y cols. Evaluation of a new measurement tool for facial paralysis reconstruction. Plast Reconstr Surg. 2005;115(3):696–704.
2. Slattery WH 3rd y cols. Side-to-end hypoglossal to facial anastomosis with transposition of the intratemporal facial nerve. Otol Neurotol. 2014;35(3):509–13.

3. Biglioli F y cols. Masseteric-facial nerve anastomosis for early facial reanimation. J Craneomaxillofac Surg. 2012;40(2):149–55.
4. Piza-Katzer H y cols. Secondary end-to-end repair of extensive facial nerve defects: surgical technique and postoperative functional results. Head Neck. 2004;26(9):770–7.
5. Falcioni M y cols. Facial nerve grafting. Otol Neurotol. 2003;24(3):486–9.
6. Kimata Y y cols. Free vascularized nerve grafting for immediate facial nerve reconstruction. Laryngoscope. 2005;115(2):331–6.
7. Koshima I y cols. New one-stage nerve pedicle grafting technique using the great auricular nerve for reconstruction of facial nerve defects. J Reconstr Microsurg. 2004;20(5):357–61.
8. Lassaletta L y cols. Anastomosis hipoglosofacial intratemporal hemiterminoterminal. Acta Otorrinolaringol Es. 2008;59(3):124–6.
9. Terzis JK y cols. The "babysitter" procedure: minihypoglossal to facial nerve transfer and cross-facial nerve grafting. Plast Reconstr Surg. 2009;123(3):865–76.
10. Terzis JK y cols. "Babysitter" procedure with concomitant muscle transfer in facial paralysis. Plast Reconstr Surg. 2009;124(4):1142–56.
11. Collar RM y cols. The subzygomatic triangle: rapid, minimally invasive identification of the masseteric nerve for facial reanimation. Plast Reconstr Surg. 2013;132(1):183–8.
12. Frey M y cols. Functional upgrading of partially recovered facial palsy by cross-face nerve grafting with distal end-to-side neurorrhaphy. Plast Reconstr Surg. 2006;117(2):597–606.
13. Koshima I y cols. Prophylactic cross-face nerve flap for muscle protection prior to facial palsy. JPRAS. 2011;64(2):185–8.
14. Labbé D y cols. Lengthening temporalis myoplasty and lip reanimation. Plast Reconstr Surg. 2000;105(4):1289–97.
15. Labbé D. Myoplastiedállongement du temporal V.2 et reanimation des levres. Ann Chiru Plast Esthet. 2009;54:571–6.
16. Rodriguez Lorenzo A. Anatomy of the motor nerve to the gracilis muscle and its implications in a one-stage microneurovascular gracilis transfer for facial reanimation. J Plast Reconstr Aesthet Surg. 2010;63:54–8.
17. Bianchi B y cols. Facial animation in patients with Moebius and Moebius–like syndromes. Int J Oral Maxillofac Surg. 2010;39:1066–73.
18. Biglioli F y cols. Double innervation in free-flap surgery for long-standing facial paralysis. J Plast Reconstruct Aesthet Surg. 2012;65(10):1343–9.
19. Harii K y cols. One-stage transfer of the latissimus dorsi muscle for reanimation of a paralyzed face: a new alternative. Plast Reconstr Surg. 1998;102(4):941–51.
20. Koshima I y cols. One-stage reconstruction of established facial paralysis using a rectus abdominis muscle transfer. Plast Reconstr Surg. 1997;99(1):234–8.
21. Hayashi A y cols. Neurovascularized free short head of the biceps femoris muscle transfer for one stage reanimation of facial paralysis. Plast Reconstr Surg. 2005;115(2):394–405.
22. Kumar PA y cols. Cross-face nerve graft with free-muscle transfer for reanimation of the paralyzed face: a comparative study of the single-stage and two-stage procedures. Plast Reconstr Surg. 2002;109(2):451–62.
23. Berghaus A y cols. The platinum chain. Arch Facial Plast Surg. 2003; 5:166–70.
24. Kao CH y cols. Retrograde weight implantation for correction of lagophthalmos. Laryngoscope. 2004;114:1570–5.
25. Kim DW y cols. Modified retrograde approach to upper eyelid static loading. Laryngoscope. 2007;117:2110–4.
26. Krastinova D y cols. Rehabilitation of the paralysed or lax lower eyelid using a graft of conchal cartilage. Br J Plast Surg. 2002;55:12–9.
27. Breslow GD y cols. Selective marginal mandibular neurectomy for treatment of the marginal mandibular lip deformity in patients with chronic unilateral facial palsies. Plast Reconstr Surg. 2005;116(5):1223–32.

Index

C. Navarro Vila (ed.), *Reconstructive Oral and Maxillofacial Surgery*,
DOI 10.1007/978-3-319-20487-1

MIX
Papier aus verantwortungsvollen Quellen
Paper from responsible sources
FSC® C105338

If you have any concerns about our products,
you can contact us on
ProductSafety@springernature.com

In case Publisher is established outside the EU,
the EU authorized representative is:
Springer Nature Customer Service Center GmbH
Europaplatz 3, 69115 Heidelberg, Germany

Printed by Libri Plureos GmbH
in Hamburg, Germany